HAPPY BIRTH

TO

....

WITH LOVE FROM

....

And Audrey

HAPPY BIRTHDAY—LOVE . . .
Complete Series

Jane Austen

Joan Crawford

Bette Davis

Liam Gallagher

Audrey Hepburn

John Lennon

Bob Marley

Marilyn Monroe

Michelle Obama

Jackie Kennedy Onassis

Elvis Presley

Keith Richards

Frank Sinatra

Elizabeth Taylor

Oscar Wilde

HAPPY BIRTHDAY
Love, Audrey

ON YOUR SPECIAL DAY

ENJOY THE WIT AND WISDOM OF

AUDREY HEPBURN

THE WORLD'S MOST ELEGANT ACTRESS

Edited by Jade Riley

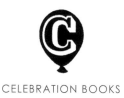

CELEBRATION BOOKS

THIS IS A CELEBRATION BOOK

Published by Celebration Books 2023
Celebration Books is an imprint of Dean Street Press

Text & Design Copyright © 2023 Celebration Books

All Rights Reserved. No part of this publication may be reproduced, stored in or transmitted in any form or by any means without the written permission of the copyright owner and the publisher of this book.

Cover by DSP

ISBN 978 1 915393 60 9

www.deanstreetpress.co.uk

HAPPY BIRTHDAY—LOVE, AUDREY

The ballerina with the funny face, Audrey Hepburn brought joy to legions of fans for decades both in her iconic cinematic career and, later as Goodwill Ambassador for the United Nations. She understood early, from a difficult youth spent growing up in Nazi occupied Holland, that life ought to be filled with love and happiness. After the war, she moved to London, the city of her father, where she worked hard to become a dancer and an actress. After a few films for Ealing Studio, she was snatched up by Hollywood and, in 1961, she became the most famous party girl of all time, Holly Golightly, in *Breakfast at Tiffany's*.

Audrey was never known for wild excess but she did love fun. She even brought her adopted baby deer, Pippen, to parties with her. Always happy to celebrate others, Ms. Hepburn also sang "Happy Birthday" to John F. Kennedy the year after Marilyn Monroe! This is not surprising given that the two briefly dated while the President was an unmarried Senator. But Audrey was more likely to be found celebrating special events and birthdays surrounded by her children. For the world's most elegant woman and muse to Parisian fashion designer Hubert de Givenchy, her pleasures were remarkably simple. Things like walking her pet Yorkie, Mr. Famous, around Rome or hiking near her retreat in Switzerland were to her "the good things in life."

Being a Mother was Audrey's most sought after role in life. Her son, Luca Dotti, recalls his Mom having just a little dark chocolate everyday as her pick-me-up. And whipping up her famous flourless chocolate cake was the usual treat for birthdays and special occasions. Despite her lean frame, Hepburn never denied herself her favorite pasta of Spaghetti Pomodoro. She would even pack her suitcase with spaghetti, olive oil and cheese! Now that's the way to celebrate *la dolce vita*.

Happy Birthday from Audrey Hepburn and . . . remember always to enjoy life's simple pleasures.

Audrey Hepburn

"Let's face it, a nice creamy chocolate cake does a lot for a lot of people; it does for me.

"Paris is always a good idea."

"Life is a party. Dress for it."

If I'm honest, I have to tell you I still read fairy tales and I like them best of all.

Some people dream of having a big swimming pool. With me, it's closets.

Elegance is the only beauty that never fades.

Success is like reaching an important birthday and finding you're exactly the same.

Anyone who does not believe in miracles is not a realist.

For me the only things of interest are those linked to the heart.

They say love is the best investment; the more you give, the more you get in return.

I heard a definition once: happiness is health and a short memory! I wish I'd invented it, because it is very true.

> "I believe in kissing, kissing a lot."

Water is Life. And clean water means health.

I love people who make me laugh. I honestly think it's the thing I like most, to laugh. It cures a multitude of ills. It's probably the most important thing in a person.

As you grow older you will discover that you have two hands. One for helping yourself, the other for helping others.

Good things aren't supposed to just fall into your lap. God is very generous, but He expects you to do your part first.

Never regret anything that makes you smile.

Ever since I was a child I loved babies.

To plant a garden is to believe in tomorrow.

> It is too much to hope that I shall keep up my success. I don't ask for that. All I shall do is my best—and hope.

The more there is, the less I want. The more man flies to the moon, the more I want to look at a tree.

Whatever a man might do, whatever misery or heartache your children might give you—and they give you a lot—however much your parents irritate you—it doesn't matter because you love them.

Take care of the small circle around you. When you have succeeded with them, then move outwards, one small step at a time.

I can testify to what UNICEF means to children, because I was among those who received food and medical relief right after World War II. I have a long-lasting gratitude and trust for what UNICEF does.

When you have found it, you should stick to it.

Well it's nice being top banana in the shock department.

You can only hope to get a combination of happy work and a happy life.

Pick the day. Enjoy it—to the hilt. The day as it comes. People as they come . . . The past, I think, has helped me appreciate the present—and I don't want to spoil any of it by fretting about the future.

I had to make a choice at one point in my life, of missing films or missing my children.

For beautiful eyes, look for the good in others; for beautiful lips, speak only words of kindness; and for poise, walk with the knowledge that you are never alone.

I believe in being strong when everything seems to be going wrong.

"True friends are families which you can select.

The beauty of a woman is seen in her eyes, because that is the doorway to her heart, the place where love resides.

> I believe in pink.

You can always tell what kind of a person a man really thinks you are by the earrings he gives you.

Who thinks you're as fantastic as your dog does?

We all want to be loved, don't we? Everyone looks for a way of finding love. It's a constant search for affection in every walk of life.

I don't want to be alone, I want to be left alone.

There are more important things than outward appearance. No amount of makeup can cover an ugly personality.

"I've been lucky. Opportunities don't often come along. So, when they do, you have to grab them.

My greatest ambition is to have a career without becoming a career woman.

The most important thing is to enjoy your life, to be happy, it's all that matters.

On the one hand maybe I've remained infantile, while on the other I matured quickly, because at a young age I was very aware of suffering and fear.

When you have nobody you can make a cup of tea for, when nobody needs you, that's when I think life is over.

The best thing to hold onto in life is each other.

Since the world has existed, there has been injustice. But it is one world, the more so as it becomes smaller, more accessible. There is just no question that there is more obligation that those who have should give to those who have nothing.

I'm not beautiful. My mother once called me an ugly duckling. But, listed separately, I have a few good features.

I believe that laughing is the best calorie burner.

> "If I get married, I want to be very married."

You can tell more about a person by what he says about others than you can by what others say about him.

Actually, you have to be a little bit in love with your leading man and vice versa. If you're going to portray love, you have to feel it. You can't do it any other way. But you don't carry it beyond the set.

I never think of myself as an icon. What is in other people's minds is not in my mind. I just do my thing.

"I tried always to do better: saw always a little further. I tried to stretch myself.

Why change? Everyone has his own style. When you have found it, you should stick to it.

For my whole life, my favorite activity was reading. It's not the most social pastime.

Dress like you are already famous.

A woman can be beautiful as well as intellectual.

I believe that happy girls are the prettiest girls.

> "I'm not a born actress, as such, I care about expressing feelings."

We can all help others.

Sex appeal is something that you feel deep down inside. It's suggested rather than shown. I'm not as well-stacked as Sophia Loren or Gina Lollobrigida, but there is more to sex appeal than just measurements. I don't need a bedroom to prove my womanliness. I can convey just as much sex appeal, picking apples off a tree or standing in the rain.

Not to live for the day, that would be materialistic—but to *treasure* the day. I realize that most of us live on the skin—on the surface—without appreciating just how wonderful it is simply to be alive at all.

> Remember, if you need a hand you'll find it at the end of your arm.

"I don't believe in collective guilt, but I do believe in collective responsibility.

People, even more than things, have to be restored, renewed, revived, reclaimed, and redeemed; never throw out anyone.

I believe that tomorrow is another day, and I believe in miracles.

I probably hold the distinction of being one movie star who, by all laws of logic, should never have made it. At each stage of my career, I lacked the experience.

> Giving is living. If you stop wanting to give, there's nothing more to live for.

"There is one difference between a long life and a great dinner; in the dinner, the sweet things come last.

"There is a science of war but how strange there isn't a science of peace.

A quality education has the power to transform societies in a single generation, provide children with the protection they need from the hazards of poverty, labor exploitation and disease, and given them the knowledge, skills, and confidence to reach their full potential.

I decided, very early on, just to accept life unconditionally; I never expected it to do anything special for me, yet I seemed to accomplish far more than I had ever hoped. Most of the time it just happened to me without my ever seeking it.

My only religion is a belief in nature.

Two things I never talk about are salary and religion.

Beauty is being the best possible version of yourself. Inside and out.

I was born with an enormous need for affection, and a terrible need to give it.

The 'Third World' is a term I don't like very much because we're all one world. I want people to know that the largest part of humanity is suffering.

> Living is like tearing through a museum. Not until later do you really start absorbing what you saw, thinking about it, looking it up in a book, and remembering—because you can't take it in all at once.

> My own life has been much more than a fairy tale. I've had my share of difficult moments, but whatever difficulties I've gone through, I've always gotten the prize at the end.

The beauty of a woman is not in a facial mole, but true beauty in a woman is reflected in her soul. It is the caring that she lovingly gives, the passion that she knows.

"Don't be like the rest of them, darling."

I lack self-confidence. I don't know whether I shall ever get it. Perhaps it is better to be unsure of yourself, as I am. But it is very tiring.

> It's that wonderful old-fashioned idea that others come first and you come second. This was the whole ethic by which I was brought up. Others matter more than you do, so don't fuss, dear; get on with it.

I believe, every day, you should have at least one exquisite moment.

> "If my world were to cave in tomorrow, I would look back on all the pleasures, excitements and worthwhilenesses I have been lucky enough to have had. Not the sadness, not my miscarriages or my father leaving home, but the joy of everything else. It will have been enough."

And I think that's what Life's all about, actually, about children and flowers.

Audrey Hepburn

ABOUT THE EDITOR

Jade Riley is a writer whose interests include old movies, art history, vintage fashion and books, books, books.

Her dream is to move to London, to write like Virginia Woolf, and to meet a man like Mr. Darcy, who owns a vacation home in Greece.

Modeling Cities and Regions as Complex Systems
From Theory to Planning Applications

Roger White, Guy Engelen, and Inge Uljee

The MIT Press
Cambridge, Massachusetts
London, England

© 2015 Massachusetts Institute of Technology

All rights reserved. No part of this book may be reproduced in any form by any electronic or mechanical means (including photocopying, recording, or information storage and retrieval) without permission in writing from the publisher.

MIT Press books may be purchased at special quantity discounts for business or sales promotional use. For information, please email special_sales@mitpress.mit.edu

This book was set in Sabon LT Std by Toppan Best-set Premedia Limited. Printed and bound in the United States of America.

Library of Congress Cataloging-in-Publication Data
White, Roger, 1941 December 1-
  Modeling cities and regions as complex systems : from theory to planning applications / Roger White, Guy Engelen, and Inge Uljee.
      pages cm
  Includes bibliographical references and index.
  ISBN 978-0-262-02956-8 (hardcover : alk. paper) 1. City planning. 2. Regional planning. I. Engelen, Guy. II. Uljee, Inge. III. Title.
  HT166.W5134 2015
  307.1'216—dc23
                              2015009381

10 9 8 7 6 5 4 3 2 1

Contents

Acknowledgments vii

1　Introduction　1

2　Theory and Consequences　13

3　Approaches to Modeling Cities and Regions　43

4　Urban Systems and Spatial Competition　65

5　The Fractal Forms of Urban Land Use Patterns　87

6　Urban and Regional Land Use Dynamics: Understanding the Process by Means of Cellular Automaton–Based Models　103

7　The Bigger Picture: Integrated Multiscale Models　141

8　The Cellular Automaton Eats the Regions: Unified Modeling of Activities and Land Use in a Variable Grid Cellular Automaton　175

9　Issues of Calibration, Validation, and Methodology　213

10　Emerging Theory　235

11　Modeling in Support of Spatial Planning and Policy Making: The Example of Flanders　251

12　Paths to the Future　295

References　305
Index　323

Acknowledgments

Much of the work reported in *Modeling Cities and Regions as Complex Systems* was carried out at the Research Institute for Knowledge Systems (RIKS) in Maastricht, Netherlands, with the encouragement and enthusiastic support of Paul Drazan, its first director. We are grateful to him and the rest of the group at RIKS for their support. Ton de Nijs, of the Netherlands National Institute for Public Health and the Environment (RIVM), was also an early and enthusiastic supporter of our work; his engagement with its approach helped shape its development, and he ultimately went on to make important contributions of his own. Elías R. Gutiérrez, economist and planner, was equally an enthusiastic supporter and, as head of the Graduate School of Planning at the University of Puerto Rico, was instrumental in facilitating the comprehensive, integrated nature of the models. Tomas Crols of the Vrije Universiteit Brussel and the Flemish Institute for Technological Research (VITO) not only produced the figures illustrating the use of network distances; he first developed the network-distance algorithms. Bev Brown of St. John's, Newfoundland and Labrador, produced the drawings illustrating the effects—both structural and emotional—of bifurcations; she also provided intelligent proofreading. Charlie Conway of the Department of Geography, Memorial University of Newfoundland, generously sacrificed more than one night in order to produce most of the other figures. Finally, April Wolff of New York was a champion of this book for years, until it was finally written.

# 1
Introduction

Cities and their regions, viewed over long historical timescales, seem to be in constant turmoil. They grow, decline, grow again, and continuously transform themselves. Over shorter timescales, the changes seem more measured and perhaps more orderly, but they occur continuously and they must either be accommodated or directed. This book is about modeling the spatial dynamics of urban growth and transformation. The aim is to achieve a better understanding of the evolving patterns of land use, population, and economic activity and to use that knowledge—and the models themselves—to increase the effectiveness of planning.

Our starting point is the observation that, in some sense, cities generate themselves—they are complex, adaptive, self-organizing systems. Of course, it is actually people who create cities, either individually or as organized into businesses, governments, and other institutions. But, for the most part, they do so inadvertently and unintentionally as they go about their daily lives. They aim to satisfy immediate needs—drop the children off at school, get to work, find a location for a new branch office, build a house to live in. They do not intend to build a city; that just happens. Even though, along the way, there are many acts of planning, these tend to be local, temporary, or incomplete. So, ultimately, a city emerges as the collective result of many individual events, most of which are not intended to be city building. But the acts of planning *are* intended to guide the development of the city, and these, to be successful, must rely on an understanding of the processes by which the city generates itself. Good models can help us to understand these processes and to work with them to create better cities.

If cities do in fact generate themselves, then the appropriate modeling framework is one based on the theory of self-organizing complex adaptive systems. This approach is already widely used in a number of fields from physics to ecology in order to model systems in which highly ordered structures appear spontaneously and then maintain themselves. Because the focus is on the dynamics of the systems being modeled, the approach is algorithmic. An algorithm can capture the step-by-step idiosyncratic process by which a city creates itself because an algorithm is an inherently executable description of a process. Furthermore, the description can be made as specific and detailed, and hence as realistic, as desired.

One of the most powerful algorithmic techniques for modeling dynamical systems is the cellular automaton (CA). The CA is an extremely simple and computationally efficient technique developed specifically to model spatial dynamics. It is also one of the most widely used platforms for research into the nature of complex self-organizing systems. The models that constitute the heart of this book are all developed within this framework, and most of them are CA based. They are, first of all, land use models: they show the evolution of land use at resolutions of tens to hundreds of meters, depending on the application. But the more advanced models also handle the dynamics of population and economic activities, either at the same resolution as the land use or at the scale of statistical or administrative regions. In addition, these models are commonly linked to or integrated with domain-specific models, such as economic, demographic, or hydrological models. The result is a family of models that give rich and realistic representations of the spatial dynamics of a number of urban phenomena.

More generally, the models in effect constitute a theory of cities as self-organizing systems. Because the models are relatively detailed and domain specific, they can function as serious scientific tools—tools that permit a confrontation of the implicit theory with reality in a detailed and rigorous way. These confrontations permit the models to be progressively improved and thus to provide a deeper, but also more practical, understanding of the spatial dynamics of cities and regions. Because of their power and realism, the models are now beginning to be used in a variety of situations as spatial decision support tools. They currently represent the most fully developed, detailed, and widely used tools for modeling urban and regional dynamics in a relatively realistic way.

Their very realism makes them seem mundane and straightforward. But under that realism lurks the wild and wonderful behavior that is characteristic of complex self-organizing systems. For example, like real cities, the models have open futures: they do not predict the future urban structure of a city, but rather an ensemble of possible urban structures, some of which may be quite different from others. Although spatial structure may appear straightforward, in fact, it is a complicated issue. It is not what you see on a map; it is *some* of what you see on a *set* of maps, and what you see depends on who you are. In other words, the self-organizing complex systems approach problematizes spatial structure. What at first seems simple is revealed to be complex, multifarious, and difficult to pin down. The underlying methodological and philosophical issues made explicit by working within the self-organizing systems framework are an important theme in this book because they underpin our understanding of the models themselves.

Spatial Structure

Cities are intricate socioeconomic entities dependent for their existence on their links with the natural environment. To fully understand them, we would need a socioeconomic-ecosystem theory of everything. Various disciplines are attempting to make progress toward this goal, but what is striking from our point of view is that most of them, whether in the natural or human sciences, consider spatial structure to be unimportant or incidental, if they recognize it at all. Perhaps spatial structure is not noticed because it is rather like the air we breathe: we are always and inescapably in it, so we take it for granted. We tend to notice these things only when something is wrong with them: we notice the atmosphere when it is polluted, and we notice the spatial structure when we can no longer function in it in the way we are accustomed to, as when we are routinely caught in traffic jams, or someone threatens to disrupt our neighborhood with a noxious facility. For most people, and most disciplines, the spatial structure is simply the setting and therefore unworthy of further consideration.

Nevertheless, cities *are* spatially structured, and clearly they function by virtue of that structure. The structure facilitates the economic, social, and cultural life of the city, and when the urban form becomes inadequate in some respect, so that it no longer acts as a smooth facilitator, the problem is noticed immediately by residents, businesses, and governments, who demand action. People think of their city in terms of spatial structure, often with a strong visual element, as described in Kevin Lynch's seminal book *The Image of the City* (1960). They map the city mentally into functional areas—industrial or residential areas, commercial strips, and so on. But they also map it in terms of social characteristics—rich and poor areas and ethnic neighborhoods. They map it, too, in emotional terms—threatening areas, areas of anomie, pleasurable areas. And they map it in terms of aesthetic characteristics—beautiful areas, ugly areas, districts redolent of history. All of these mental mappings affect the way people behave in the city—where they go, what routes they choose to get there, where they decide to establish businesses and public facilities, and where they decide to live and work. And these behaviors, in turn, affect the evolution of the spatial structure. This is the process of self-organization.

Continuous change of the urban spatial structure is certainly a prominent characteristic of cities, and one that is important to planners. But is it of any deeper significance? The answer would seem to be yes. Spatial structure seems to be an essential aspect of the emergence of complex, functional systems of every sort. The original work in the theory of self-organizing systems, Ilya Prigogine's investigation, during the 1950's and 1960's, of far-from-equilibrium chemical systems, focused on the appearance of macro-scale—that is, visible—spatial structure in reacting chemical systems. The canonical example is the Belousov-Zhabotinsky reaction, in which a variety of visible patterns—concentric circles, spirals, or multi-armed spirals—can appear when a reaction takes place in a shallow dish and the relative concentration of chemicals is maintained far from equilibrium (Nicolis and Prigogine, 1989). As Prigogine's group and others extended their work to examine the phenomena of self-organization in other fields, from biology to urban systems, they continued to focus on spatial structure. The implicit message is that spatial structure is both a defining characteristic and an essential factor in the emergence of complex systems, whether physical, chemical, biological, social, or economic, and this is certainly the case with cities. All of these systems come into existence by virtue of processes that create a spatial structuring of their constituent elements; their functionality depends on the pattern of that structuring, and different patterns yield different systems with different functions.

Of course, the constituent elements are also important. The people, businesses, and institutions that collectively constitute the spatial structure have their own characteristics and dynamics that are essential to the system, and these are the characteristics that are studied by the corresponding disciplines—demography, sociology, economics, organization theory, and so on. As much as possible, we need to incorporate the domain knowledge from these other disciplines into our models of spatial dynamics. Doing so not only improves the richness and reliability of the models; it has the bonus of integrating these other domains with one another through the spatial dimension because interactions are almost always locationally specific. Similarly, models of spatial structure enable a fully integrated treatment of natural and human systems, something that has otherwise proven difficult to achieve except in very crude ways.

Historical Studies of Urban Form
The dynamical, complex systems approach to spatial structure has only been possible since computer-based modeling became feasible. Before that, studies focusing on spatial structure were necessarily descriptive, although they occasionally included a diachronic component or simple static models—the Chicago school of urban ecology, for example, was known for its formal models. An additional problem was that location-specific data were largely unavailable until well into the twentieth century. Essentially, the only urban spatial data available for most past periods consist of street maps from historical documents or archaeological excavations. Studies of the long-term evolution of urban spatial form therefore tend to be restricted to the evolution of the pattern of streets and roads, although it is not necessarily easy to assemble these data: the work of Bernard Rouleau (1967) on the history of the Paris street network bears witness to this. This approach is, of course, methodologically quite different from the one we follow using dynamic models, and substantively it is different in its focus on street patterns rather than land use and socioeconomic

distributions. Nevertheless, for the very reason that it is eccentric to our concerns, it provides a way to see our modeling approach in a broader context, so that we can understand more clearly what is present only implicitly in our models, and what is not present at all.

Studies of urban form based on historical street patterns have for the most part been carried out by architects with an interest in the city, such as Spiro Kostof (1991), A. E. G. Morris (1972), and Aldo Rossi (1982), or by urban historians like Lewis Mumford (1961). A recurring theme of these writers is the influence of belief systems on the patterns that appear in street networks. Although the network of streets and roads serves the need for mobility, the form of that network is not simply functional; in many cases, it also expresses cultural values. For example, in Paris, beginning during the Renaissance and continuing into the baroque period, characteristic squares (*places*) appeared, along with radial streets and the beginning of the Axe historique running west from the Tuileries Palace; these new geometric patterns, contrasting with the irregular street pattern inherited from the medieval period, reflected the ideals of order and rationality that characterized the Renaissance. Ideals of the ordered landscape have continued to surface in urban planning projects, for example, in the City Beautiful movement in the United States during the first part of the twentieth century, in the design of new capital cities like Brasilia, and in the extension of existing ones, like the prolongation of the Axe historique, with its visual and symbolic importance to Paris, into the new business center of La Défense, beyond the city of Paris proper.

The desire for a landscape that reflects cultural ideals is perhaps seen most clearly in the rationalized landscape of the then-rural areas west and south of Paris, where in the seventeenth and eighteenth centuries the landscape architect André Le Nôtre and others created a network of rigidly straight *allées* to give structure to the countryside, supplementing the axial gardens and the ornamental canals that surrounded the palaces of the great nobles (figure 1.1). Some of the geometry of this landscape, such as the radiating allées of the *pieds d'oie*, echo the geometry of the techniques used to implement the newly discovered laws of perspective. These laws also served to impose a kind of structural rationality on the visible world by providing a geometrical method for modeling visible reality in two dimensions. The geometrical nature of the relationship was implicitly taken to mean that the natural world itself had a hidden geometrical order. This conflation is explicitly displayed in Paolo Ucello's famous painting the *Battle of San Romano*, where the positioning of the spears expresses both a geometrical order inherent in the battle and the laws of perspective used to create the painting. In this connection, the camera obscura, another Renaissance invention, can be considered an early modeling technology, analogous to a computer, one that projected the three-dimensional world onto two dimensions in conformity with the laws of perspective and thus permitted an accurate

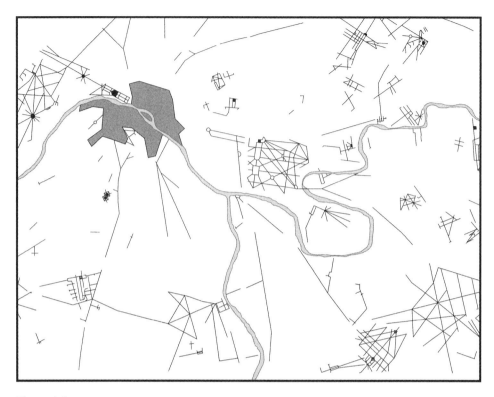

Figure 1.1
Baroque landscape of the Île-de-France; the shaded area is Paris. (Adapted from data in Benevolo, 1980)

representation of the visible world to be created in the form of a painting. It has even been suggested that the camera obscura has implicitly served as a paradigm of the positivist worldview that reality can be represented unambiguously and accurately—in other words, objectively—by means of a mechanical or formal model.

In the sense that our approach is concerned with models and theory, it might be considered neopositivist. Unlike architects and urban historians, however, we do not deal explicitly with cultural values and worldviews. But, ultimately, we should. We know from the work of both these groups that values and worldviews play a role in shaping the city. To point to a mundane contemporary example, the widespread urge in Anglo cultures to live in a single-family house surrounded by an extensive lawn contributes in a major way to low-density development and urban sprawl. Socioeconomic and demographic patterns are known to be affected by cultural values as well, though often in more indirect and subtle ways. In fact, it is likely that these factors are already present implicitly in our models because they are almost certainly among the determinants of the values of several of the parameters. A shift in social values would therefore be reflected in a need to recalibrate the models, with a consequent change in model behavior. A deeper and more explicit understanding of the relationship between cultural values and model structure, especially as expressed by parameter values, would at the very least allow us to make better judgments about the circumstances under which the models are likely to become unreliable. Explicitly including cultural effects might also enable us to make the models more widely applicable.

Since the time of classical Greece, the most common planned urban form has been the rectilinear grid. New cities in the Greek and Roman Empires, bastide towns in medieval Europe, and cities established in recent centuries in European colonies have all commonly been laid out on a grid. At times, the grid has had symbolic value, as in Chinese administrative centers, but, for the most part, it seems to have been adopted as a matter of convenience. In any case, like the elaborate Baroque geometries, it is a signature of the planned city. By the twentieth century, however, some architects concerned with urban form had begun to idealize the organic form of unplanned cities and to wonder how it could be achieved by design. The project to achieve an unplanned effect by planning was of course paradoxical. But the focus on organic form was a recognition of the fact that even unplanned cities are not formless, but are in fact highly structured in a way that cannot be captured by Euclidian geometry. In spite of their diversity, cities with an unplanned street pattern have a recognizable style that is somehow the result of incremental growth in the absence of a master plan.

In this contrast between the planned, Euclidian urban form and the unplanned, organic form, we see the opposition between planning and self-organization—between top-down and bottom-up processes. Much of the literature on urban form, especially that produced by architects, emphasizes the planned elements of urban form for obvious reasons: the planned elements are explicit and can be related to the cultural characteristics and historical events of the period, whereas organic form can at best be tracked diachronically, but always seems essentially contingent and accidental; in other words, little can be said about it. Many cities seem to have forms that are largely unplanned, even if, like Paris, they have planned inclusions. Even in North America, where the grid is considered the norm, if we zoom out to the metropolitan scale, the urban area as a whole is almost always "organic" in form, consisting of an irregular patchwork of different street patterns—grids, various curvilinear layouts, and unplanned networks—all held together by a system of major arterials that were either preexisting roads or later additions planned not to express a particular geometry, but rather to optimize traffic flow and connectivity at minimal cost. Thus, even though almost all urban areas have a form that reflects planning activities to varying degrees, globally, that form tends to be unplanned, organic, and self-organized. It is the self-organization of urban form that is the focus of this book.

Modeling in Context

Though we have been discussing urban form in terms of the pattern of streets and roads, that is not the focus of our treatment in this book. For the long sweep of urban history, the street layout is essentially the only aspect of urban form for which data are still available. Over the past century or so, however, with the appearance of cadastral and taxation records as well as census data, it has become possible to examine other aspects of urban structure, such as patterns of population density, ethnicity, income, and land use. Land use has been a particular focus of interest in recent years, largely because of the widespread availability of remotely sensed data, and it is the starting point for the models discussed in this book. But we go on to include population and economic activity in subsequent models, in order to arrive at a more comprehensive treatment of the evolution of urban form—a treatment that should also be more useful for both planners and others who must deal with the growth, organization, and reorganization that constitute every city's ongoing history.

Ironically, even though the availability of remotely sensed data was one of the main drivers of a surge of interest in developing models of urban land use change, such data are almost useless for distinguishing various urban land use classes. On the other hand, they do permit a number of rural land use and land cover classes to be distinguished. This provides an opportunity to model the city in its rural context—that is, to treat an entire region as the single, integrated system that it is. Cities and countryside are almost always treated as separate, unrelated phenomena, studied by different disciplinary specialties. If they are brought together in a single study, they tend to be treated as oppositional phenomena, as in Raymond Williams's book *The Country and the City* (1973). Yet each depends on the other, and some of the most pressing planning, political, and social problems arise from this interdependency. The loss of agricultural land to urban expansion, the intensification of agriculture in response to higher land prices in highly urbanized regions, and the loss of affordable housing for rural families as houses are converted to cottage use by urban families—all are manifestations of this interdependency. In fact, around large cities the distinction between urban and rural begins to break down as periurban land uses such as golf courses, rural recreation areas, and hobby farms come to dominate the countryside. As the models described in this book are extended to include rural phenomena explicitly, they will become increasingly useful for understanding and dealing with the problems arising from the urban-rural interdependency.

The progression from modeling land use to modeling land use together with the associated demographic and economic phenomena to modeling all of these plus agricultural activity and natural phenomena may seem like a grandiose project to create a model of everything, but that is not the case. Although modeling is a scientific tool, the activity of modeling is more an art than a science. When beginning to develop a model of some phenomenon, the most important step is deciding what to include. A model that includes too little is in a sense blind. It lacks information about factors that have a significant effect on the phenomenon being modeled. However well it may seem to perform in a specific situation and over the short run, such a model is not robust; it is unable to take into account ongoing changes in the situation to which it is being applied. On the other hand, including too much makes a model cumbersome and difficult both to apply and to understand. The art of model building lies in understanding how to include just enough, but no more. Of course, the judgment should be informed by knowledge of the situation; typically, there is at least some relevant research to suggest which additional phenomena may have an important influence on the ones being modeled and should therefore be included. But, ultimately, the knowledge base is never sufficient in itself to ensure the quality of the model. The quality depends on the informed intuition of the modeler, working with a deep understanding of both the situation being modeled and its wider context.

In almost every application of a model, the user has a particular focus of interest that is somewhat different from that of other users making other applications. In order to accommodate the widest range of applications, a model needs to be generic but customizable. Such a model is able to handle a wide variety of situations, as a very comprehensive model would, but to remain relatively simple in each individual application by giving minimal or no treatment to phenomena that are of little interest or importance in the particular case. For example, in the case of a comprehensive model that includes land use, population, economic activity, and agriculture, if the current application is focused on urban density, then the agricultural module can remain passive since there is no need to model agricultural dynamics. On the other hand, if the application is directed at understanding the impact of urban expansion on agriculture, then the agricultural dynamics module can be fully implemented, while the urban module can be simplified by using fewer economic sectors. Further flexibility can be achieved by using the core model as a platform for integrating standard preexisting models from other disciplines as necessary for specific applications. For example, the basic land use model described in chapter 6 has at various times been linked dynamically with an input-output model of the economy, a hydrological model in which infiltration and runoff depend on land use, and various traffic and transportation models. Since these linked components are typically well tested and well understood, they augment the capabilities of the land use model while contributing only a small amount of extra uncertainty about the performance of the full integrated model.

The models that are the focus of this book have been developed over a period of twenty-five years and are the product of the modeling approach just described. Although closely related—they are variations on a theme—they share a common core. Because their development was driven by the requirements of a variety of end users—clients in need of a model to assist them in addressing particular problems—they evolved as a family of models; the core model has therefore been repeatedly extended or modified, or linked dynamically to other models in order to meet the varying requirements of particular end-user applications. In every case, however, the models are based on the best domain knowledge available from urban and economic geography, regional science and transportation engineering, with models from other fields such as economics and hydrology borrowed as required. The aim is to keep the models rooted in the appropriate science even as their focus is determined by the needs of end users.

Of course, one of the goals of the modeling program is to extend the science—to deepen our understanding of cities and regions. Most of the existing analysis and theory in this area is static, and thus can tell us little about why and how cities and regions change. Since our models incorporate much of this theory but do so in the context of a complex self-organizing systems approach, a new, dynamic, theory begins to emerge, one that offers insights into the way cities structure and restructure themselves as they grow. From this perspective, it might seem that having clients determine the problems that the models address would interfere with the scientific goal. For the most part, however, this seems not to be the case. In a pure research setting—that is, in the absence of clients with often complex problems—it is easy to simplify the problems unduly in order to deal with them in a clean, precise, and apparently scientific fashion. The result can be a rather artificial, sterile treatment. Client-driven research keeps the research in contact with real, complex situations, and thus forces attention on unanticipated but useful problems. The research is messier, but the results, in the end, are better.

Modeling for Complex Self-Organizing Systems

Classical science values simplicity in theory backed up by rigorous testing, but this is an untenable position in the disciplines that deal with complex systems. Indeed, disciplines that have opted for simplicity or mathematical rigor in theory, such as economics, have effectively abandoned empirical testing. The only serious scientific alternative, as we will argue in the chapter 2, is to immerse the theory and the models in empirical complexity. Though it seems messy and its results often inconclusive, this approach reflects the nature of the phenomena that we are trying to understand. Formal complexity theory offers some hope for simplicity amid the complexity. A basic premise is that complex structures can be generated by simple processes; in principle, therefore, we might hope for a simple model that can generate a complex city. In fact, we find that this is indeed possible—up to a point. Or, really, up to two points. The first qualification is that the simple model generates not just a complex city, but many complex cities, which, according to the standard interpretation, represent the many possible cities the current city could become. If we assume that the future is open, that is, constrained but not entirely determined, then the fact that the model generates many possible futures for the city is not a fault but a strength: the model captures not just the complexity of the city but also the openness of its future. The second qualification is that real cities are not just complex, but complicated. They integrate many different phenomena, any one of which might be modeled as a complex self-organizing system. But if we hope to understand real cities through our models, then the models must include at least several of the most important phenomena. That makes them complicated. Both the open futures and the multiplicity of relevant phenomena mean that rigorous tests of the models are impossible. Results of validation tests are indicative, but usually not conclusive. Given this situation, multiple applications and multiple tests are the best approach to building confidence in a model—in other words, we need to keep the model immersed in empirical situations and see how it works. In this approach, we build individual models, but, over the long run, taking into account past experience and new situations, we create one model after another; the models essentially evolve. Modeling thus mirrors the processes by which cities are structured: acts of model design are carried out on a continual basis, but, in the end, the model, like the city, largely structures itself in response to the empirical constraints encountered in the course of many applications.

Because an appropriate methodology for the complex self-organizing systems approach is still emerging, modeling in this context is a process of exploring new methodological territory. For example, what does it mean to validate a model of a system with open futures? We do not quite know. As yet, there are no well-tested standards, nor a fully developed logic of the situation. These issues are important, and good modeling requires that we be aware of them and work through them as reasonably as we can. When possible, we may even take a step or two toward resolving them.

Ultimately, then, when we work within the framework of complex self-organizing systems theory, we find ourselves traveling through the land of the Spanish poet Antonio Machado (1989), the land where

Traveler, there is no path to follow.
The path is made by walking.

In this land, it is important to keep looking around, to see as much as possible, so that as we travel we will make a path that is interesting and useful.

2
Theory and Consequences

World is crazier and more of it than we think,
Incorrigibly plural. I peel a portion
Of tangerine and spit the pips and feel
The drunkenness of things being various.

—Louis MacNeice (1907–1985)

Cities are complex. They are also self-organizing. The complexity is obvious to anyone who has any experience of a city, even though it is usually just as obvious that the complexity is highly organized and more or less functional. It may be less obvious that cities are self-organizing since we who live in them create them, and do so with a high degree of intentionality. Through our individual, purposeful decisions, and especially through the collective decisions of developers, governments, planning departments, and special-purpose agencies like transit authorities, we intentionally modify and extend our cities so that they satisfy our various needs and desires. But it is precisely the number and variety of agents involved that means that the city is, in the end, largely self-organized. Each individual decision is made in the context of the situation existing at the time, so that each is guided and constrained by the cumulative result of previous decisions. As a result, even though individual features of the city reflect the intentions of the individuals and organizations responsible for them, the structure of the city as a whole emerges largely without anyone having decided it. For this reason, it makes sense to think of the city as emerging from an endogenous process of self-organization: the city creates itself. This view is well represented by Aldo Rossi, an Italian architect who was concerned with urban form and who, following the French urban geographer Georges Chabot, maintained that "the city is a totality that constructs itself and in which all the elements participate in forming the *âme de la cité*" (Rossi, 1982, p. 55).

We know and understand cities by living in them. Occasionally, this understanding is made explicit, as in Jane Jacobs's classic book *The Death and Life of Great American Cities* (1961), a work that has had a lasting influence, most likely because it seems to capture some useful truths about the way cities work. Although the "data" consist largely of her own observations and lived experiences in New York, and thus reflect the real complexity of that particular city and its âme, Jacobs was able to generalize, to draw lessons from the changes she observed over the years and to show why loss of complexity means death for any neighborhood, or even for an entire city. Her approach has a deep resonance with the theory of complex self-organizing systems because she recognized the irreducible role of idiosyncratic detail, the functional role of complexity, and the necessity of a diachronic approach, that is, a focus on change.

The vast literature on cities produced by historians and sociologists, as well as by planners, geographers, and others, has greatly extended and contextualized our indigenous knowledge. This literature is mostly rooted in a humanistic tradition that includes the softer social science approaches, and thus retains a wealth of detail and nuance reflecting the richness of the city itself. Standing in contrast to this tradition is one that has been characterized as scientific. Though grounded in neoclassical economics, this more recent approach encompasses urban and regional economics, and it also involves urban and economic geography, transportation engineering, and several other fields. Its aim is to produce a formal theory of urban form and structure, one that is deductive in nature and based on a few postulates of human behavior such as utility maximization and rational choice. Its language is mathematics, although it places increasing importance on inferential statistics. Despite its notable success in several specific domains such as traffic prediction and the spatial behavior of retail customers, it is increasingly marginalized as a mainstream approach to understanding urban systems because most of its theoretical results are unrealistic and unusable. As a case in point, the mathematical treatment of the spatial pattern of urban land uses has become increasingly sophisticated, but the outcome continues to be a city of concentric zones, each with a single land use; all detail, all complexity, and all realism are lost (see, for example, Alonso, 1964; Angel and Hyman, 1976; Fujita, 1986, 1989; Papageorgiou, 1990). Indeed, social scientists, except for economists, have for the most part rejected this approach as a way of understanding cities.

Applying the theory of complex self-organizing systems to cities is, in a sense, an attempt to generalize and formalize the qualitative understandings developed within the framework of the humanities and social sciences. This essentially scientific approach aims to capture the inherent complexity of the city, including the continual transformations by which the city makes and remakes itself; despite its formal methodology, however, it shares several essential properties with the approaches of the soft social sciences and humanities. Specifically, it generates and works with histories, it recognizes and relies on the fundamental role of context in explanation, and its predictive power is inherently limited. In these respects, it is much closer to qualitative methodologies than it is to the classical scientific approach dedicated to the search for universal laws. On the other hand, since its foundations are in formal, computable systems, this approach retains the logical rigor and explicitness of the classical "hard" sciences. In this sense, its theories are objective: their logical consequences can be examined explicitly and extensively.

The complex self-organizing systems approach has its roots in two schools. The first is the Brussels school, growing from the work of Ilya Prigogine at the Université Libre and the Solvay Institute, both in Brussels (the synergetics approach, originating in the work of Hermann Haken at Stuttgart, is broadly similar). The second is the Santa Fe school, associated with the Santa Fe Institute in New Mexico, founded by physicists from the Los Alamos labs. Although both schools share the same underlying philosophy, the emphasis and methods of their approaches are somewhat different. Prigogine's approach is anchored in the natural sciences, specifically, in the behavior of systems driven by an input of energy—in other words, essentially all of the systems we are concerned with on this planet, from purely physical ones like the weather to biological, ecological, and social systems. The Santa Fe approach, on the other hand, centers on the use of relatively abstract computer models and seeks to understand in a general way how complex systems self-organize and adapt. In other words (and exaggerating the differences), the Prigogine approach investigates the behavior of real systems, whereas the Santa Fe school investigates the algorithmic logic of model systems. In fact, both approaches are useful, especially when combined. Although the focus of this book is on real systems—cities and regions—our methods involve simulation models.

Far-from-Equilibrium Systems

"From being to becoming" is the expression Prigogine (1980) used to describe the emergence of the science of self-organizing systems—the science of becoming—from the classical science of universal laws describing the behavior of entities that already exist—the science of being. The phrase nicely emphasizes the fundamental problem that classical science ignores: where do new things come from? How is novelty possible? The problem involves time.

Classical science largely involves laws that are time reversible, which means in effect that, by observing the system through the lens of the laws, we step outside time and see the entire system, past and future, all at once; in other words, for us, the observers, time does not exist. As long as the laws can be expressed adequately using the language of logic and mathematics, the world we know through them will be one of being rather than one of becoming, because logic and mathematics are themselves without time (see box 2.1).

As Ilya Prigogine and Isabelle Stengers (1984) point out, however, the development of thermodynamics in the nineteenth century—and in particular, the

Box 2.1
The Crack in the Timelessness of Mathematics

Although a thermodynamic system may take time to reach its equilibrium state, once there, if not disturbed, it stays there, and is thus effectively timeless. This equilibrium state is the state of maximum entropy or, equivalently, minimum potential energy, and it can therefore be defined as the state in which the derivative of the potential energy function with respect to time is equal to zero. In other words, the mathematics of the situation is calculus.

Calculus, like all analytical mathematics, is timeless in the way that logic is: since the whole system is effectively a tautology, it does not in itself imply time in any essential way. A particular application may include a variable t representing time, but for the mathematics as such, t is just another variable, like x, y, or z. The discovery of chaotic behavior has put a crack in the timeless structure of mathematics, however, and computer-implemented algorithms have opened up a gaping hole to reveal a formal world that includes analytical mathematics as a special case.

The crack in timelessness can be illustrated with a system of at least three differential equations, or more simply by a single difference equation. Though analogous to differential equations, difference equations treat time as discrete rather than continuous. They are appropriate for treating systems where events happen at discrete times, or as an approximation where differential equations would be too cumbersome to work with. Our example is the discrete logistic equation

$$X_{t+1} = rX_t(1 - X_t) \tag{2.1.1}$$

where $0 < r < 4$, $0 \leq X_0 \leq 1$, and the subscript t indicates the time period.

Equation 2.1.1 describes a series of changing values of X; but does the value settle down to a stable, equilibrium value? Setting $X_{t+1} = X_t$, we can solve for the equilibrium value X^*:

$$X^* = 1 - \frac{1}{r} \tag{2.1.2}$$

For $r \leq 3$, this is in fact the equilibrium value of X (since we do not allow negative values of X, for $r < 1$, we set $X^* = 0$). But, at $r = 3$, the solution of equation 2.1.2 bifurcates, so that, for $r > 3$, X^* is an unstable solution, and if r is not much greater than 3, there are two stable solutions, with the equation oscillating between them: the equilibrium or attractor is a period-two cycle. As we increase the value of r, the period-two cycle bifurcates to a period-four cycle, then a period-eight cycle, and so on; and after all even-period cycles have appeared, odd-period cycles also occur. Eventually, for r greater than approximately 3.57 the cycle becomes chaotic—that is, its period is infinitely long and apparently random, and the values are extremely sensitive to the initial value, so that, except for the first few values, it is impossible to calculate them. In other words the solution seems random and unpredictable, yet the equation is deterministic, involving only multiplication and subtraction.

The attractor, unlike the now-unstable equilibrium X^*, cannot be derived analytically and stated as an equation with X^* as a function of t. It must be calculated, time step by time step, yet even that approach will fail after a relatively small number of steps (the

Box 2.1 (continued)

> actual number depending on the computer we use), so that the system really is unpredictable. The reason that the attractor (the solution) cannot be expressed analytically is that it is a fractal and thus infinitely complex. And the reason that the system is unpredictable is that, since the attractor is infinitely complex and we lack infinite precision, we can never know exactly where on the attractor we are starting out, or exactly where we are going on it.
>
> The discrete logistic equation is a deterministic chaotic system. The system is deterministic, but the outcome is, for us, undetermined. From our point of view, the system is creative. In the words of Melanie Mitchell, James Crutchfield, and Peter Hraber (1994, p. 499): "A deterministic chaotic system...can be viewed as a generator of information."

formulation of the second law, the law of increasing entropy—brought time into physics in an essential way. The second law holds that, in the kinds of systems treated by statistical mechanics, time is *not* reversible: there is an arrow of time. Although the second law once violated the sensibilities of many physicists, it has endowed statistical mechanics with a characteristic essential to sound theory: the ability to generate testable predictions. Any isolated thermodynamic system can be predicted to evolve to the state of maximum entropy possible given the system's environment. Thus, for example, if you do not drink your cup of coffee, it will cool to room temperature; if you do, it will cool in your stomach to your body temperature.

Prigogine asked what happens when energy is pumped into a system to push it ever farther away from its thermodynamic equilibrium. The answer is that it will organize itself into macro-scale structures. If the cold coffee is poured back into the pot, the molecules of liquid, which at this point have only Brownian (i.e., random) motion, will, when the pot is heated, organize themselves into macro-scale convection cells of organized flows. Of course, since the second law still applies, there must be a corresponding, though greater, increase in entropy elsewhere, in this case, in generating and transmitting the power used to heat the pot and in heating the pot itself (Prigogine and Stengers, 1984). The price of self-organization (lower entropy) is always higher entropy elsewhere, often in a form we refer to as "pollution." Self-organizing systems structure themselves by exporting entropy.

The process of self-organization that occurs as a system is pushed farther from thermodynamic equilibrium by greater energy inputs can be illustrated in a literal example that also has a broader metaphorical value. Think of a river system draining into the sea. If we put a canoe into one of the headwater streams, we can drift downstream with no effort, letting the current carry us. Our lazy holiday trip comes to an end when we reach the mouth of the river because there is no more current to carry

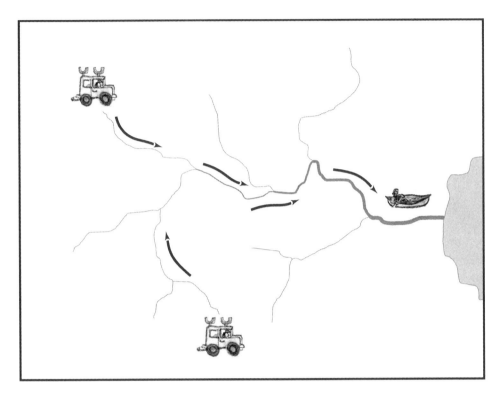

Figure 2.1
Equilibrium location for the canoe is the mouth of the river regardless of the starting point; it is thus predictable.

us (figure 2.1). At this point, we have reached thermodynamic equilibrium. Having started the trip from a position of high potential energy—i.e., low entropy—we have been carried along as the system evolved toward its maximum entropy, equilibrium state. Wherever we start our trip, in whichever tributary, we will always end up at the same spot—the mouth of the river. In other words, this entropy maximizing system is predictable, as we would expect since it is an instantiation of the second law of thermodynamics.

Now, having arrived at the mouth of the river, we turn the canoe around and head upstream. Suddenly, everything is different. First, in order to move at all, we must paddle hard; laziness is no longer an option. Then, as we move upstream, we continually come to choice points—do we take the right fork or the left? Do we have a particular goal in mind, like the headwater where we left our car? And if so, do we have a map and know how to use it? Or are we just exploring? In other words, as we put energy into the system by paddling and move ever farther from thermodynamic equilibrium, we find an increasing number of possible system states—that is,

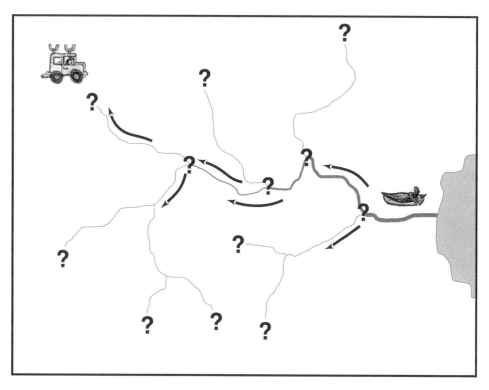

Figure 2.2
When the canoe is paddled upstream, away from its equilibrium position, its final location cannot be predicted.

tributaries in which the canoe could be located (figure 2.2). The system state is no longer predictable by a simple law. Rather it depends on a history of choices made at the bifurcation points, that is, points where one possible system state splits into two. What determines the choice? Perhaps pure chance; but as long as we are paddling the canoe, the choice may be guided by a goal and constrained by the limits of knowledge (do we have a map? If so, how good is it?), competence (can we read the map?), and physical ability (is the fork we want to take navigable, or is the current too swift for us because of flood conditions?). The system thus seems quite different. It is no longer predictable. Given the initial state, we can no longer say what the final state will be. The final state is the result of a particular contingent history, the history of our choice at each bifurcation point. Consequently, explanation by universal physical covering law must be replaced by historical explanation, and that can become quite complicated as various relevant factors are included, factors that were not relevant when the system was moving toward its maximum entropy, equilibrium state.

The physics of these two types of situations is closely tied to the mathematics used to analyze them. In the downstream case (figure 2.1), a potential energy function can be defined over the area of the river basin and differential calculus used to find the minimum of this potential function and show that it corresponds to sea level. In the upstream case (figure 2.2), the potential function will show all the local minima corresponding to a given energy input, but will give no indication as to which solution will be chosen—hence the unpredictability.

Pushing the example of a far-from-equilibrium system well into metaphorical territory, if we send many canoes upstream from the mouth of the river, we may find that the various headwaters each collect roughly the same number of canoes; or we may find that many headwaters collect just a few canoes, a smaller number collect a larger number of canoes, and a very few headwaters collect many canoes. In other words, this far-from-equilibrium system can generate a variety of possible patterns of canoe clusters. We might whimsically think of these clusters as canoe cities, and the ensemble as a regional system of such cities (figure 2.3). Of course, real systems of cities, and the cities themselves, are also far-from-equilibrium systems in that they depend on a constant inflow of energy in the form of food, gas, electricity, and so on. They construct and maintain themselves by dissipating the energy in higher-entropy forms such as sewage, garbage, and greenhouse gases.

In general, then, when we inject energy into a thermodynamic system, we convert simple, law-like, predictable behavior into complex, unpredictable, but increasingly ordered behavior. Nevertheless, it is the *same* system. The only difference is that, instead of taking free energy out of the system, we are putting energy into it. And if it is the same system, if our study of it as it moves to equilibrium is characterized as science, then our study of it as it moves away from equilibrium must also be characterized as science, though a different kind of science—one with more complications and less certainty, but one yielding just as much understanding.

All of the global systems of interest to us are far from thermodynamic equilibrium and are undergoing continuous self-organization in the sense described by Prigogine. Tectonic processes that shape the surface of the earth are driven by heat from radioactive decay in the interior of the planet. Surface processes, from ocean and atmospheric circulation to biosphere dynamics, are driven by continuing inflows of energy from the sun. And human societies, with their increasingly elaborate economies, are also ultimately dependent on the flux of solar energy, as well as on fossil fuels. Of course, ecosystems and human societies are more than just physical systems. Unlike the purely physical systems, which are simply collections of blind molecules, they are composed of goal-directed entities, that is, living organisms. In the case of a bacterium, the goals may be simple, whereas at the other extreme, the goals of human beings and their organizations are multifarious and complicated. But in both cases, as physical systems far from thermodynamic equilibrium, they undergo a process of

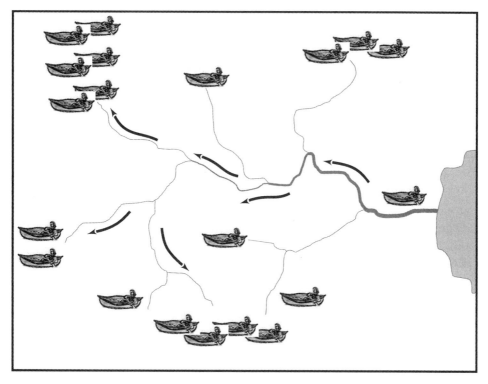

Figure 2.3
If many canoes are sent upstream, they will map out all of the possible final locations—the far-from-equilibrium steady states—and will collectively constitute a system of "canoe cities," analogous to an urban system, with many small aggregations of canoes and a few large ones.

self-organization. The goals and intentionality found in living systems simply serve to mediate and direct the process, as when, paddling our canoe upstream, we have to decide which fork to take. Of course, in modeling cities, we will be focused on the mediation process—the culture-based tastes and desires, the economics, the politics, and the planning—rather than the physics. But it is important to recognize that at the most fundamental level we are dealing with a physical system. This perspective may ultimately lead us to deeper insights into the relationship between the natural environment, on the one hand, and our economy and society, on the other.

The Algorithmic Approach

The key to modeling cities as self-organizing systems is to treat them not as artifacts but as processes—which means embedding the model in time. From this perspective, the natural language of modeling is the algorithm, since an algorithm is a representation of a process. An algorithm must normally be executed in time, step by step. Although some special algorithms can be "solved" to find the outcome without executing them, much as a difference or differential equation can be solved to find the value of the variable as a function of time (e.g., equation 2.1.2 in box 2.1), the halting theorem shows that, in general, this is not possible. The output of most algorithms can only be known by executing them, step by step, *in time*. This is the truly revolutionary aspect of the computer: the program, while executing, is an algorithm embedded in time, from which it cannot be removed. It thus allows us to treat far-from-equilibrium systems formally since these systems are also inextricably embedded in time as they organize or create themselves. The phenomena emerging in far-from-equilibrium systems are the ones that have always resisted treatment by conventional scientific laws. Because far-from-equilibrium systems have open futures, they are *creative*; therefore, universal laws can have little to say about them.

On the other hand, algorithms can represent far-from-equilibrium systems, thus permitting us to explore the possibilities inherent in them. But what kind of algorithms? For insights into the basic nature of complex self-organizing systems—insights that are in a sense analogous to the universal laws of classical science—simple algorithms that capture the generic behavior of such systems are appropriate. The original algorithm of this kind was the cellular automaton (CA), conceived by Stanislaw Ulam in the late 1940s at the Los Alamos National Laboratory as a simple tool for exploring the nature of dynamical systems (see box 2.2). Since then, CA have been ever more widely used to explore the general nature of dynamical systems because computationally they are highly efficient—they run fast. This is important because it means that a wide variety of situations can be investigated quickly to give comprehensive results; Michael Batty (2013) emphasizes this point as well.

When it was proved that the Game of Life, an extremely simple CA with two cell states and three transition rules, was capable of universal computation (Poundstone, 1985), CA quickly became a favored technique for investigating the nature of complex self-organizing systems. Later, other types of algorithms useful for investigating complex adaptive systems were developed, such as classifier systems, artificial neural networks, and random Boolean networks. The algorithmic approach is associated with the Santa Fe Institute since much of the generic, abstract work on the nature of complex systems has been carried out there. If the Brussels school was instrumental in developing a natural sciences–based theory of complex systems, researchers at the Santa Fe Institute were in effect working toward a formal theory. Although there is no fully developed formal theory as yet, there are strong suggestions of basic principles, which appear most centrally in the work of Christopher Langton and Stuart Kauffman.

Langton approached complex adaptive systems by examining the behavior of a simple generic model—a one-dimensional CA, but one with a relatively large cell

Box 2.2
Cellular Automata

The mathematicians Stanislaw Ulam and John von Neumann conceived cellular automata (CA) in the late 1940s to provide a simple, easily computable formalism for studying the dynamics of nonlinear systems. In particular, von Neumann was interested in the problem of self-replication and wanted a formal way of modeling the problem. CA have since been widely used to study a variety of problems in nonlinear dynamics, especially those involving self-organization because they are the prototypical systems that can generate patterns of any degree of complexity by the repeated application of very simple rules. They are also inherently spatial, which is a major advantage when they are used to model geographical phenomena.

A classical CA is defined by the following characteristics:

Cell space This is typically a grid of square cells, usually two-dimensional, but also frequently one-dimensional in purely abstract theoretical investigations of emergence and self-organization.

Time step Time is treated as discrete: the dynamics on the cell space proceed step by step.

Cell states A set of two or more categorical states is defined, and, at any particular time, each cell is characterized by one of these states.

Cell neighborhood The neighborhood of a cell is defined as a certain set of cells around the cell. The classical cell neighborhoods are the von Neumann neighborhood, consisting of the four cells adjacent to the given cell in the rook directions, and the Moore neighborhood, the eight cells surrounding the given cell in the queen directions, but neighborhoods may be much larger.

Transition rules One or more transition rules relate the state of each cell in the cell space to the states of the cells in its neighborhood. The neighborhood each cell is evaluated according to the rule set to determine what its state should be, and then all cell states are updated simultaneously.

Of course, when a CA is designed to model a particular phenomenon such as urban growth, these conventional CA characteristics must be modified as appropriate. For example, cell space may be inhomogeneous, or the raster irregular, consisting of cadastral plots; cell states may be continuous rather than categorical; the cell neighborhood may be larger or irregular; and the cell state updates may be sequential rather than simultaneous. We will consider many modifications like these in the models discussed in the following chapters.

Interest in CA became much more widespread after it was proved that the Game of Life, a CA developed by the mathematician John Conway, is formally equivalent to a Turing machine; that is, it is capable of universal computation. Game of Life is a two-state ("live" and "dead") cellular automaton with an eight-cell (Moore) neighborhood and simple rules: if a cell is alive and has either two or three live neighbors, it stays alive; if it is dead and has exactly three live neighbors, it comes to life; in all other cases, it will be dead. This CA is able to act as a Turing machine because, starting from a sufficiently dense random scatter of live cells, it quickly organizes itself into (1) local stable structures that in effect act as memory (figure 2.2.1a), but that can also be deleted (figure

Box 2.2 (continued)

2.2.1b); (2) structures that are mobile and can thus communicate with and act on the memory structures (figure 2.2.2); and (3) structures that are transforming themselves and thus, in effect, actually carrying out computation (figure 2.2.3). These transforming structures often arise when a mobile structure collides with a memory structure, and the result may be several new memory structures as well as one or more mobile units, heading off to possibly collide with other structures.

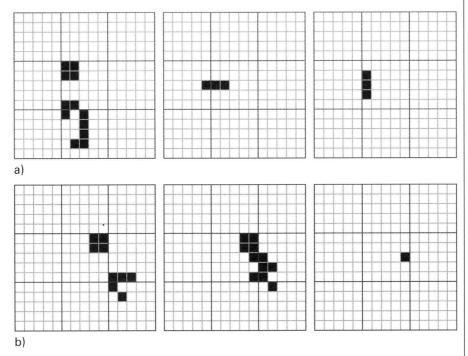

Figure 2.2.1
(a) Game of Life: Storage (memory) configurations: (1) two stable structures; (2 and 3) the blinker, a period-one configuration. (b) Game of Life: Deletion: (1) the stable square of four cells is approached from lower right by a glider; (2) the situation three iterations later; (3) the situation after six iterations. The single black cell will disappear at the next iteration.

Box 2.2 (continued)

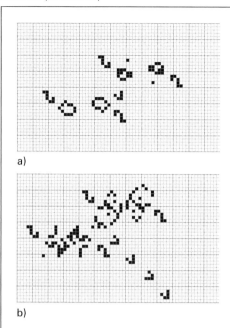

Figure 2.2.2
Game of Life: Glider gun and gliders. (a) Glider gun; (b) glider gun eighty iterations later, with a stream of gliders moving off to the lower right.

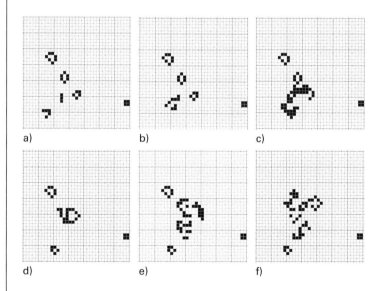

Figure 2.2.3
"Computation": (a) Glider gun approaches a cluster of storage structures from the lower left; (b) at iteration 10, after the glider has collided with the blinker, a more complex dynamic configuration appears; (c) at iteration 20, the first stable structure is about to be engulfed; (d) at iteration 30, the CA dynamics have created a new stable structure in the lower left, that is, they have "stored information in memory"; (e and f) the "computation" continues.

Box 2.2 (continued)

> Although urban and regional CA-based models are not formally equivalent to Turing machines, they do suggest that we consider a self-organizing city to be an information-processing structure, and that tempts us to raise strange questions: just what is a city computing? What is it thinking?

neighborhood as well as a relatively large number of cell states (therefore it is actually a class of CA). Since the state of a cell in a CA depends on the configuration of cell states in its neighborhood, this generic CA has a large number of possible transition rule sets. Each rule in a rule set specifies which cell state will be the outcome of a given neighborhood configuration, with one of the states designated as the "quiescent state." The many different possible sets of transition rules can then be characterized by the proportion, λ, of rules in a rule set that leads to the quiescent state. Langton showed that lower values of λ result in a steady state or simple limit cycle equilibrium, whereas higher values lead to a chaotic churn of cell states. Between these two regimes, however, values for λ near a critical value, λ_c, generate extremely long, highly structured transients, and the transient length increases exponentially with the size of the cell space. These transients have fractal properties and are apparently capable of computation. Interestingly, they have intermediate values of Shannon entropy. Computation requires (1) information storage, which is possible only with the stability and order characterized by low Shannon entropy; (2) information transmission, which raises entropy; and (3) the apparent randomness or chaos of information transformation itself, corresponding to high entropy, so that the required dynamical balance occurs at an intermediate level of system entropy (Langton, 1992). In other words, the CA generates interesting, complex configurations—dynamic structures that are capable of computation—when it is poised on the boundary between simple order and chaotic behavior. Langton says of this, "Life exists at the edge of chaos."

Stephen Wolfram, a pioneer of systematic research on CA properties, had earlier discovered similar complex behavior (his class IV behavior) in simple one-dimensional CA (Wolfram, 2002), but Langton's results provide a much richer understanding of the phenomenon. Langton has shown similar behavior in another class of CA, and it has been noted that the Game of Life also has a rule set with $\lambda \approx \lambda_c$ (Mitchell, Crutchfield, and Hraber, 1994, p. 508). Of course, as Langton himself recognizes, none of these results prove that a CA with $\lambda \approx \lambda_c$ will *necessarily* support universal computation, and Mitchell, Crutchfield, and Hraber (1994) pose some qualifications to Langton's hypothesis; but the results are very suggestive. In any case, for purposes of modeling actual complex systems, it is probably not important that the algorithm being used is strictly capable of universal computation as long as it is able to generate sufficiently rich behavior. What is important is that it can capture the phenomena being modeled. Indeed, although the CA used for most of the urban models described in this book are *sub*critical ($\lambda < \lambda_c$) in their deterministic form, they are augmented by a random perturbation so that, in effect, they function as edge-of-chaos models. As we will see in chapter 5, this feature of the model structure seems to reflect a real duality in the way cities function.

Also at the Santa Fe Institute, Stuart Kauffman (1993) used random Boolean networks rather than cellular automata to investigate the behavior of complex systems. Kauffman pursued this research program intensively over several decades, and his work, along with Langton's, is responsible for many of the deep insights into the nature of complex adaptive systems. He chose to work with Boolean networks because, unlike the cell neighborhoods of CA, they place no restriction on the pattern of connections, although, otherwise, they are quite similar to Langton's CA. As a biologist, Kauffman seeks to understand life—any possible life, not just the life we know on this planet. His aim therefore is a formal understanding of adaptability and evolvability, the two characteristics he considers essential for life.

The Boolean network models are quite general: they consist of a network of N nodes, each of which can be in one of two states, with each node connected, on average, to K other nodes. As in a CA, the state of a node depends on the state of the nodes in its neighborhood—that is, those nodes to which it is directly connected. Connections and initial node states are assigned randomly. In Kauffman's interpretation, the nodes represent genes, the node states, alleles, and the whole network, the genome of an organism.

Node states, like alleles, depend on one another. For example, a node may be turned on or off depending on the on or off state of the nodes it is connected to. Given a set of rules specifying how a node's state depends on those it is connected to, it is possible for a set of nodes to become frozen in a given configuration, so that the states of these nodes cannot be affected by nodes outside of the frozen set, even though they are connected to those nodes. For large values of K, that is, for highly connected systems, the states of nodes in the network fluctuate chaotically. As K becomes smaller, isolated frozen sets appear. For $K = 2$, the frozen set percolates through the whole network, leaving isolated regions of chaotic dynamics that cannot communicate with one another since no signal can cross the frozen structure. In this regime, the system has a relatively small number of attractors, good resistance to perturbations, and, when fitness values are assigned to the node states, an ability to adapt by hill climbing on the associated fitness landscape. In other words, the behavior of the system is, in a sense, optimally complex, consisting of a mix of ordered and chaotic dynamics that gives it the ability to adapt, which is similar to the ability to compute. $K = 2$ is therefore apparently a critical value analogous to Langton's

$\lambda \approx \lambda_c$. For $K = 1$, the system is functionally modular, consisting of a number of isolated subsystems that cannot affect one another (Kauffman, 1989); these are analogous to the simple patterns that appear in Langton's low-λ CA, or to the patterns generated by Wolfram's class I and II CA.

Assigning fitness values to alleles (node states) means that each network has an associated fitness landscape that is a function of the network structure and the individual allele fitness values. The organism represented by the network can then move about on the fitness landscape by flipping alleles. This allows it, in principle, to improve its fitness by climbing the peaks on the landscape. When several species of interacting organisms are involved, the fitness landscape is a function of the coupled Boolean networks. In this case, as one species climbs a peak on its fitness landscape, that landscape is being deformed by the adaptive behavior of another species climbing on its own landscape. For lower values of K, the deformation is slower than the movement uphill, so that adaptation is possible, but the peaks are lower, so mean fitness is relatively low. For higher values of K, the peaks are high, but the deformation is so rapid that it is not possible to climb them before they move, so in this case too, mean fitness is low. Separating these two regimes is a critical value of K at which hill climbing is just possible, and mean fitness is maximized (Kauffman, 1994). In the vicinity of the critical value, avalanches of coevolutionary change propagate through the system in response to even minor changes in alleles. These avalanches have a power law distribution.

Cities, too, may be thought of as consisting of a collection of "species": families, convenience stores, supermarkets, manufacturers, transit systems, and so forth, competing for resources such as land, access, customers, and money. For a city to function successfully, these species must coadapt toward a state where their mean fitness is optimized. Although in the urban models described in this book we do not model coadaptation explicitly, it is present implicitly in the calibration: the models are calibrated to produce results that have the characteristics of successfully coadapted cities. Coadaptation could be introduced explicitly by embedding a market model for land and by modeling the individuals (people, businesses, organizations) that make up the populations of the "species." The models would then be (in part) self-calibrating.

Candidate Principles and Domain-Specific Models

Kauffman's results using Boolean networks are similar to Langton's findings using CA. In both cases, it seems that complex, highly structured behavior emerges at a boundary between simple order and chaotic churn. Furthermore, the complex behavior has the capacity for a rich functionality that both the ordered and the chaotic regimes lack: the ability to compute or the ability to adapt and evolve toward an optimum state, which is also, in effect, computation. Kauffman (1994, p. 84) suggests that this is a candidate principle (a "putative principle" in his words), and candidate status is perhaps as much as we can hope for at present. If there are no covering laws for the behavior of far-from-equilibrium systems, then it seems likely that there are no universal principles describing the behavior of formal complex adaptive systems. On the other hand, the halting theorem is such a principle, and so others may exist.

Another quasi-principle that has been proposed is that far-from-equilibrium, self-organizing systems produce fractal structures (see box 2.3). In Langton's CA, the long transients appearing at the critical value of λ usually contain fractal patterns, as do Wolfram's class IV CA; and the power law avalanches of coevolutionary change in the critical regime of Kauffman's Boolean network are also a fractal feature. It is significant that fractal structures emerge along with complexity in these model systems (indeed, they characterize the complexity) because far-from-equilibrium natural phenomena also typically have fractal properties. Coastlines (Mandelbrot, 1982), river systems (Mandelbrot, 1982; Huang and Turcotte, 1989; Thornes, 1990; Maritan et al., 1996), riverbeds (Montgomery et al., 1996), and pulses of contaminants in rivers (Kirchner, Feng, and Neal, 2000); trees (Mandelbrot, 1982), lungs (Mandelbrot, 1982), and extinctions in the fossil record (Solé et al., 1997); the distribution of marine species (Haedrich, 1985), the distribution of marine prey as well as the movements of their predators (Sims et al., 2008), and the size of clusters of ant colonies (Vandermeer, Perfecto, and Philpott, 2008); human travel (Brockmann, Hufnagel, and Geisel, 2006), the pace of life and innovation in cities (Bettencourt et al., 2007), and the growth of corporations (Stanley et al., 1996)—all have a fractal structure. And so do cities. All of these phenomena are generated and maintained by a constant flux of energy. There is movement toward a consensus, although no proof, that all complex self-organizing, far-from-equilibrium systems are characterized by fractal structure. Per Bak has developed this point most thoroughly, and refers to it as the "principle of self-organized criticality" (Bak, 1994, 1996).

For many systems, the fractal structure may take the form of a power law distribution of some quantity, where the frequency of the phenomenon is inversely proportional to a power of its size. For example, the number of species on an island as a function of island size, the number of trips to the downtown of a city as a function of distance, and the number of patches of residential land use in a city as a function of size of patch are all described by an equation of the form $y = ax^n$. But in spatially extended systems like cities, the fractal nature often appears as a characteristic form, for example, an extremely convoluted edge; the edge of a city, like a coastline, is typically a fractal, and its form can be represented as a power law.

Another general feature of self-organized far-from-equilibrium systems is that the self-organization emerges from a series of bifurcations, where the system must

Box 2.3
Fractals

Fractal structures involve an enormous richness of detail. They are complex—infinitely complex in the mathematical limit—in the sense that they have similar features across a wide range of scales (Mandelbrot, 1982; Lauwerier, 1991; Schroeder, 1991). In other words, they are self-similar: their structure appears similar regardless of the scale at which it is examined. For this reason, they are often referred to as "scale-free structures." Discovered as mathematical entities at the end of the nineteenth century, they were quickly put aside as "monster curves" (Mandelbrot, 1982) because it was impossible to say much about them analytically. They were implicitly rediscovered, this time as both natural and political phenomena, in the twentieth century by the physicist Fry Richardson (1926, 1961), who, despite his original and imaginative efforts, found the problems they posed as difficult as the mathematicians had (Mandelbrot, 1982). It was Benoit Mandelbrot (1975, 1982) who finally put fractals on the map and named them. He called them "fractals" to emphasize the fact that these structures have noninteger—that is, fractional—dimensions. He had the essential tool that the earlier researchers had lacked: a computer. To actually work with a fractal, given its complex, recursive nature, requires a means of executing an algorithm, which the computer provided. Generating a fractal with an algorithm is essentially an exercise in self-organizing a complex structure.

The recursive process of generating a fractal is often illustrated by generating one of the "simple" geometric fractals. The fractals relevant to urban models, however, are those which involve a random process, like diffusion-limited aggregation (DLA). The simple example shown here (figure 2.3.1) is generated on a raster by a process in which a single "particle" is placed in the center of the area to constitute the seed of a nucleating structure. A number of other particles are then placed at random on the raster, and each follows a random walk until it encounters the nucleating structure, at which point it sticks to it. In the early stages, the growing structure is compact, but any slight protuberance is more likely to be encountered by a random walker, so the protuberances will grow longer, and, at some point, branch for the same reason. The result is a dendritic structure with a dimension less than 2 but greater than 1. This fractal dimension expresses the fact that if we take the seed as the reference point, the area of the structure (the area actually occupied by the individual filled squares) increases with *less* than the square of the radius of a circle drawn around the seed as we increase the radius of the circle.

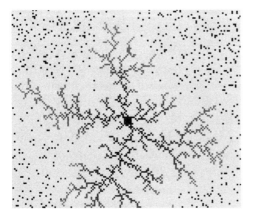

Figure 2.3.1
Structure generated by diffusion-limited aggregation (DLA). The particle density is 10%.

choose one of the possible states that open up to it as energy is put into the system. Bifurcations are often discussed as phenomena arising in natural systems, but of course they are mathematical phenomena as well, where the number of possible solutions to an equation may increase as the value of a parameter becomes larger. A classical geographical example is the spatial cost function, $C_j = \sum r_i w_i d_{ij}^n$, which gives the total cost, C_j, of shipping products to the destination, j, from a number of origin points, i, where r_i is the rate charged on the route from i to j, w_i is the amount shipped, and d_{ij} is the distance; the parameter n represents the fact that shipping costs are usually not strictly proportional to distance. If we are looking for the location j that will minimize the total shipping costs, the problem is unambiguous for $n \geq 1$: the equation has a single solution, that is, a single minimum. But $n = 1$ is a bifurcation point. For $n < 1$, there are a number of solutions, that is, a number of local minima (see box 3.2). These minima are analogous to the fitness peaks in Kauffman's Boolean network models; thus, when Kauffman finds that the number of peaks grows as the mean number of connections increases, he is describing a bifurcation phenomenon. In many cases, for example, urban land use patterns, self-organization occurs as a result of the system passing through a series of bifurcations. The bifurcation structure itself may be a fractal, as in upstream travel on the river system of figure 2.1, and the result may then be that the self-organized system has a fractal structure.

The candidate principles that apparently govern the behavior of complex self-organizing systems and the quasi-universal attributes that describe them have emerged in the course of the last forty years as a result of work with relatively simple, highly generic models such as those we have discussed. These principles, though interesting in their own right, also provide support for more realistic, domain-specific models, including models aimed at practical applications. This is not to say, however, that the lessons of the generic models can be applied directly in these more specific models. The candidate principles, even if we are eventually able to drop the qualifier "candidate," remain principles rather than covering laws. Even in the simple generic models we have discussed, in any one run of the model, they may not be manifest, or they may appear only as a weak tendency, or with a long delay. The same is true of the fractal characteristics. Nevertheless, the principles can help in the verification of a model's structure: if a detailed model of a particular complex self-organized system is not compatible with the principles, that is, if it can never manifest them, then it is probably not the right model. Similarly, to the extent that the phenomenon being modeled exhibits various fractal characteristics, the model must be able to reproduce them; fractal measures thus contribute to model validation.

More generally, the formal knowledge we have of generic complex self-organizing systems provides guidance in formulating appropriate models in specific domains such as urban spatial structure. It tells us, for example, not to build an equilibrium model of urban land use like the Alonso-Muth model (Alonso, 1964; Muth, 1969). Even though the urban land market generally clears and is thus apparently in equilibrium at any particular time, this in itself tells us little about how actual land use patterns are established and evolve. On the other hand, it is often useful to embed equilibrium models like a land market model as elements in a dynamic model. In this context, the equilibrium models represent mechanisms operating in the real system and help structure the dynamics of the larger model. They are analogous to the frozen structures in Kauffman's Boolean networks operating in the critical regime. In fact, those structures are limit cycles on an attractor—that is, they represent equilibrium behavior embedded in the nonequilibrium dynamics of the global model.

As a matter of practical convenience it is often useful to design a model so that it *emulates* a model operating in the critical regime between order and chaos, rather than designing it so that it actually possess such a regime. For example, the urban land use models discussed in this book would, if treated as deterministic, operate far into the ordered regime and produce unrealistic, simple land use maps having no fractal characteristics, whereas, with a random element, they produce complex, realistic maps characterized by fractal properties. The random element is, in effect, an efficient way of generating a large number of deterministic transition rules that together produce critical regime dynamics. From another point of view, the random element can be looked at as a simple way of emulating a heterogeneous population of agents (individual people, businesses, etc.) each with a land use decision rule; without this emulation, the deterministic model has only a few agents—one for each active land use—and a correspondingly small set of rules.

Techniques for Modeling Cities and Regions

All of the models presented in this book are simulation models of dynamical systems. Most are based on cellular automata. But as we have seen, alternatives to CA exist, and the choice of technique depends on what is to be modeled. In principle, Boolean networks could be used to model urban systems; indeed, for some particular problems, they might be quite appropriate. But, in general, it is not clear how to align the structure of a Boolean network with the urban phenomena that we might be wanting to model, such as land use or the spatial distribution of employment. Artificial neural networks have occasionally been used (e.g., White, 1989), but, again, their structure is not easily aligned with the structure of most urban phenomena. Ideally, the modeling tool we use should be one that can represent directly and explicitly the important elements—the phenomena and the relations among them—of the system we wish to model. The closer we come to a one-to-one relation between the elements of reality and the model, the less the model is a black box and the greater the confidence we can have that it is an appropriate representation and can be relied on to give us useful insights into the behavior of the real system.

Cellular automata, Boolean networks, and artificial neural networks can all be viewed as agent-based systems, where the agents collectively constitute a computational technique, as in Langton's swarm intelligence (Minar et al., 1996), but they do not necessarily represent any actual individuals. In contrast, in individual-based models, the agents *do* represent real individuals in the system being modeled—for example, real people, real businesses, or real houses; or, in the case of the nodes in Kauffman's Boolean models, real genes. The advantage of using individual-based models to model complex systems is that they permit a system to be represented explicitly in as much detail as required, with the self-organizing macrostructure emerging bottom up by means of interactions among the individual agents. The results are rich and detailed, and our confidence in them depends not just on validation testing of model output, but also on the fact that we can see a one-to-one relationship between the model structure and the structure of the system being modeled: if the model looks like reality, then it is more likely that it functions like reality and has similar outcomes.

In principle, therefore, individual-based models are the most appropriate basis for simulating urban systems, and they have in fact been fairly widely used for that, either by themselves or in combination with cellular automata (see, for example, Filatova, Parker, and Van Der Meer, 2009; Parker and Filatova, 2008; Parker, Berger, and Manson, 2002; Parker et al., 2003; Portugali and Benenson, 1997; Portugali, 2000; Marceau and Benenson, 2011; Jin and White, 2012; Power, 2009, 2014). There are important practical considerations that limit their usefulness, however. The first is the apparently banal issue of run time. Because the urban models of interest here are all complex systems models of far-from-equilibrium systems, their behavior, as we have seen, is not entirely predictable, either because of chaotic dynamics or because of sensitivity to random perturbations in the initial conditions or behavioral rules. The self-organized structures that they generate emerge through a series of bifurcations, where the system must choose between two possible futures. In other words, these model systems have open futures. In order to calibrate an individual-based model and then to map out its possible behaviors and their relative probabilities, the model must be run many times. For this to be practical, the run time should be short, ideally, minutes. A model with many agents, perhaps millions in the case of an urban model, each with relatively realistic (i.e., complicated) behavioral rules, is not fast. Furthermore, there may be an aggregation problem since generally we are not interested in individual agents, but rather in the meso- and macro-scale patterns that emerge from their collective behavior and interaction. A related problem is that it may be difficult to link the emergence of particular patterns to specific features of the model. In short, individual-based models are ideal for modeling systems of modest size, or systems in which it is not possible to simplify or generalize the representation of agent behavior without losing essential characteristics of the system. But they are cumbersome for very large systems or systems where agent behavior can reasonably be generalized to some degree.

Cellular automata are ideal for modeling many urban phenomena because they have two great advantages: they are inherently spatial, and they are fast. A CA is by definition spatial, and therefore spatial phenomena can be mapped directly onto the cell space. In fact, a two-dimensional CA can be seen as a dynamic geographic information system (GIS): a map in a raster GIS is indistinguishable from the state of a CA at a particular iteration. In a sense, a CA simply adds a process to a raster geographic information system so that maps evolve in response to the rules of the process given their current state. The raster structure, together with the fact that the cell neighborhood and the transition rules are fixed, means that the execution time is typically very fast. In contrast, in an individual-based model, the "neighborhood" of an agent consists of the set of all those agents with which it interacts. That set is not in general fixed, but rather changes from agent to agent, and from one time period to the next because it is determined in part by the behavior of the agents.

Of course, it is possible to define a CA cell space that is not a raster of square cells. An isotropic CA in which each cell is represented by coordinates chosen at random within it has been used to eliminate the geometric artifacts that can be generated by a regular raster (Markus and Hess, 1990), and in the name of realism, cadastral maps and maps of land use polygons have replaced the raster of square cells in some models. These alternate specifications of the cell space certainly have advantages and can be justified in the name of realism—of building a model that replicates the actual system. But, typically, they severely degrade run time. One model using land use polygons to define the cell space required several hours to calculate one time step in a typical application. At that speed, it was impossible to run the model enough times to ever develop a comprehensive picture of its behavior. On the other hand, not all cell space modifications degrade run time. In fact, some, like the variable grid raster described in chapter 8, are introduced specifically to maintain fast execution times when other modifications to the CA would otherwise seriously slow run times.

Modifications to cell space are just one way that the classical CA as described in box 2.2 has been altered. In fact, researchers have tortured it almost out of recognition in the name of building realistic models of particular phenomena, and we are as guilty of this as anyone. No defining CA characteristic has been spared:

- *Cells* As already described, regular grid cells have been replaced by other polygons, both regular and irregular.
- *Cell space* Homogeneous cell space has been replaced by inhomogeneous space.

- *Cell states* Discrete cell states have been replaced by continuous quantitative states, and even by vectors of states containing both discrete and quantitative representations.
- *Cell neighborhood* The small local neighborhood has been replaced, in some cases, by a scattered, noncontiguous set of cells and, in others, by a contiguous but very large neighborhood, in at least one case covering the entire modeled area.
- *Transition rules* Simple rules have given way to elaborate, and occasionally model-generated ones.
- *Updates* The simultaneous update rule for cell transitions has been replaced by asynchronous updates.
- *Dynamics* Even the autonomous dynamics of the classical CA have been reined in by imposing exogenous constraints.

As we have mentioned, the two key considerations when modifying the classical CA are realism and run time. Unfortunately, these goals are often in conflict, so that there is a trade-off between them. In too many cases, however, the trade-off is ignored and realism is optimized at the cost of increased run time. Collectively, the models discussed in this book make use of cellular automata that have been altered in most of the ways listed, always in the name of realism, but always in a way that does not degrade run time. The variety of ways that CA can be modified enhances their power and versatility, and this has ensured that CA remain the technique of choice for many spatial modeling problems.

Methodological and Epistemological Issues

Whatever technique we choose for modeling complex self-organizing systems, we find ourselves up against a number of methodological and epistemological issues that have not yet been fully resolved. In this respect, it seems that the science of these systems is indeed, as some have claimed, a new kind of science because it is giving rise to a new kind of philosophy of science. Traditionally, science has relied on the principles of reproducibility and predictability. Within this convention, scientific theories are verified through empirical testing, which requires that the theory make predictions that can be compared with data from actual observations. But what if the theory, for any specific application, predicted a variety of possible outcomes? If the theory predicted that these were the *only* possible outcomes under the specified conditions, and our empirical data did not correspond to any of them, then we would conclude that the theory was wrong. On the other hand, what if the data supported one of the predicted outcomes? Although the theory would have passed the test for that particular outcome, the other predicted outcomes might be ones that could never actually occur. If we had some way of knowing this to be so, then we would conclude that the theory was wrong in spite of its success on the particular test. Or if there were many *more* possibilities than those predicted by the theory, and we were able to know this, we would again conclude that the theory was defective.

One way around this problem is to make many tests, to see whether, in aggregate, the empirical observations do correspond to each of the predicted alternatives, and to no others. But this approach raises other questions. Are the various tests really comparable? Or are they instead tests of somewhat different theories? The problem is clear in the case of an urban land use model. When the model is applied to a specific test city, it will generate a large set of possible land use maps, and most of these will fall into one or another of a small set of classes of maps that are quite similar to one another; these similarity classes represent bifurcations. But there is only one empirical land use map, and we cannot rerun the real city many times to generate an ensemble of them to compare with the ensemble of maps generated by the model. If the empirical map falls into one of the high-probability similarity classes, our confidence in the model is strengthened; but we still have no way of knowing whether the other predicted classes are real, or only artifacts of a bad model. One way around this problem is to apply the model to other cities. But the maps of the other cities will be completely different, so the similarity classes, and even the number of these classes, will also be different. Furthermore, we will be testing a slightly different model for each city because the model will have to be recalibrated for each one and thus will have different values for some parameters; furthermore, the land use categories will typically be defined somewhat differently for each city, and even for apparently equivalent classes, there may be differences due to different data sources or classification algorithms. In short, the situation is messy, and clean tests are not possible.

On the other hand, messiness is not the same as complexity, and the nature of complexity opens the way to a partial solution to these problems. The classical scientific paradigm developed in a context in which theories were deterministic and data could either be collected clean in the laboratory or cleaned up by statistical means. In the inductive quantitative social sciences, the working assumption is that there are underlying laws, or at least regularities, at work, but that these are hidden by the messiness—usually characterized as "noise"—that is to be found in almost all data sets. The laws are to be found by using statistical techniques to clean up the empirical data and extract the regularities. Cleaning up the data means that the many data points are replaced by a representative value such as the mean, and the "noise" thus eliminated is quantified by a measure such as the variance. The essence of this approach is to seek laws by destroying data.

The complex self-organizing systems view of this situation is quite different. The messiness in the data is most likely not noise, but rather an expression of the complexity generated by self-organizing systems. However, because in these systems a single process can generate a large number of possible outcomes, it is generally not possible to discover the underlying process (or "law") inductively from empirical data. A powerful example of this is provided by Daniel Brown and colleagues (2005). Using a CA with a given set of parameter values to model land use, they generated two land use maps from the same initial conditions. Because of the bifurcation phenomenon, these maps were noticeably different: one had a large cluster of a particular land use in the northwest part of the map; the other had a similar cluster, but in the southeast. They treated one of these maps as an actual land use map and used it to calibrate the model. When the calibration was optimized, the model performed well at reproducing the map used to calibrate it but could not produce the other map. On the other hand, the original, correct, model—correct in the sense that it was the one that produced the "observed" landscape—did not perform as well as the model derived inductively because it frequently produced patterns that were quite unlike the "observed" one. In other words, the inductive procedure produced an incorrect model, and the correct model seemed to perform suboptimally.

Since, in general, it is not possible to generate good models of complex systems inductively, they must be created a priori. For human systems like cities, this is usually not such a difficult task because complex systems models are, as we have seen, bottom up: they generate the complexity from relatively simple local rules, and we often have relatively direct access to these rules because we can observe them in our daily lives. In other words, our experience can frequently guide us as we formulate a model, and our intuition about whether the structure of a model is a reasonable representation of the system we are trying to understand is often reliable. Of course, we cannot be satisfied with intuition. We must test the model, and at this stage, the complexity becomes useful. Unlike statistical models, which destroy data, complex self-organizing systems models generate data—often enormous amounts of data—although, of course, it is artificial data. As a consequence, there are many ways to characterize the output, and thus many measurements that can be made, and this increases the testability of the model.

For example, we may test a land use model by comparing an output map with the corresponding map of the actual land use. In many cases, this is done by making a cell by cell comparison and calculating a statistic like Kappa. For many purposes, including those for which Kappa was developed, this is an appropriate procedure. But, for evaluating a complex self-organizing systems model of land use, it is not. Because the model produces not one map but many, the appropriate comparison at the cell level would be between the *probability* of a particular land use and the actual use. But more relevant are comparisons made at the level of land use polygons because it is the *patterns* of land use that are important, and there are very many ways that patterns can be characterized. For example, there are measures of polygon shape such as those found in the FRAGSTATS software, measures of contiguity of polygons of different land use, wavelet-based measures, various local and global measures of fractal dimension, and so on. This is an active area of research, with new techniques appearing regularly (see Boots, 2006; Hagen-Zanker, 2008). But most of these measures are based on pattern characteristics that would be quite similar across all of the maps produced when a single application is rerun many times. For example, if we rerun the model repeatedly, we will get many maps, some of which will appear quite different from one another; but they will all have very similar values for the fractal dimension describing the patch size frequency distribution, even though the actual location of patches may be quite different on the various maps. Most of the other measures of pattern will also have this property: a given measure will yield very similar values across the range of maps.

To a significant degree, these various measures are independent of one another. Consequently, a model may perform very well on some of them and poorly on others. Although it is relatively easy to calibrate even a bad model so that it will perform well according to one or two measures, only a model that is both essentially correct in its structure and a relatively realistic representation of the system being modeled will be able to give good results according to a larger number of measures. Thus, although the Alonso-Muth land use model, a neoclassical equilibrium model that predicts concentric, single-use zones around the center of the city, passes one test—empirically, the various land uses do in fact differ in their mean distance from the center, so that there is in effect a statistical tendency toward concentric zones—it fails almost any other test. By not treating the self-organized city as a complex system, it fails to generate complex results—the concentric zones have no complexity, no patches of various sizes, no irregularities, no fractal properties. In contrast, complex self-organizing systems models of a city generate complex land use maps that can be tested in a wide variety of ways, and that therefore have a wide variety of ways in which they can succeed—or fail. According to Karl Popper's falsifiability principle, this is a strength.

Traditionally, tests of theories are thought of in binary terms: either the test supports the theory or it refutes it, although it has long been recognized that the world, even the world addressed by science, is messy, and one test is rarely enough to make or break a theory. Popper (1959, 1963) proposed a more nuanced criterion for evaluating a theory: the more powerful a theory's predictions, that is, the more improbable they are a priori, the more confidence we can have in the theory if the predictions are not falsified in a test. Since complex systems models produce voluminous, complex output that can be characterized in many ways, they can also be subjected to many independent tests. The greater the number of tests, the less probable it is a priori that the model will pass all of them. Therefore, the more tests and the greater the proportion of tests that the theory passes, the greater the confidence we can have in it. The multiple test approach also provides a partial solution to the dilemma posed by Brown: that the model that most reliably reproduces the actual land use map may well be the wrong model. Often the model calibration that appears optimal by a standard map similarity measure like Kappa fails other tests of pattern, such as those involving fractal dimensions. Calibrating the model to balance the optimization over a range of tests reduces the risk of a spurious calibration, though it does not eliminate it.

In his first book, Popper (1959) privileged falsification over verification on the grounds that strict verification of a universal statement is logically impossible outside the realm of mathematics and logic. In subsequent decades, he continued to develop the point of view implicit in this position, so that he ultimately arrived at an idea of science that could hardly be described in terms of logic: evolution would be the more appropriate word. In this view science, like the world it seeks to understand, is open, creative, undetermined. Ideas—and the theories and models that may express them—are just as much a part of the world as physical objects, and just as capable of acting as causal agents. This conception of the world and science is very much in harmony with the complex self-organizing systems approach, and it poses many of the same methodological questions. It is the beginning of a broader view of science, and of scientific methodology. It has already given rise to an appropriate philosophical basis—evolutionary epistemology. The root of the scientific imperative for definitive tests, for verification, was the desire to have certain knowledge and to know that it was certain. Perhaps the basic problem in the philosophy of science was to show that this was possible. Popper showed that it was not. Evolutionary epistemology develops the position that what it is logically possible to know evolves with the world and our knowledge of it. In a strange way, this position embeds epistemological philosophy in the real physical, biological world and makes it contingent on the state of that world. In other words, evolutionary epistemology does not stand outside the world, examining it from the outside; it is inside the world, examining it from the inside. It parallels the discovery that algorithms are necessarily embedded in real time, in the world; they do not stand outside and independent of it, as mathematics does. This is a form of realism.

Implications for Planning

Urban and regional models based on a complex self-organizing systems approach are significantly more realistic than other types of urban models. This gives them the potential to evolve into a powerful tool for planners, although it is not always obvious to planners why such a tool would be useful. Planning practices vary widely around the world. Some countries practice a relatively comprehensive and technocratic form of planning to guide future spatial development. Others, however, do not attempt to determine the future pattern of land use; their planners focus instead on general characteristics like densities or technical specifications such as those required for the provision of streets, and thus have little interest in a land use forecast. But even in the countries where spatial planning is practiced seriously, planners may question the need for a land use forecasting tool since the point of their plans is to specify what the land use will be. In the Netherlands, for example, a CA land use model being considered for adoption was criticized on the grounds that it forecast a land use pattern that did not match the official plan. It was assumed that the future land use would be as shown in the plan.

Indeed, there is a real question as to whether planning is actually effective or merely illusory. Nurit Alfasi, Jonatan Almagor, and Itzhak Benenson (2012) examined the effect of the 1980 comprehensive land use plan for the area surrounding Tel Aviv. The plan specified in detail both the areas that could be developed for residential, commercial, and industrial uses and the areas that were to be retained as agricultural and natural areas. The authors found that, by the year 2000, 65% of all development and 75% of residential development did *not* conform to the 1980 plan because of variances and modifications made during the implementation period. On the other hand, in some cases land use restrictions have been effectively enforced. The London greenbelt, for example, has been maintained for more than sixty years, though at the cost of unplanned-for development beyond it. The lesson is that it is difficult to comprehensively override the intrinsic dynamics of urban or regional development by means of a prescriptive plan, although it is feasible to *guide* development if the process is understood and if there is a way of testing the effects of various interventions. As a planning tool, an urban or regional land use model can play a significant role in providing such guidance.

Whereas comprehensive land use planning may be absent or relatively ineffective in many places, infrastructure planning is universal and always has a major impact, whether anticipated or not. Here the need for reliable estimates of future development patterns is widely recognized since new infrastructure is typically planned to meet anticipated needs. In the case of highways especially, there is a recognized need for planning with integrated models, since the introduction of new transport elements into a region will alter the development pattern, and this will in turn modify future infrastructure needs. This problem led to the first integrated dynamic models of urban regions in the 1960s. For example, the Penn-Jersey model for the Philadelphia area modeled the relationship between extensions of the transportation system, changes of population and employment by zone in the metropolitan area, and zonal changes in demand for transportation capacity. Although the same general approach was used in models developed for several other metropolitan areas, ultimately it passed from the scene. Today there is a resurgence of interest in land use–transportation interaction (LUTI) models because the need for them is widely recognized and because the required resources in terms of data, modeling techniques, and computing power are now widely available. Complex systems models based on CA bring new capacities to the LUTI models. In particular, they model demand with much higher spatial resolution than conventional approaches, and because of the multiple outcomes that characterize these models, they give a better idea of the uncertainty inherent in the system being modeled.

The complex self-organizing systems perspective suggests that effective spatial planning should be based on a realistic understanding of the spatial dynamics of urban and regional development. Successful planning would then consist of guiding that development in directions that are both feasible and desirable. The models embodying this perspective provide a way of investigating the likely effects of various policies that might be implemented to guide development in the desired direction. For example, what would be the effect of building a new ring road (beltway or loop in the United States)? Would the road be likely to increase the pressure to develop a particular area of productive agricultural land? The complex systems approach offers the possibility of reducing reliance on prescriptive land use regulations while increasing the effectiveness of land use planning. It may also improve the effectiveness of infrastructure planning by bringing about a better match between infrastructure needs and provision. One barrier to its more widespread adoption by planners, however, is the presence of multiple outcomes due to bifurcations.

Although planners are used to working with various scenarios, a complex systems model will produce a range of outcomes, many of them quite similar, but some quite different, even when applied to a single scenario. This can be confusing to end users, who, experience shows, tend to treat the output of *one* model run as the predicted outcome and to ignore the others. On the other hand, the prediction of multiple possible outcomes is potentially the most valuable feature of a complex systems model for many planning problems. Given that it is not possible to predict the future absolutely, the most important prediction is the qualitative one. What are the major possibilities, and how likely are they to occur? The many runs of a complex systems model together map out the bifurcation tree and, to the extent that the model is correct, give us this information. The model can then be used to run "what if" experiments on various policy options to find ones that increase the probability of arriving at one of the more desirable possible futures, and thus reduce the likelihood of ending up with an undesirable one. This is a relatively abstract way of looking at the planning problem, but nevertheless an important one because it emphasizes getting the big picture right.

Moving complex systems models into planning applications promises not just to give planners a new tool, but also to deepen our understanding of cities and broaden our knowledge of the possibilities and limitations of the models themselves. With repeated applications in a variety of cities and regions, and with consequent modifications and extensions, we should acquire a nuanced sense of the degree of confidence that we can have in these models under various circumstances. This amounts to evolving more successful models, models in which we can have ever greater confidence. The process is very much in the spirit of evolutionary epistemology. Complex self-organizing systems have been characterized as embodying both contingency and necessity. In treating the models as part of the system that is evolving them, we have added a third element—intentionality.

3
Approaches to Modeling Cities and Regions

Thus, many an idea which helped me progress…gave me the happiness of a discoverer; it was connected in my memory to some forest path…where the sun cast its light patches through the foliage on the earth…. Then, I was able to drink contentedly a glass of wine.
—Walter Christaller, *How I Discovered the Theory of Central Places*

Over the last half century, researchers have followed a variety of approaches to build models of cities and regions. Regrettably, most of them were not as enjoyable as Christaller's. The approaches range from the static, optimizing, mathematical framework of microeconomic theory to inferential statistics applied to spatial data sets, and from the dynamical mathematical framework of systems theory to cellular automata and individual-based modeling. Although all of these approaches continue to be used, for the most part, they define user communities that have little interaction with one another. They tend to be seen as competing approaches or even, in some cases, as incompatible with one another, rather than as complementary. This is a problem in a field with so few researchers because research based in the different methodological paradigms tends not to be mutually reinforcing. Yet the approaches can be complementary when they are brought together. This is the implicit theme of this chapter, and it is made more explicit in the models discussed in later chapters.

Here we focus on two of these approaches: system dynamics modeling and modeling based on cellular automata (CA), with an emphasis on the latter. In fact, both of these approaches deal with dynamical systems, and there are large overlaps between them, as well as with other approaches, such as those using individual-based models and artificial neural networks. The choice of which technique to use depends on what is being modeled, the purpose of the model, and practical considerations such as data availability or run time. Their roots are in different research communities: system dynamics techniques were developed largely by physicists and engineers, whereas CA originated with mathematicians working in a computational context, and both individual or agent-based modeling and artificial neural networks are techniques created by computer scientists.

Although these techniques have only recently been adopted by the urban and regional modeling community, the history of urban and regional modeling stretches back almost two centuries. It provides a useful perspective on the current state of the field and strategic guidance as we continue to extend and develop our models and the techniques we use to build and test them.

An Historical Overview

The modern history of urban and regional modeling began in the first part of the nineteenth century with Johann von Thünen, a Prussian social theorist who hoped that a deeper understanding of human society, including economics, would lead to an improved quality of life. Two aspects of von Thünen's thinking stand out. First, he believed in formulating social and economic principles mathematically—indeed, his equation for the just wage for agricultural labor is engraved on his tombstone. Secondly, he was an empiricist; he even bought a farming estate where he could test his ideas—he saw the estate as a microcosm of society. In *The Isolated State* (von Thünen, 1966), originally published in 1826, he developed a theory that related land use to the value of what could be produced on it: each parcel of land would be devoted to the crop or other use that maximized the net revenue from it. The net revenue that could be obtained from each crop depended not only on the productivity of the land for the crop, but also on the price received at the market where the crop was sold net of the transport cost to get the crop to market. Thus the land use of each parcel was ultimately a function of the distance to the market, the transport rate, and the productivity of the land. In the ideal case of spatially uniform productivity and a radially uniform, market-centered transportation system, the overall land use pattern would be one of concentric zones of different crops or activities around the market center. Of course, in a less ideal setting, the concentric zones would be distorted or even fragmented.

A century later, again in Germany, August Lösch, an economist, and Walter Christaller, a geographer, independently developed theories to explain the location of central places, that is, towns and cities that provide goods and services to a surrounding area (in other words, they are not primarily manufacturing centers). These models assume that the economics of supplying the good or service requires a minimum or threshold size of operation, and hence that the area served must be large enough to support an operation of that size. The customers are assumed to be distributed uniformly throughout the area and always to get a good or service from the nearest center offering it—the classical isotropic plane postulate. Although these assumptions imply that the centers will be located in a hexagonal configuration, a number of different hexagonal arrangements are possible, depending on the details of the model (box 3.1). These models are, in a sense, precursors of the dynamic

Box 3.1
Central Place Theory

Developed in the 1930s in Germany by Walter Christaller and by August Lösch, both classical central place frameworks were formal geometrical systems interpreted in terms of economic, geographic, and political principles in such a way as to constitute theories of the location of towns and cities providing goods and services to a surrounding area. Both theories made the initial assumption that the landscape on which the centers were located was an isotropic plane: customers were distributed with uniform density and travel was by Euclidian shortest paths, with travel between all pairs of points on the plane possible at the same speed and cost per kilometer.

Christaller (1966) assumed that there are five types of goods. For each type, firms offering the good have a characteristic minimum or *threshold* size of operation, which, given the uniform density of the spatially distributed customers, implies a minimum size of market area. (The assumption of a threshold size, like that of the isotropic plane, was implicit on Christaller's part; these assumptions were made explicit by later writers [e.g., Beavon, 1977]). Goods of the lowest order have the smallest threshold size, and progressively higher-order goods have larger thresholds. Each class of goods also has a *range*, a maximum distance that customers are willing to travel to get it; this defines the maximum possible radius of the market area. Looking at just one class of goods and assuming that just a few firms offer those goods, there may be unserved areas. In this case, more firms will appear because there are profits to be made, and this competitive situation will lead to still more firms appearing until all firms have been reduced to their threshold size. The firms will be arranged in a regular hexagonal array, each firm surrounded by a hexagonal market area of threshold size because this is the configuration that permits the maximum number of firms to exist. Moving up the hierarchy of goods, the hexagonal market areas are progressively larger. Here is the first difficulty for Christaller's theory: it does not explain how the presumably immobile firms achieve this locational pattern.

Next, firms offering lower-order goods are assumed to colocate with those offering higher-order goods, so that a nested hierarchy of centers emerges, with each center of a given order also offering all goods of lower order. In other words, the hexagonal nets of market areas of the various orders are superimposed in such a way that higher-order centers always coincide with centers of the next lower order. And here is the second difficulty: although the colocation of firms seems intuitively plausible, Christaller proposed no mechanism to ensure that this result does not contradict either the isotropic plane or the fixed-range assumption. The most obvious reason for firms of a lower order to colocate with higher-order firms is that their customers would make multipurpose trips, which would increase the firms' turnover. This would increase the effective range of the lower-order goods, but it would do so at the cost of lost market share for firms located in lower-order centers. That lost business would put those firms below their threshold size and they would disappear, thus destroying the regular hexagonal network of market areas for that order of good. Another incentive to colocate would be economies of agglomeration—that is, a lowering of operating costs because of colocation. But because this would increase profitability, it would allow the range to expand, with the same consequences as in the case of multipurpose trips.

Box 3.1 (continued)

Christaller proposed three schemes by which the hexagonal networks could be superimposed. In the first, each lower-order center lies at a corner point of the hexagonal net of market areas of the next higher order (figure 3.1.1a). Thus each higher-order center is surrounded by six lower-order centers, but shares, so to speak, each one with two other centers of its own level, and, counting the lower-order center that coincides with the higher-order one, the ratio of lower- to higher-order centers is 3:1. This pattern is called the "market principle" because it maximizes the relative number of higher-order centers. The second scheme has each lower-order center located at the midpoint of the line connecting two adjacent higher-order centers (figure 3.1.1b). This gives a ratio of 4:1 and is called the "transportation principle" because the lower-order centers are on the direct routes between higher-order centers, thus maximizing the efficiency of the transportation network. In the third and final scheme, called the "administrative principle," each lower-order center is located entirely within the market area of the higher-order center, giving a ratio of 7:1 (figure 3.1.1c). Note that under any of these three schemes, not just the transportation principle, the presence of a transportation network would violate the isotropic plane assumption.

August Lösch (1954) developed a somewhat similar central place model as part of his larger work on spatial economics. Although he also postulated an isotropic plane and businesses offering goods or services to a surrounding population, he assumed that the number of different types of businesses, as determined by the minimum required customer base, was much larger. He also dropped the requirement that the hierarchy of centers be nested, so that centers of the same hierarchical level as defined by the number of different activities would in general have different sets of activities. The scheme Lösch used for colocating the centers of the hexagonal nets of the various sizes (he spoke of "rotating the nets") produces alternating 60-degree sectors, with "city-rich" sectors (ones with relatively more centers of larger size) alternating with "city-poor" sectors. He suggested that the city-rich sectors were associated with major transportation routes. Once again, however, if he had explicitly introduced transport routes the isotropic plane assumption would have been violated and the hexagonal geometry destroyed.

Both Christaller and Lösch were clear that their formal models were intended as aids to thinking about the complex problems presented by the spatial distribution of economic activity—not as substitutes for thinking. In their view, the contradictions noted above simply represent the point at which the models must be augmented with the more powerful and flexible resources of human thought. By the 1960s, however, when their models were revived in North America, formal models such as theirs tended to be taken literally as objective statements about the nature of a central place system. In this role, it was not clear in practical terms how to validate them, or how to apply them to real systems without violating the isotropic plane assumption. Rather than reformulate them as computational models, however, most spatial economists and economic geographers chose to abandon formal theory in favor of inferential statistics.

Box 3.1 (continued)

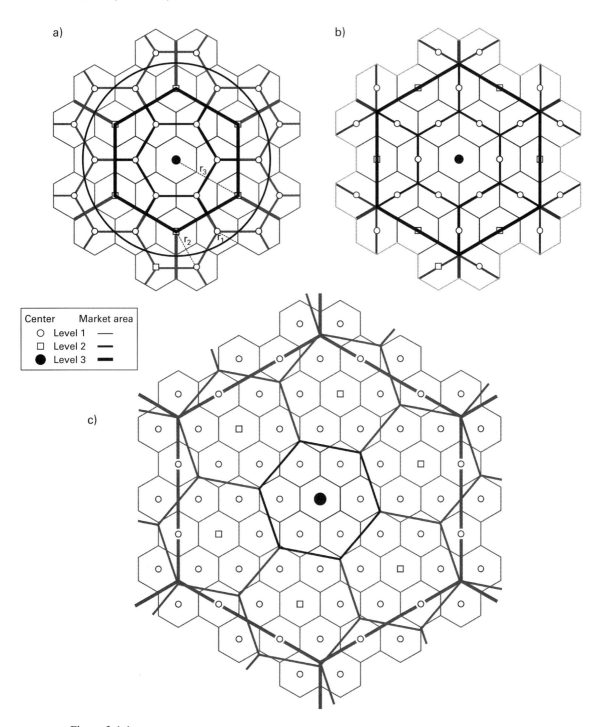

Figure 3.1.1
Christaller central place systems reflecting (a) the marketing principle; (b) the transportation principle; (c) the administrative principle.

central place model discussed in chapter 4. In *The Economics of Location* (1954), originally published in 1940, Lösch was attempting to understand the spatial implications of economic theory, but his book is sprinkled liberally with ideas and insights that go beyond the formal framework. Christaller's view was also broad. His major work, *Central Places in Southern Germany* (Christaller, 1966), originally published in 1933, was inspired by the regularities he saw in the patterns of cities and towns and transportation routes of southern Germany as he stared at his atlas, and by the thoughts he had about these patterns as he roamed the countryside on weekends, occasionally stopping on a hilltop to admire the view (see Christaller, 1972). His model of central place systems constitutes only a single chapter of the 1933 book; the others are devoted to his insights into the nature and causes of the settlement landscape that are too rich and nuanced to fit into the formal model. Both men were attempting to reconcile what, at the time, was the necessary simplicity of a formal model with their more comprehensive knowledge of a complex reality.

The fourth major theorist modeling the spatial structure of the economy was Alfred Weber, also working in Germany in the first half of the twentieth century. In 1909, Weber (1957) published a model for the optimal location of manufacturing establishments. At its core was a mathematical model (box 3.2) that stated that the optimal location was the one that minimized the total cost of shipping inputs in from various source locations and shipping products out to various markets. Space was again assumed to be isotropic. The problem has a graphical solution as long as there are no more than a total of three input and output locations. Otherwise, the solution has to be approximated, which was not practical at the time, although a mechanical device, a Varignon frame, was used in special cases for this purpose. Like the central place theories of Christaller and Lösch, Weber's theory was much richer than what could be captured in the equations of his model. For example, he discussed phenomena such as the effects of spatially varying labor costs and the conditions under which agglomeration economies would arise in local clusters of industries.

In the 1950s and 1960s, these three models from the first half of the twentieth century, together with von Thünen's model from the first half of the nineteenth century, were adopted as the foundations of the emerging fields of location theory, quantitative geography, and regional science. Because they were formulated mathematically (or at least geometrically) and seemed to generate testable hypotheses about location patterns, they were taken as the starting point for what was to be a scientific theory of the spatial structure of the economy and society. Von Thünen's model, which formed the basis of Ricardian rent theory, reappeared in modern times in the theories of urban land use proposed by William Alonso (1964) and Richard Muth (1969), theories that are extensions of neoclassical economics, and, more recently, in the new urban economics (e.g., Fujita, 1989; Papageorgiou, 1990; Angel and Hyman, 1976). These modern theories, though much more sophisticated in their

Box 3.2
The Weber Model

Weber's theory of industrial location is based on the assumption that the facility should be put at the location that minimizes the total cost of producing and distributing the product. This cost has several components—most notably, transportation (to assemble the inputs at the facility and distribute the product to the market sites) and labor—and it may be altered by externalities, especially agglomeration economies. Weber dealt first with the issue of transportation costs, and then introduced the other effects as modifying factors. Transportation costs are modeled on an isotropic plane; in other words, transportation can occur between any two points on the plane and costs are always directly proportional to the Euclidian distance between the points. The heart of Weber's theory, finding the location that minimizes total transportation costs (figure 3.2.1), is then deceptively simple:

$$\text{minimize } C_j = \sum_i r_{ij} w_{ij} d_{ij} , \; i = 1...n \tag{3.2.1}$$

where

C_j = total cost of shipping inputs into and product out from site j;
    i indexes the input and market sites
r_{ij} = the rate charged on shipments between i and j
w_{ij} = the amount to be shipped
$d_{ij} = \left((x_i - x_j)^2 + (y_i - y_j)^2\right)^{\frac{1}{2}}$ = the Euclidian distance between i and j.

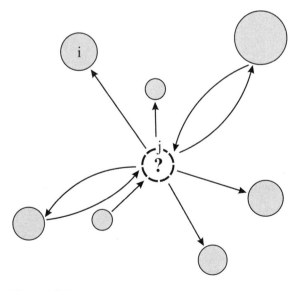

Figure 3.2.1
Schematic diagram illustrating Weber's theory of industrial facility location.

Box 3.2 (continued)

All the input and market sites are known and their locations are fixed; the amount to be produced, the quantity of inputs required from each site, and the amounts to be shipped to each market are also fixed. Therefore, the only unknown in equation 3.2.1 is the location of the production facility, represented by its coordinates (x_j, y_j). Taking the partial derivatives with respect to the coordinates, the solution is given implicitly by the simultaneous equations

$$0 = \sum_i r_{ij} w_{ij} (x_i - x_j)^{-\frac{1}{2}} \qquad (3.2.2a)$$

$$0 = \sum_j r_{ij} w_{ij} (y_i - y_j)^{-\frac{1}{2}} \qquad (3.2.2b)$$

Although a solution to these equations exists, it cannot be found analytically, and an exact geometrical solution is known only for the case where there are at most three points i. To approximate the solution, Weber used a sort of special-purpose analog computer known as a Varignon frame, which consisted of a large board, like a tabletop, with holes drilled through it at the appropriate spots to represent the locations of the n sites. A string was passed through each of the n holes, and the ends on the table top were tied together. On the other end of each string, a weight proportional to w_{ij} was attached. With the weights all pulling according to their different masses, the knot is pulled into the position that represents the solution to the equations. However, because this device has no representation of rates, it only gives the solution when all rates are constant. Weber was lucky: in Germany at the time he was writing, that was the case. But that situation was extremely unusual. Almost always and everywhere, rates are tapered, that is, they are less than proportional to distance, a situation that can be represented, for example, by raising d_{ij} to a power less than one. (Incidentally, if we use d_{ij}^2 in equation 3.2.1, then the problem becomes one of finding the center of gravity, and the equations 3.2.2 are easily solved.)

With the advent of computers, it became simple to approximate the solution and Varignon frames around the world were discarded or converted to other uses (the one in the Department of Geography at the Memorial University of Newfoundland became a display board for the departmental squash ladder). To replace the frames, most researchers used a gradient descent algorithm, like the one published by Harold Kuhn and Robert Kuenne (1962), applied to the transport cost surface. In the only realistic case, however, that of tapered rates, there are in general multiple local minima on the cost surface; therefore the algorithm must be run a number of times from different initial trial points in order to locate these minima, although there is no assurance that all of them will be found. The lowest of the minima is then chosen as the global optimum. From another point of view, this procedure can be seen as a sensitivity analysis of a simulation model.

As mentioned in the main text, once the Weber model was put into a computational context, it evolved in two quite different directions. Luc-Normand Tellier (1992, 1993) used it as the basis of a dynamic model for the evolution of regional spatial structure. In his model new facilities were introduced one at a time, and clusters of facilities

Box 3.2 (continued)

> appeared and grew as each newly located facility became a possible input or market site for facilities located subsequently. But other researchers discretized the problem by replacing continuous space with a network, and Weber's single solution point was generalized to the location-allocation problem of locating p facilities and assigning to each one a catchment area in order to optimize access to the facilities according to a performance criterion and subject to various constraints. For a number of years, Michael Goodchild and Dominique Peeters engaged in a friendly competition to produce the fastest solution algorithm.
>
> The bifurcating evolution of the Weber model is interesting because, in the first case, it led to an explanatory theory of the spatial structure of urban systems, but one with few practical applications, whereas, in the second, it led to a useful technique for solving practical problems, but one with few theoretical or explanatory implications. Nevertheless, both branches illustrate a way to break the impasse that was faced by much of location theory: do not simplify in order to solve equations; instead, keep the realism and compute.

mathematical formulation, produce essentially the same highly schematic result: concentric zones. Largely because of economists' commitment to a classical idea of science, there is general agreement that models should be formulated in such a way that the equations can be solved analytically, the assumption being that if they cannot, there is no way of knowing what the theory predicts. The problem with this position is that, in the case of most spatial systems, it is impossible to formulate analytically tractable models unless they are restricted to one-dimensional space—hence the proliferation of results characterized by radial symmetry. Furthermore, the requirement for analytic tractability means that, in almost every other respect, the models are unable to represent complex reality in any but the most caricatural way. One consequence of adopting such an approach was a lack of interest in empirical tests on the part of those developing the models. Another was a growing belief, outside the community of those modelers, that such models are uninteresting and of no use.

The central place models of Christaller and Lösch, on the other hand, were adopted more or less in their original form. Neither their originators nor later modelers fully formalized them; had they done so, they would have discovered several hidden internal inconsistencies. Instead, the major effort was a laudable attempt to provide empirical support. Geographers went to places like Iowa that best approximated an isotropic plane to collect data and analyze them for the relevant patterns (see, for example, Berry, 1967). Because isotropic planes exist only in Flatland, the problem of transforming a nonisotropic distribution to an isotropic one spawned one of the first major efforts to introduce statistical techniques into theoretical geography and regional science. Although the transformation problem was never satisfactorily solved, partly as a result of the efforts to do so inferential statistics came to dominate work in regional science and quantitative geography, essentially to the exclusion of formal models and theory. The last systematic treatment of central place theory as such was by Brian Berry and John Parr (1988). The fields of spatial and land economics, on the other hand, remain engaged with formal theory, although they also have a substantial commitment to empirical data.

Weber's industrial location theory was the most successful of the classical theories in terms of its impact on modeling in the last third of the twentieth century. The great practical difficulty with the Weber model when it was developed was that there was no way (other than a Varignon frame) to solve for the optimal location—a difficulty that disappeared with the advent of computers and the solution algorithm based on gradient descent developed by Kuhn and Kuenne (1962). At that point, the model evolved in two quite different directions. On the one hand, Tellier (1992, 1993) iterated solutions, with each newly located point becoming a possible source or destination point for the next facility to be located. In this way, he created a model of a growing, self-organizing landscape of facilities or, more generally, urban centers. On the other hand, researchers such as John Hodgson (1981), Michael Goodchild (1984), Avijit Ghosh and C. Samuel Craig (1984), Pierre Hanjoul and Dominique Peeters (1985), D. Peeters, Jacques-François Thisse, and Isabelle Thomas (1998), Anthony Yeh and Man Hong Chow (1996) and Vladimir Yasenovskiy and John Hodgson (2007), discretized the Weber model, removing it from isotropic space and transforming it into the location-allocation problem, where the goal is to find the optimal location of p points to serve n users distributed realistically, with movements to the p locations constrained to a network (see Brimberg et al., 2008, for a review). This descendant of the Weber model has a number of practical applications and is widely used.

Another area of spatial modeling, one that has only become important since the 1950s, is spatial interaction theory. The theory had its origins a century earlier in the work of Henry Carey (1858) as an analogy with the Newtonian theory of gravitation, but it quickly developed into a rich collection of models driven by empirical studies. Although the original formulation stipulated that the movement of people, goods, or information between two locations would be proportional to the product of the size of the two locations and inversely proportional to the square of the distance between them, this equation ultimately became more elaborate and application specific. The exponent on distance became a parameter to be calibrated; distance was measured not in miles or kilometers but rather in travel time, travel cost, or some more elaborate composite. In addition, an alternative form of the equation, the negative exponential, was proposed and widely adopted. This was partly the result of attempts by Alan Wilson (1970) and others (Niedercorn and Bechdoldt, 1969;

White, 1976; Timmermans, 1984) to provide a theoretical foundation by deriving the spatial interaction relationship from more fundamental principles—entropy maximization in the case of Wilson, utility theory in the case of John Niedercorn and Burley Bechdoldt on the one hand and Roger White on the other, and discrete choice theory in the case of Harry Timmermans. As the theory became both more rigorous and more general and the applications more numerous, spatial interaction theory, codified by Stewart Fotheringham and Morton O'Kelly (1989), became the most advanced and successful branch of location theory and spatial analysis. The field continues to evolve, with a self-organization approach to traffic flow and network problems becoming increasingly significant (see, for example, Helbing, 2001; Helbing and Tilch, 1998; Torrens, 2012).

Spatial interaction modeling is important for everything from marketing to congestion forecasting to infrastructure planning, and the approach has become essentially a discipline of its own. Since the emergence of spatial structure requires interaction, however, an explicit treatment of the phenomenon is necessary in almost any spatial model. One of the fundamental weaknesses of both the central place models and the land use models of the Alonso-Muth type is that they do not have an explicit and realistic representation of the spatial interaction that is driving the formation of the structures they are concerned with.

By the 1980s, the research community using mathematical models to develop a general theory of the spatial structure of the economy and society (see, for example, Isard, 1956; Isard and Smith, 1969) had begun to fragment. One group intensified its commitment to inferential statistics and largely turned its back on formal theory and models. The result was a growing collection of studies that established very narrow hypotheses in very specific or local contexts, but that failed to cohere into a general explanation of spatial structure. A second group, the location theorists, sought refuge in economics departments or business faculties and continued working along traditional lines, building and analyzing mathematical models without much concern for empirical content. And a third group, dissatisfied with the disconnected and apparently trivial results of the statistical approach, left the theory and modeling community altogether and adopted various postmodern approaches. The three groups did, however, have one thing in common: they all failed to recognize the opportunities offered by computing.

The increasing availability of computing resources at this time made simulation modeling a practical possibility. But almost no one working in the area of urban systems, quantitative geography, regional science, or location theory was using it, despite its being the most appropriate technique for modeling spatially extended systems. The lone exception was Torsten Hägerstrand, a Swedish geographer. Long before others, Hägerstrand introduced process models and simulation techniques to geography, referring to this approach as "time geography"; he also pioneered a focus on individuals that foreshadowed individual-based modeling (Hägerstrand, 1952, 1967, 1970, 1975). Eventually, researchers from other disciplines who had expertise in simulation modeling saw the absence of process modeling in urban and regional studies as an opportunity and began to move into the field. Physicists, chemists, computer scientists, engineers, and, finally, geographers, especially those specializing in remote sensing and geographic information systems (GIS) began modeling urban and regional systems with much success. Their varied backgrounds brought new techniques as well as new ideas and perspectives to the problem of modeling these systems.

What was missing was domain knowledge. Most of these disciplinary immigrants adapted very quickly, acquiring a solid knowledge of the phenomena they were modeling, and frequently a good domain intuition as well. But some did not. For example, modelers with a background in GIS or remote sensing—fields defined by techniques rather than domain knowledge—frequently develop CA-based land use models in which the transition rules are extracted from the land use data with techniques such as logit analysis applied to land use changes. The implicit assumption is that land use determines land use, and no other explicit knowledge is required to specify the transition rule: all necessary information such as personal preferences, commercial requirements, or cost of travel is implicitly expressed in the land use transitions themselves. This assumption is true to a certain extent, and it has the advantage of furthering the search for an automatic calibration technique. But, in the end, it is inadequate because other knowledge *is* required to more fully understand the land use transition process, and thus to find realistic transition rules.

The significance, then, of location theory models as they developed in the 1960s and 1970s resides not so much in the models themselves as in the useful domain knowledge they often embody, knowledge that is mostly absent from current complex systems models. Thus there are real gains to be made from uniting the two approaches in order to bring the richness of domain knowledge embodied in location theory into the powerful and flexible modeling framework of the complex self-organizing systems approach. In chapter 4, we discuss an example of a model that does just that—one that treats a central place system as a self-organizing landscape. And in later chapters, we will continue to incorporate relevant domain knowledge and classical models into our approach.

The necessity of taking domain knowledge seriously is one lesson to be learned from the history of urban and regional modeling. Another, related, lesson is to retain as much as possible of the "incorrigible plurality" of reality. The pioneers of modeling in the nineteenth and early twentieth centuries were aware of the richness and complexity of the phenomena they were modeling and never lost sight of the importance of that reality; they kept their models immersed in that context. The modelers who followed them tended to downplay the importance of the phenomena and focus on the models themselves, emphasizing elegance, simplicity, and analytical tractability. Even the statistical modelers were committed to treating the world as simple; their world was one that could be completely described by simple relationships between independent and dependent variables, relationships established by rejecting null hypotheses. Complex causal structures, and especially those involving feedback, were inadmissible. In short, the importance of domain knowledge was diminished, the richness of reality disappeared, and the models, whether mathematical or statistical, turned out to be of little relevance or use and thus were widely abandoned, especially within geography.

Modeling Spatial Complexity: System Dynamics and Cellular Automata

Parallel to the theoretical developments we have been discussing, several large land use–transportation modeling projects were undertaken in the 1960s by planning agencies in the United States in an effort to improve the forecasting of future transportation infrastructure requirements. The models that resulted from these projects were focused on spatial interaction. As systems developed to serve specific planning needs, these equation-based computational models required extensive data as input. In the end, they were not widely adopted by planning agencies, but they did stimulate the further development of spatial interaction theory and associated modeling and calibration techniques (Fotheringham and O'Kelly, 1989), as well as the development of related urban and regional models (Batty, 1976). In certain ways these later models, although not dynamic, are the precursors of the models discussed in this book, and, indeed, we have incorporated some of them into our models. Preceding this work and then paralleling it was a program to develop a mathematical theory of geographical systems—both natural and human—within the framework of general systems theory (see, for example, Bunge, 1966; Warntz, 1965, 1967, 1973–1974; Coffey, 1981). This stream of research, although never widely influential, anticipated the models described in this book; its underlying philosophy is broadly similar to ours.

One model developed at this time was, however, dynamic. Based on several interacting sectors—housing, labor, and industry—with a tendency to growth but subject to a limits-to-growth constraint, Jay Forrester's urban dynamics model (1969) generated widespread interest in dynamic modeling, but it was criticized for being too abstract and embodying too little knowledge of the way cities function to be of any real interest as an urban model. The approach, sometimes known as the "system dynamics approach," was echoed a decade later in a new class of urban and regional models.

The common characteristic of models using a system dynamics approach is, of course, the dynamics themselves. Rather than focusing exclusively on the equilibrium or steady state of the system as the traditional approaches do, such models follow the path of the system as it moves toward the equilibrium. The equilibrium state itself is often of little interest, the assumption being that long before equilibrium is attained, the system will have been perturbed, or even restructured into another system, one with another equilibrium.

Another common characteristic of spatially explicit dynamic models is that they have a core consisting of a classical spatial interaction model, and the pattern of spatial interaction shapes the dynamical self-organization of the system. Unlike the traditional models of von Thünen, Christaller, Lösch, Weber, and their followers, or even more recent models such as those of William Alonso (1964) and Yorgos Papageorgiou (1990), dynamic models discretize space, so that it consists explicitly either of points or of zones, with zones usually being represented as points. The spatial interaction flows are a function of both the inherent attraction of the destination and the inhibitory effect of distance and are expressed in relative terms: the proportion of interaction originating in zone i going to zone j is calculated as a proportion of all interaction originating at i, including interaction from i to i itself:

$$I_{t,ij} = \frac{f(S_{t,j}, D_{ij})}{\sum_j f(S_{t,j}, D_{ij})} \tag{3.1}$$

where

$I_{t,ij}$ = the flow from i to j at time t
$S_{t,j}$ = the attractivity of j at time t
D_{ij} = the distance from i to j
n = number of zones
$j = 1...i...n.$

Attractivities are usually represented by some measure of the size of the destination: for example, population, employment, or retail floor space, in which case the attractivities also, in effect, represent the system structure. Distance is measured in any appropriate way—for example, as miles or kilometers, travel time, cost, or some composite of these. The spatial interaction function $f(S_{t,j}, D_{ij})$ represents flows from i to j; it may take various forms—usually either an inverse power (gravity) or a negative exponential form. Because it now appears in a dynamic context, it must be subscripted for time. The sum in the denominator is the *potential* at i; it is a measure of accessibility to the entire system. Since $I_{t,ij}$ is a proportional measure, to find absolute volumes of interaction, it must be multiplied by the total outflow from i.

Flows may be measured in any relevant way. They may represent high-frequency (e.g., daily) flows of people, money, or information—flows that will ultimately affect the restructuring of the system as measured by the sizes of the origins and destinations; or they may consist of low frequency movements, the migration of the activity itself—for example, people changing their place of residence, or businesses relocating. The dynamic model, then, will consist of equation 3.1 augmented with equations translating the interaction effect into changes in the S_i, followed by an update of the S_i as the dynamic cycle proceeds. In this case, the model will simply relocate the activity represented by S_i. But if, in addition, there is a growth function that forces S_i, then the model must allocate the new activity as well as relocate existing activity. Both the dynamic central place model presented in chapter 4 and the regional model introduced in chapter 7 are of this type. So are the models of Peter Allen and colleagues (Allen and Sanglier, 1979, 1981; Allen et al., 1984; Allen, 1997), although they are more complex and are aimed at capturing a wider variety of phenomena.

Peter Allen and his team—including Guy Engelen—were part of Ilya Prigogine's Brussels group, and their models were developed explicitly to represent the process of self-organization of urban and regional systems. Although these models have equation 3.1 at their heart, their forcing function is a logistic equation, introduced to represent the effect of technological change:

$$\frac{dP_i}{dt} = bP_i(P_{ci} - P_i) - mP_i \qquad (3.2)$$

$$P_{ci} = N_i + \sum_j r_j S_{ij} \qquad (3.3)$$

where

P_i = population of region i
P_{ci} = carrying capacity population of i
S_{ij} = size of economic sector j in region i
b = combined rate of births and in-migration
m = the combined rate of deaths and out-migration
r_j = the rate at which economic sector j supports population
N_i = the "self-sufficiency" carrying capacity of region i.

Notice that the technology change is region specific, so that it represents not only innovation, but also the introduction to region i of an activity that already exists elsewhere. New economic activities are introduced in a stochastic manner across regions and through time, so that, for any particular region, the forcing function is, in a sense, a cumulative series of logistic functions. Thus, when a region acquires a new type of activity, it undergoes a wave of growth that begins slowly, then accelerates, and finally tapers off at the level defined by the carrying capacity. A region may undergo repeated waves of growth of this sort. In the complete model, equation 3.1 is introduced through the parameters b and m, which are thus not parameters at all, but functions capturing both the natural demographics and the migration of people from one region to another in response to competition among regions as represented by equation 3.1. The fact that the complete model (actually, a family of models) was relatively complex and difficult to calibrate hindered its widespread adoption, although it saw several different applications in the 1980s. For example, it was applied in the United States for the Department of Transportation using the fifty states as the regions, and in Senegal to that country's ten regions. The version of the model used in Senegal was unusual in that it included natural environmental factors.

Although Denise Pumain and her group in Paris worked with Allen's model (Pumain, Saint-Julien, and Sanders,1986), they later developed their own urban system modeling framework based on a multiagent approach: towns and cities are treated as agents with certain attributes, and the various levels of the urban hierarchy are modeled as different classes of agents. On the basis of spatial interactions in which they exchange economic activities, agents experience differential rates of growth and become more or less specialized, and some change class as a result of their growth—that is, they become cities of a different type at a different level of the urban hierarchy. In some versions of the model, agents (i.e., cities) are able to innovate, and possess a degree of intentionality. This is a novel application of the agent-based approach, where large aggregates of activities like cities are treated as individual agents interacting with others. In terms of the level at which the modeling is carried out—that of cities in the urban system—it resembles a classical system dynamics approach, but it benefits from the flexibility inherent in the use of agents (Bretagnolle, Daudé, and Pumain, 2003; Pumain, 1997, 2006).

In the end, very few system dynamics models of cities and regions were ever developed or applied. Although models like Allen's embody good insights into the processes driving spatial dynamics, when they are sufficiently detailed to be realistic, they are difficult to implement in large-scale applications. But perhaps more important, potential end users seem to have relatively little interest in an overall view of the future of their region. They tend to be much more focused on immediate, relatively local or specific problems, which often seem to be handled better, or at least more conveniently, by existing tools such as geographic information systems, statistical analysis, or data mining, or by extensions of these techniques. Also, with geographic information systems now the universal basis for storing, presenting, and analyzing spatial data, users expect high-resolution results, and, in this context, region-based system dynamics models look crude and clumsy.

Cellular automata are the obvious solution to the problem of implementing realistic dynamic models in large-scale applications. They were originally developed to model dynamical systems in the abstract, for theoretical purposes, but since they are typically defined on a regular grid, they are immediately compatible with both pixel-based remotely sensed land use or land cover data and raster-based geographic information systems. A CA is, in a sense, simply a way of introducing dynamics to a geographic information system. The similarities are probably the reason that many

CA land use modelers have moved into the field from backgrounds in remote sensing or GIS. Perhaps because of the technical background, there has been much experimentation with modifications of the basic CA framework. For example, cell neighborhoods have been made larger (White and Engelen, 1993), variable in size (Pinto and Antunes, 2010), or even defined on a network (O'Sullivan, 2001). Cell states, classically categorical, have been defined as densities or even as combinations of categories and densities (White, Uljee, and Engelen, 2012). Transition rules have been made fuzzy (Al-Ahmadi et al., 2009; Al-Ahmadi, See, and Heppenstall, 2013). And cells have been made irregular: Michael Batty and Yichun Xie (1994) have used cadastral units; Nuño Pinto and António Antunes (2010) have used census blocks to combine data and form; and Niandry Moreno, Fang Wang, and Danielle Marceau (2010) have used land use polygons that capture the dynamics by changing size and shape rather than state. Almost without exception, however, the world of CA is populated with models containing only two dynamic states: rural and urban. Again, this may be a consequence of relying on remotely sensed data: it is difficult to distinguish among various urban land uses.

Cellular automata are currently the most widely used technique for modeling land use. However, in spite of the number of modelers involved, because there are few sustained research efforts, the cumulative results are characterized more by breadth than by depth. One of the few continuing programs aimed at developing the approach is that of Xia Li and colleagues. For a number of years, they have explored the possibilities of CA-based land use modeling in the context of rapidly growing urban areas in China (Li and Yeh, 2000). And because their interest is clearly framed by planning issues, their focus is on advances that will improve the reliability of these models and facilitate their use. In practice, this means that, among other aspects of the problem, they have emphasized calibration techniques. They first investigated the use of an artificial neural network (ANN) approach in order to capture the nonlinear nature of the CA dynamics in the calibration (Li and Yeh, 2002). They later examined error propagation in CA (Yeh and Li, 2006) and the use of kernel-based learning techniques to extract nonlinear transition rules for the CA, showing, in a test application to Guangzhou, that these techniques gave similar results to the ANN approach in terms of accuracy, but with greater transparency in the rules themselves (Liu et al., 2008).

Recently, Li and colleagues have investigated the use of genetic algorithms applied to landscape metrics and have found that the results are superior to those of approaches using other optimization criteria (Li et al., 2013). They have hypothesized that transition rules may be local, that is, different parts of a city or region may be characterized by different transition rules (Li, Yang, and Liu,2008; Li and Liu, 2006). If this is the case, then calibrations that yield a patchwork of local rules or period-specific rules would be more accurate—and more useful for planners. They have shown how the various local rules may be interchanged to produce a rule set that will optimize a desired characteristic, in this case, compact development (Li, Yang, and Liu, 2008). But the major unexamined question here is whether locally specific rules simply represent another form of overcalibration. Further pursuing the link with planning, Li and colleagues have combined a CA-based land use model with an optimization technique to produce an optimized zoning scheme for protecting natural areas (Li et al., 2011). They have also combined a CA-based model with an artificial immune system that modifies the operation of the CA to represent the effect of planning policies on the urban dynamics (Liu et al., 2010).

Another sustained research program is that of Juval Portugali, Itzhak Benenson, and colleagues (Portugali, 2000; Portugali and Benenson, 1994, 1995, 1997; Portugali, Benenson, and Omer, 1994, 1997; Benenson, 2007; Benenson and Torrens, 2004). They developed a series of models to investigate the self-organization of the city as a sociocultural entity. Each model built on the previous ones by incorporating phenomena explicitly that had earlier been treated only implicitly. The first in the series was essentially just a CA-based model, but later models introduced agents acting in the CA space, and the agents became increasingly complex, so that, in the end, the agents themselves became to some extent self-organizing entities. The cellular space represented the urban matrix in which the agents moved around, acted, and evolved. The agents were endowed with ethnic, cultural, economic, and other characteristics. On the basis of their interactions within a local neighborhood, their cultural or ethnic characteristics could evolve, or they could decide to move to a cell with different neighborhood characteristics. In this way, not only did the spatial structure of the city evolve, but so did the agents themselves, so that, for example, new, hybrid ethnicities emerged. In other words, in what represents a higher-order self-organization, some of these models produced not just a new spatial arrangement of what was already there, but new types of entities.

These models are exceptional in several ways. First is their resolution, which, in some cases, was to the level of individual buildings. Second, and more important, is their use of agents in a CA context. Though not the only ones to do this, Portugali, Benenson, and colleagues carried the integration farther, so that, in their final models, the CA dynamics were dominated by the agent-level processes. Finally, the most unusual aspect of the models was their focus on sociocultural characteristics. These are probably the most important aspect of a city, but they are largely ignored by contemporary urban modelers, who tend to focus on land use. These models are not only built with real technical virtuosity; they are also developed in a rich and nuanced interpretive context, something rarely seen in the modeling world.

One of the most widely applied CA-based models of urban growth is SLEUTH, developed by Keith Clarke and colleagues (1997; Clarke and Gaydos, 1998; Silva and Clarke, 2002). It was first applied to the San Francisco Bay Area to simulate the urbanization of that region over the period 1900–1990. Like most CA-based land use models, it deals with only two categories: urban and rural. Unlike most, however, and more realistically, its dynamics unfold on an inhomogeneous cell space: the topography (specifically, the slope of the land) and highways both influence the probability of a cell transition from rural to urban. In other respects, the model resembles a combination of a diffusion-limited aggregation (DLA) model with a conventional CA. Rather than working through the raster cell by cell, determining the future state of each cell on the basis of the state of its neighborhood and the transition rules and then updating all cells simultaneously, the procedure in SLEUTH is to choose a rural cell at random to initiate a local cascade of urbanization events according to a set of rules applied sequentially.

The model defines four types of growth a priori: spontaneous, diffusive, organic, and road influenced. Each type of development has its own growth rate, so that the growth rate of the urbanized area is the sum of these four individual rates. Spontaneous growth occurs if the randomly chosen cell has at least one urban neighbor, or has a sufficiently low slope value; this growth may thus result in isolated urban cells. Diffusive growth occurs when the selected cell is within a defined buffer of an urbanized area and the slope is sufficiently low; in this case several other cells within the neighborhood of the newly urbanized cell are then also urbanized to create a new urban cluster sufficiently large to initiate organic growth. Organic growth is the conversion to urban of all cells with at least three urban neighbors, up to a certain limit. Finally, highway-influenced growth takes place when the randomly selected cell lies within a certain distance of a highway. A location along the highway is then selected and that cell is urbanized, together with a sufficient number of cells around it to ensure that organic growth will be possible. The rules for spontaneous, diffusive, and organic growth can be considered reasonable representations of an actual growth process. The deterministic nature of the organic growth criterion proved problematic and was modified in later versions of the model. As for the treatment of highway-oriented growth, the rules clearly bear little resemblance to any actual decision process. Nevertheless, the four sets of growth rules, taken together, do produce good simulations of actual urban growth patterns.

A unique feature of the SLEUTH model is that the parameters governing the amount of growth that occurs each year are self-modifying. As the city grows, the inhibitory factor of steep slopes becomes less and the attractive factor of highway-oriented growth grows. Furthermore, the growth rate itself, calculated as the ratio of newly urbanized cells—the result of the four individual growth processes—to the total number of urbanized cells, evolves. Upper and lower limits of "normal" growth are specified as parameters, and when the growth produced by the model breaches one of those limits, the growth rate is modified. If growth exceeds the upper limit, for example, the growth rate is increased, but in each subsequent year there is a small decrement; the result is a spurt of exponential growth that then tapers off. Having the growth rate determined endogenously has the advantage of capturing the internal feedback effects of urban growth. But the procedure ignores the larger context: the growth of any urban area is only partly generated endogenously; the most important determinant of growth is the city's role in the larger regional, national, and global urban systems.

The growth rates of SLEUTH are determined by a set of parameters that have as their primary role the determination of the spatial behavior of the urbanization process. These parameters—the dispersion, breed, spread, slope resistance, and road-gravity coefficients—control, respectively, the degree of dispersion, the amount of new growth around urbanization seeds, the contiguous spread of existing urban areas, the extent to which slopes are avoided, and the amount and location of road-oriented growth. These, together with the parameters involved in the self-modifying growth rates, are calibrated by an automatic calibration routine to give the best representation of both the historical growth rate trajectory of the urbanized area and its spatial form.

Over the past decade and a half, SLEUTH has been regularly modified and improved (Dietzel and Clarke, 2006). Most of the improvements involve the substitution of more efficient calibration routines, although some modifications have been made to the structure of the model itself in order to correct problems such as too much edge growth (Jantz, Goetz, and Shelley, 2003; Jantz and Goetz, 2005). The model has had many applications in the United States, a lesser number in China, and a scattering elsewhere (Chaudhuri and Clarke, 2013). The fact that all applications are calibrated automatically, with many calibrations based on the same multicriterion measure (the target measure has changed several times over the years), means that the results are standardized, and thus support comparison. Such a comparison was undertaken with a sample of fifteen applications from the United States and six from other countries (Clarke, Hoppen, and Gaydos, 2007) to see if there were in fact commonalities among the cities, or variations among them that were correlated with other factors. The five spatial parameters—dispersion, breed, spread, slope resistance, and road gravity—were examined. Although in a few cases the results were as expected—for example, Atlanta and the Denver–Rocky Mountain front had very high values for the road-gravity coefficient—for the most part, the values differed widely from one city to another and few patterns were evident. In fact, the relative sizes of the diffusion, breed, and spread parameters varied dramatically from one city to another for no apparent reason, suggesting that the values are unstable and, to a large extent, substitutes for one another. For example, the diffusion, breed, and spread values for Houston are 1, 3, 100, and for Seattle, 87, 60, 45, although both cities are known for a high degree of sprawl. Thus it seems that the collection of SLEUTH applications is not able to reveal much about what Elisabete Silva (2004) has called the "DNA" of cities. This is unfortunate because the numerous standardized applications of the model gave us our best opportunity to date to gain some insight into the possibility of universalities in the processes of urbanization. We will return to this issue in chapter 10.

The modeling history recounted here is to some extent embodied in the models presented in the following chapters. Thus the system dynamics model of retail centers within an urban area described in chapter 4 is essentially an integration of several of the older modeling approaches within a dynamical framework. And chapters 6–8 show how a spatial interaction–based system dynamics model of activity location is first linked interactively to the CA-based land use model and then, in a later version, absorbed into the structure of the CA itself. The implicit lesson is that the various approaches to modeling cities and regions are not so much alternatives to one another as they are mutually supportive, and the more closely they can be integrated with one another in order to exploit their complementarities, the more powerful the resulting models will be.

4
Urban Systems and Spatial Competition

Individual cities everywhere are integrated into larger urban systems. As a result, their success, or lack of it, depends on their synergetic and competitive interactions with other cities, as well as on their interactions with the rural hinterland. In this chapter, we discuss an urban system model that captures some aspects of the spatial competition among cities. Moreover, it can also be applied to spatial competition among retail centers within cities. Unlike the models discussed in later chapters, it is not based on a cellular automaton (CA), although it makes use of cell space. It represents an integration of economic theory with spatial interaction theory, but, unlike those theories, it is dynamic and, for that reason, represents an excursion of location theory into the realm of complex self-organizing systems.

The model can be seen as an update of the classical central place theories of August Lösch and Walter Christaller; like those theories, it seeks to explain the location and size of central places competing with one another to serve a dispersed population of consumers. Central place theories are essentially theories of the spatial structure of the wholesale and retail system. They do not include a treatment of primary goods since such goods are either highly dispersed in their production (e.g., agriculture) or highly localized (e.g., mining). Manufacturing is also excluded, since both production and customers tend to be highly localized—as, for example in the case of the fuselage section of an airbus, although some manufacturing activities, such as soft drink bottling, behave much like a typical central place activity. Indeed, some urban systems, such as those which make up the hierarchy of market centers in agricultural regions, do consist largely of central places and thus can appropriately be covered by a central place theory. Most urban systems, however, have too much activity in the manufacturing and specialized services sectors to be treated purely as central place systems. Furthermore, whereas the traditional theories of Christaller and Lösch were explicitly developed for systems of market towns, a generic theory should be equally applicable to the system of retail centers within an urban area. The model presented here can be applied to classical central place systems, although it is perhaps more relevant and useful when applied to the system of retail centers within an urban area.

The key difference between the model and those of Christaller and Lösch is that this model is dynamic. It includes an explicit process by which the competing centers grow or decline depending on the outcome of their competition with one another; thus its output is not a static equilibrium configuration, but rather a time series of maps. It also includes a somewhat more realistic microeconomic representation of the central place activities, and describes the behavior of the customers with a standard spatial interaction model rather than a simple go-to-the-nearest-center rule. Modelers can change components of the model at will to make it more realistic or more applicable to a particular situation. Because it is never necessary to be able to derive a final equilibrium result, but only to be able to calculate the state of the system at the next time step, elements of the model can be made as complicated—in other words, as realistic—as desired without increasing the difficulty of working with it.

The model and its applications are described by Roger White (1974, 1975, 1977, 1978), by Jun Ren and White (1995), and by Ngiap-Puoy Koh (1990). At about the same time, several other similar models of the competitive dynamics of urban and retail systems were proposed. Alan Wilson and colleagues (Wilson, 1976, 1977; Coelho and Wilson, 1976; and Poston and Wilson, 1977) advanced such a model. T. R. Smith (1977) published one in a study of the New York banking industry. More significantly, the model developed by Peter Allen, Michèle Sanglier, and colleagues (Allen and Sanglier, 1979, 1981; Allen et al., 1984; Allen, 1997) and described in chapter 3, though similar in many ways to the model discussed in this chapter, had a much more elaborate representation of the economics of the centers and thus could reasonably be applied to urban or regional systems of any kind, not just to true central place systems. Some years later, Paul Krugman (1998) also began developing dynamic location models of this kind, which he referred to as the "new economic geography." However, his were toy models that were neither applied to real systems nor investigated for their theoretical implications; they thus added little of interest to the field.

The Basic Model

The basic model (White, 1977) starts with the idea that, at any particular time, the observed structure of the central place system is the result of the differential histories of growth and decline of the centers that make it up, including the appearance of new centers and the elimination of centers that failed. In other words, the urban system is the scene of ongoing spatial competition, where some centers are more successful than others, and some may be failing. In this competitive scene, the success or failure of a center depends on its ability to attract customers (or, more specifically, revenue) from the surrounding region, but since there are also other centers in the region competing for the money that will be spent by those customers, revenue flow to the center is essentially a competitive spatial interaction phenomenon. Although the costs to be covered by the centers— infrastructure, facilities, wages, and so on— will scale with the size of the center, they will not always do so linearly: there may be economies or diseconomies of scale or agglomeration. The greater the difference between the revenue flowing into a center and the costs of building, maintaining, and operating the center, the more rapidly the center grows; if the difference is negative— if, that is the center is running at a loss—then the center shrinks. Depending on the application, these notions of revenue, cost, profit, and loss may be interpreted literally, as in the case of a commercial retail center, or notionally, as in the case of an entire city.

The heart of the model is a growth equation, with the growth of a center assumed to be a function of its profitability:

$$S_{t+1,i} = S_{t,i} + g(R_{t,i} - C_{t,i}) \tag{4.1}$$

where

$S_{t+1,i}$ = size of center i at time $t + 1$
$S_{t,i}$ = current size of center i
$R_{t,i}$ = current revenue received by centre i
$C_{t,i}$ = current cost of operation of center i

and g is a function relating profit to growth.

In the basic version of the model, the centers are assumed to be located in a cell space that is isotropic except for the presence of the centers themselves, which serve their own population as well as a rural population distributed evenly over the cells not containing a center. They compete with one another for the revenue that they can earn from this population. Each center may contain a number of economic sectors, each characterized by a growth equation like equation 4.1, so that the center size is the sum of the sizes of the sectors that are present. In greater detail, the model is as follows.

The population P of the cell containing center i is a function of the amount of activity in the various sectors k present there:

$$P_{t,ki} = \sum_k a_k S_{t,ki} \tag{4.2}$$

where a_k is a parameter, and the sector size $S_{t,ki}$ is measured in some unit appropriate to the application, such as number of establishments, square feet or square meters of floor space, or, for urban systems applications, the population of the urban center.

The proportion of revenue flowing from a cell to a given center is calculated by a spatial interaction equation of the proportional form, which takes into account the fact that, for each center, every other center acts as a competing destination. The total revenue flowing to a center is then the sum of its share of the revenue from each cell.

$$R_{t,ji} = \sum_j p_k P_{t,j} f(S_{t,ki}, D_{ji}) \qquad (4.3)$$

where

$R_{t,ki}$ = revenue of sector k in center i at time t
p_k = per capita expenditures on goods or services of sector k
$P_{t,ij}$ = population of grid cell j
D_{ji} = distance from cell j to center i

and $f(S_{t,ki}, D_{ji})$, as the spatial interaction function giving the proportion of flows from cell j that go to center i, takes one of the following forms:

Gravity Equation:

$$I_{ji} = \frac{(S_{t,ki} D_{ji}^{-n_k})}{\sum_i (S_{t,ki} D_{ji}^{-n_k})} \qquad (4.4)$$

Negative Exponential:

$$I_{ji} = \frac{(S_{t,ki} \exp(-n_k D_{ji}))}{\sum_i S_{t,ki} \exp(-n_k D_{ji})} \qquad (4.5)$$

where

I_{ji} = the proportion of flows from cell j that go to center i $(0 \le I_{ji} \le 1)$
n_j = an interaction parameter applying to sector j; n represents the distance elasticity of demand for spatial interaction.

Because both forms of the spatial interaction function have been popular in spatial interaction modeling and both have been widely used in empirical applications to problems in marketing and traffic forecasting, we leave open the possibility of using either one. This has the added advantage of allowing us to test the model to see whether the results are robust in the face of a change in the specification of the interaction equation.

The cost of operating each sector at each center depends on the sector size in that center:

$$C_{t,ki} = c_k S_{t,ki}^{m_k} \qquad (4.6)$$

where

b_k = fixed cost
c_k and m_k = marginal cost parameters.

For $m_k < 1$, the sector experiences economies of scale or agglomeration, and, for $m_k > 1$, diseconomies.

In this basic formulation of the model, we take growth to be proportional to current profit:

$$S_{t+1,ki} = S_{t,ki} + g_k (R_{t,ki} - C_{t,ki}) \tag{4.7}$$

where g_{ki} is a constant, and the new center size is then the sum of the sector sizes:

$$S_{t+1,i} = \sum_k S_{t+1,ki} \tag{4.8}$$

In some applications, the growth constant is replaced by a more elaborate function involving both profit accumulated over several time periods and thresholds above or below which no action is taken. Koh (1990) applied the model to the major retail system of St. John's, Newfoundland and Labrador, and experimented with a more realistic growth function, one that recognized that decisions to expand or shrink a business do not usually reflect strictly short-term considerations, but rather an evaluation of the long-term prospects. In this approach, growth or decline was based on the rate of return averaged over a longer period than a single year or time step and only took place if the mean rate of return exceeded a threshold level. Specifically,

$$r_{t,ki} = \frac{\left[\dfrac{\sum_{t-h}^{t}(R_{t,ki} - C_{t,ki})}{h}\right]}{R_{t,ki}} \tag{4.9}$$

where

h = number of time periods on which growth decision is based
$r_{t,ki}$ = rate of return for sector j in center i at time t.

If $r_{t,ki} > u_{gk}$ (for $r_{t,ki} > 0$) or if $r_{t,ki} > u_{dk}$ (for $r_{t,ki} < 0$), \hfill (4.10)

where

u_{gk} = threshold rate of return to initiate growth in sector j
u_{dk} = threshold rate of return to initiate decline in sector j,

then the size is adjusted as in equation 4.6. Otherwise, the size does not change.

Koh also made other appropriate modifications to the abstract specification of the model, for example, using census tracts rather than a regular grid and census tract income data in the revenue function, which meant that the space was not homogeneous. The ability to relax simplifying assumptions as necessary without affecting the calculability of the model avoids one of the major problems with the classical central place theories.

A Theory of Central Place Systems

Not only does the basic model allow us to calculate the growth trajectories of the centers making up a system, which can be useful in applications to regional development or retail center strategy, it also provides the basis for a theory of central place systems. Extensive sensitivity analysis shows that there are systematic relationships between several of the parameters and the type of central place system that emerges as the model runs. Since these parameters measure fundamental economic and behavioral phenomena, the model effectively produces a general explanation of the varying structure of central place systems in terms of those phenomena. To develop these theoretical results, the model is run in its simplest and most generic form: the centers are located on an isotropic plain and growth is proportional to profit. In the initial stages of generating the theory, it is also convenient to assume that there is only one sector and that centers have no population.

The most important parameter determining spatial structure is the spatial interaction parameter, n—that is, the exponent on distance in the gravity equation, or the distance coefficient in the negative exponential equation. This parameter is responsible for a bifurcation in the structure of the central place system. When n has a low value ($n < 1.2$ approximately in the gravity equation), center size depends on relative location both within the region and with respect to other centers (figure 4.1a). Specifically, the more centrally located a center is within the modeled region, and the farther it is from its nearest neighbors, the larger it tends to be. On the other hand, when n has a high value ($n > 1.7$ approximately), centrality within the region becomes unimportant as a determinant of a center's size, which is affected only by the distance to its nearest neighbors (figure 4.1b). The bifurcation appears regardless of the initial sizes or configurations of the centers, though of course those will affect the details of the central place system that evolves. The bifurcation also appears when the negative exponential interaction equation is substituted for the gravity equation, although the values of n over which the transition occurs are, of course, different. Changing the scale is equivalent to changing the value of n. For example, multiplying all distances by 0.1 is equivalent to lowering the value of n from $n = 2$ to a value approximately in the range of 1 to 1.2. If distances are measured in travel time, such a scale change would correspond to the introduction of a new transportation technology, for example, the change from travel by foot or horse-drawn vehicle to travel by automobile.

This bifurcation represents two types of spatial behavior. The low-n case corresponds to a situation in which the system is supplying a high-order good, known as a shopping good because customers want to be able to compare and choose from a wide selection. Competition with neighboring centers that also offer the good is one factor that will affect the growth of a center offering the good; the presence of

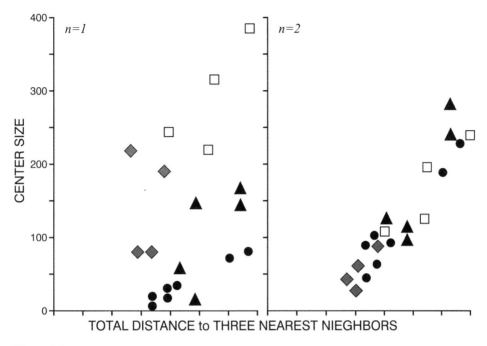

Figure 4.1
Center size versus distance to the three nearest neighbors for centers that are initially small: (a) $n = 1$; (b) $n = 2$. Distance to edge of map is shown as follows: circle, 0–5; triangle, 5–10; diamond, 10–15; square, 20–22.5. (Adapted from White, 1977)

nearby centers will tend to restrict growth. On the other hand, for high-order goods, location is relatively less important than the quality of the destination, represented in this model by center size, which is a measure of the variety or choice available. Therefore, a center that is better located for access from all parts of the region is better able to benefit from whatever size advantage it has. Somewhat paradoxically, then, the center with the best overall location in the region—that is, the most centrally located center—will tend to have a competitive advantage, even, under some circumstances, if it is not initially the largest. It is thus likely to grow to dominate or eliminate the other centers. In effect, customers bypass nearer but smaller centers to get to a larger center.

This pattern, in which the size of a major retail center (MRC) is negatively related to its distance from the center of the map, was the norm in U.S. metropolitan areas before the rise of planned shopping centers. Using the central business district (CBD) as the location of the center of the city, data from the U.S. Census Bureau (1958, 1963, 1967, 1972, 1977) for 19 Standard Metropolitan Statistical Areas, with populations ranging from 0.5 to 1.5 million people in 1960, show a negative relationship between the size of a major retail center and its distance from the central business district in both 1958 and 1963. In the latter year, the relationship was significant in all cities at the 0.10 level, and in 11 of the 19 cities, at the 0.05 level; R^2 values ranged from 0.17 to 0.94, with 12 cities having $R^2 > 0.50$. In subsequent years, the relationship became progressively weaker. By 1977, the relationship was significant at the 0.05 level in only four cases, and in only one case was $R^2 > 0.50$.

In the high-n case, the system is supplying a low-order good, a convenience good for which variety and comparison are not important. In this situation, because customers tend to go to the nearest center, the amount of revenue received by a center is essentially determined by the proximity of the nearest surrounding centers—the nearer they are, the more restricted the center's market area and therefore the smaller the center is. Relative location in the larger region is unimportant.

The parameters of the cost equation are also important in shaping the structure of the central place system. The effect of the distance parameter n as described above corresponds to the simplest possible cost equation: costs are directly proportional to the size of the center—that is, the fixed cost $b_k = 0$ and the marginal cost exponent $m_k = 1$. If fixed costs are introduced, the bifurcation governed by the distance parameter becomes even more pronounced because now some centers are eliminated. The map used as the initial distribution of centers is shown in figure 4.2a. For the low-n, shopping goods case, most centers are eliminated, and those few that remain tend to be clustered in the center of the region (figure 4.2b). The largest of these centers corresponds to the primary central business district, whereas the other, smaller centers represent cases of *forestalling*—that is, secondary CBDs that intercept customers on their way to the primary center. For the high-n, convenience goods case, fewer centers are eliminated, and those are mostly in areas that have a greater density of centers (in this case, essentially the top half of the map), so that the resulting distribution of centers is significantly more regular than the original distribution (figure 4.2c). The low-n case represents the traditional central business district, whereas the high-n case resembles the distribution of convenience stores or neighborhood shopping centers in large cities.

Introducing a nonlinear cost function, that is, one representing economies or diseconomies of scale or agglomeration, distorts the expression of the bifurcation based on n but does not eliminate it. When economies are present ($m_k < 1$), most centers are ultimately eliminated, as is to be expected, even for high-n systems. Diseconomies ($m_k > 1$), on the other hand, reduce both the range of center sizes and the number of centers eliminated, but they leave intact the concentration of centers in the central part of the area that typifies low-n systems, as well as the dispersal of centers throughout the region that characterizes high-n systems. Because, empirically, retail centers within urban areas have long experienced diseconomies of agglomeration (e.g.,

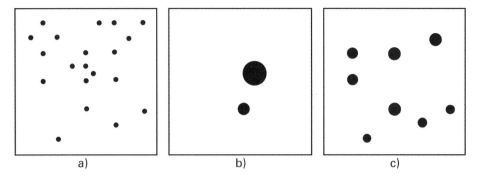

Figure 4.2
Simulation results with large initial center sizes: (a) location of initial centers; (b) $n = 1$; (c) $n = 2$. (Adapted from White, 1977)

Urban Land Institute, 1969; Kramer, Sabath, and Buchmeier, 2004), this is the relevant case in most applications.

So far we have treated the high-order and low-order sectors separately in order to discover the basic organizing principles of the spatial structure. But real central place systems have centers that contain both sectors in varying degrees. What does the model specified in equations 4.1–4.8 say about this situation? Although, in reality, there are many sectors, with each described by its own revenue and cost functions, the existence of the bifurcation dependent on the distance-decay parameter means that modeling with only two sectors—high- and low-order—is a reasonable approximation to a many-sector model. If we drop the assumption that centers have no population, then population becomes a function of the size of the two sectors, as shown in equation 4.2, with the population parameters a_j now taking on nonzero values. In other words, the population attracted by the activity of each sector—the population required to run the businesses—provides a local market for the sector itself as well as for the other sector. Together, the population parameters determine a local multiplier for the retail sector. For stability, the sum of these parameters must be less than the marginal cost of either one of the sectors.

The size distributions of these two-sector systems look much like those of some real urban systems. For reasonable values of the population parameters, the rank-size distribution of centers is linear, as is the case in many actual systems, although the slope tends to be somewhat steeper, with values of -1.37 (figure 4.3, left) and -1.2 (figure 4.3, right) for the systems shown in figure 4.3, whereas real systems with linear distributions tend to have slopes within the range of -0.8 to -1.2 (Berry and Parr, 1988). The aggregate population of the centers represents 40% of the total population for the systems shown in figure 4.3. This is similar to the ratios observed in true central place systems—that is, urban systems with centers that have only

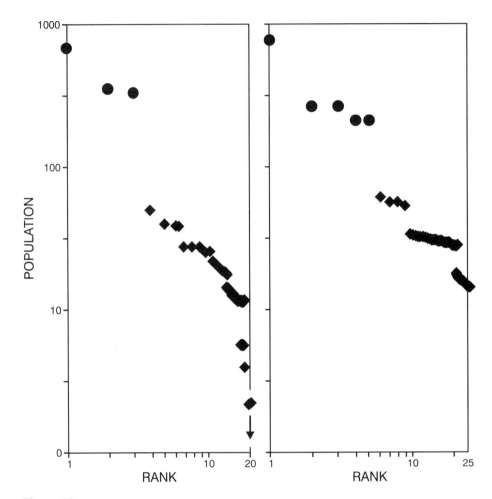

Figure 4.3
Rank size relationship for two maps of center locations: (*left*) uneven; (right) regular. For both, $a_1 = a_2 = 0.2$; $n_1 = 3$, $n_2 = 1$. Circles: two sector centers; diamonds: one sector centers. (Adapted from White, 1978)

minimal primary or secondary activity. For example, in his classic studies of the central place system of Iowa, Brian Berry found that the ratio of the population of a center to the total population served by the center is about 0.3. In an analogous Canadian case, the ratio of the urban population of Prince Edward Island to the total population is about 0.38. It is only for intermediate values of the population parameters that the model generates a linear rank-size distribution. For higher values, the system collapses to a *primate* situation, that is, a situation where one center is much larger than any of the others. This, too, is a situation observed in many real urban systems. Of course, because most actual urban systems are not simply central place systems (they include other activities, notably, manufacturing), the two cases are not strictly comparable. Nevertheless, the model does open another avenue toward explaining rank-size distributions.

The robust results from the sensitivity analysis performed on the generic specification of the model can be summarized as follows.

For the low-n (high-order) case:
1. Retail centers will be few and concentrated in the central part of the urban area.
2. Because most of the retail establishments of this type are located in these few centers, there will be a high degree of duplication, that is, each center will have many establishments of the same type.

For the high-n (low-order) case:
3. Low-order or local retail centers will be relatively evenly dispersed with respect to the distribution of population or income.
4. There will be little duplication of functions in these centers.

For two-sector urban systems:
5. When population multipliers are relatively low, so that the majority of the population remains rural, the set of urban centers will conform to a linear rank-size distribution with a slope a little steeper than -1.
6. When population multipliers are low and costs are more than proportional to size (diseconomies of scale or agglomeration), centers will show a convex rank-size distribution.
7. When the population multiplier of the low-n (high-order) sector is large enough to ensure that the majority of the regional population is urban, a primate center will appear.

These are the basic predictions of the model, and together with the model itself, they constitute a theory of central place systems. The model can be applied to individual cities, as in Koh's (1990) study of the dynamics of the major retail centers of St. John's, or to a regional system of central places as in Ren and White's (1995) study of the urban system of the Atlantic region of Canada, and if the results are reasonably good, each such application adds support to the theory. Furthermore, if the theory is sound, the robust relationships or principles emerging from the sensitivity analysis of the generic specification of the model should appear in any application, and should be observed in any actual retail or central place system. On the other hand, the generic specification is static (constant population uniformly distributed; no new centers introduced), whereas most real cities and regional systems are growing and have been doing so for centuries and are also spatially inhomogeneous. Therefore, the manifestation in real systems of the general phenomena predicted by the theory will be somewhat distorted or hidden. Of course, the theory could be made to cover the case of growing, inhomogeneous systems by extending the sensitivity analysis to include generic cases of growing cities or regions, spatial inhomogeneity of population or income, and transportation network configuration. Nevertheless, with a bit of interpretation, the basic phenomena predicted using the fixed isotropic landscape can be observed in real cities and urban systems. We have already indicated some of these correspondences between the predictions and actual central place systems, for example, in the case of two-sector systems and the rank-size distribution. But it is interesting to look further at the ways that the low-n phenomena are manifested in actual retail systems.

The major retail center of a city is typically located near the center of the city, which seems to be in line with the prediction for the low distance parameter case. In most cases, however, the central location is a historical artifact—the retail area did not move into the center of the city, the city grew up around the proto–retail center. And in port cities, the city center is usually next to the original port facilities, and thus, in effect, on the edge of the growing urban area. Nevertheless, the implications of the theory can still be observed. For example, as a city grows, it may leave its major retail center in an increasingly eccentric location with respect to the urban population or its income. If that happens, the MRC will typically follow, usually in relatively discrete jumps of about a mile (a kilometer or two). For example, the major retail center of New York City has relocated several times during the history of the city, the more recent jumps being to the 14th Street and Broadway area around 1875, to 23rd Street by 1895 (Domosh, 1990), and then to midtown (34th–42nd Streets) in the first decades of the twentieth century; currently, it may be in the process of moving again, farther to the northeast. In four centuries, it has moved approximately 4 miles (~6 kilometers) to the north, tracking the urbanization of Manhattan, the outer boroughs, and the suburbs beyond, but also following the secular movement of wealth to the north. In London, the retail center has migrated some 4 kilometers (~2.5 miles) over the centuries, from the City westward to Oxford Street. In this case, it may have been primarily following income rather than population since population is located more symmetrically around the City than is income, which is concentrated to the west.

Forestalling can occur, resulting in one or more secondary major retail centers near the primary one. This is more likely to happen when there are important transit nodes outside the central business district, or when the city is divided ethnically or culturally. In Dublin, for example, the O'Connell Street retail center on the north side of the city contrasts with the traditionally more Anglo Grafton Street center on the south side; in Montreal, until relatively recently, a secondary major retail center, one largely serving the French-speaking population, was located a few kilometers to the east of the central business district, dominated by the English-speaking business community. In both cases, historically, there was also an income difference associated with the cultural difference, and this probably facilitated the development of the secondary forestalling centers since retailers prefer to be in centers that are relatively homogeneous in terms of being upscale, midscale, or downscale.

Major retail centers have always been places where variety and the possibility of comparison shopping have been maximized by including many establishments of the same type. Traditional markets were usually organized into districts where many merchants offering the same type of good were crowded together: butcher's shops, produce stores, rug merchants, sellers of cooking pots—each group formed its own compact cluster within the market. In the central business district of a typical large city as it emerged in the second half of the nineteenth century, the segregation of different types of retail activities may have been less extreme, but there was still a high degree of duplication—*many* stores selling women's clothing, *many* selling jewelry, *many* selling shoes, and so on—which ensured variety and the possibility of comparison shopping. The multiple stores of each type clustered together in spite of the fact that they were both competing with one another and generating diseconomies of agglomeration (e.g., in the form of high land prices and rent) because, as the model shows, the spatial dynamics favor agglomeration as long as the friction of distance is low. In contrast, minor retail centers tend to have little duplication. The duplication of establishments of the same kind was noted but not considered particularly significant in the voluminous literature of urban and retail geography that appeared in the second half of the twentieth century. In a striking case, it appears as the most salient feature in Keith Beavon's (1977) statistical analysis of shopping centers in Cape Town, South Africa, the Canterbury region of New Zealand, and Snohomish County and the city of Spokane, both in Washington State, although Beavon apparently does not notice it. In his cluster analysis, two primary clusters appear: a small group consisting of major retail centers, which cluster largely because of their high duplication of retail functions, and a large group containing all other centers, which have in common, at this level, a lack of duplication of functions (figure 4.4). Beavon essentially ignores this primary division and focuses on subgroups, interpreting them in terms of the central place theories of Christaller and Lösch.

Thus, in a general way, the two robust principles concerning the behavior of activities characterized by a low distance-decay parameter (low-n) seem to manifest themselves in the historical spatial behavior of major retail centers in actual cities. But because the model presented here is a simple system dynamics representation of the retail system, in effect, it characterizes behavior as a simple mechanical reaction to the current situation. That approach seems to work well enough when the system is characterized by a number of relatively small agents (retailers in this case), as was approximately the case when the situations described in New York, London, Dublin, and Montreal were evolving. But that may have been only a long, though important,

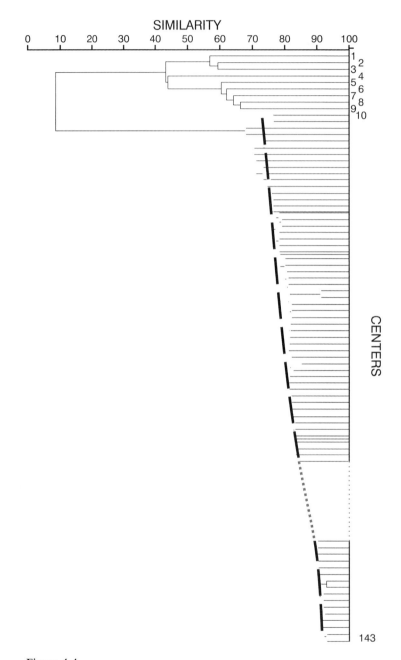

Figure 4.4
Cluster analysis of retail centers in Cape Town, South Africa. The clustering levels are generalized except for the largest centers. (Adapted from Beavon, 1977)

transitory phase. The locational principles may be valid, but it seems that whenever possible, people prefer not to be subservient to them, but to put them to use for their own ends. In this case, the end is profit.

The itinerant fairs of medieval Europe are an early example of adapting the two principles of low-n retail systems in an innovative way. Given the very low population and income density levels of most of Europe at the time, together with the extremely slow and costly nature of transportation, our model would predict that the cities would have only rudimentary retail centers and that very few high-order goods would be offered. There would not be enough purchasing power within a day's walk of any center to support a range of permanent establishments offering higher-order goods. But itinerant market fairs offering luxury goods of various types overcame these limitations. Appearing at the same location at regular intervals, such as every year or every five years, they were able to offer a sufficient variety of goods to make it worthwhile for customers to travel for many days to take advantage of the offering. Because they were able to draw from a very large market area, it was profitable to hold them. In terms of our model, the itinerant fair system was an effective scheme for increasing the size of the destination and lowering the value of the distance parameter by effectively shrinking distances, thus transforming a high-n space with small, self-contained market areas into a low-n space with nonlocal interactions—but only intermittently. However, intermittently was better than never.

As population and income density in Europe grew and mobility improved with transportation innovations, by the mid-nineteenth century the central business district emerged in its role as the primary retail center for high-order goods—the classic retail center generated and maintained by the dynamics we have described. Economically, it was highly successful, but the competition within it was intense. It was in this context that the first major intentional innovation in retail structure occurred: the department store, which first appeared in Paris in the 1860s in an attempt to capture more of the profit of the retail center by replicating the entire center in one establishment. Economically, the innovation was a success, and it spread rapidly. Rather than replace the existing, self-organized retail center, however, the department store actually strengthened it, by giving it increased visibility and making it more attractive. In the end, the department store was just another enterprise in the retail center created by the spatial dynamics of the system.

In the mid-twentieth century, a second, similar innovation appeared: the regional shopping mall. Once again, this replicated an entire major retail center, but even more comprehensively. It included a number of independent enterprises, with much duplication (e.g., many women's clothing stores), and it also included one or more department stores. Not only was this innovation profitable; it changed the spatial structure of the retail system. Shopping malls were typically built on the periphery of the urban area, where the model shows that major retail centers could not grow spontaneously and incrementally. The malls were able to succeed there for two reasons. First, because they were built as a complete major retail center, they avoided the earlier period of growth during which a smaller center would be uncompetitive in attracting customers in a low-n world (except in the relatively rare case of forestalling), so they were able to attract sufficient revenue from the beginning. This strategy is echoed in the many-mall world by the aggressive response described by William Applebaum and S. O. Kaylin (1974), in which a retail center that is facing losses reacts, not by contracting, but by expanding sufficiently to compete profitably. Second, the malls were small enough to have relatively low costs, given that major retail centers are subject to diseconomies of scale. Land costs were also lower in the peripheral locations they preferred. Of course, other factors contributed to the success of malls, such as the widespread use of the automobile, but, essentially, the mall represents a clever, if unconscious, working with the dynamic principles of low-n retail systems. In the United States, but not elsewhere, over a period of several decades, shopping malls essentially took over the system of major urban retail centers and, in most cases, relegated the retail function of the central business district to a minor role (figure 4.5). Ironically, in doing so, they turned the retail systems they dominate into high-n systems, but ones with a higher level of product diversity. Since malls are so similar to one another, they have the spatial dynamics of convenience goods: there is little reason to drive past one to reach another, more distant one. The next step in this evolution of strategies to capture profits in the low-n retail world is currently being taken by big-box stores and power centers, and malls are suffering—are they now an endangered species?

Other Theoretical Perspectives

The discussion of historical developments in urban retail systems focused on the relationship between entrepreneurialism and spatial dynamics as represented in the simulation model, essentially an economic model that abstracts from individuals, whether people or enterprises. But because entrepreneurial activity is something carried out by individuals, if we were to pursue this subject more deeply than the plausible stories we have told, it would be appropriate to use an individual-based modeling framework. The two approaches are complementary because they treat different levels of the same phenomenon: the individual-based approach focuses on the behavior of individual people and businesses, whereas the retail model treats the system-level properties of economic and spatial dynamics. Furthermore, an individual-based approach to entrepreneurial activity would permit a formal treatment of the structural evolution of the retail system through entrepreneurial innovations such as those we have just described. Structural evolution is the transformation of one system into a different, often more complex system. The system consisting of

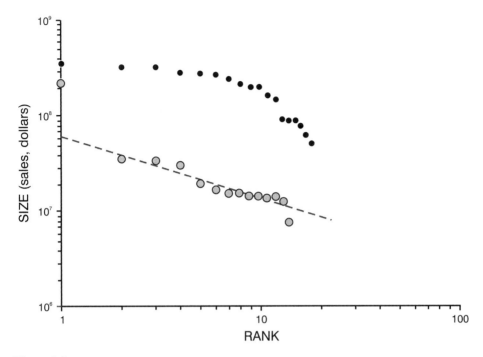

Figure 4.5
Rank-size relationship of major retail centers, Seattle, 1963 (gray circles) and 1982 (solid circles). (Source: Calculated from data in U.S. Census Bureau, Census of Retail Trade, 1963 and 1982.)

both unplanned retail centers and malls is a different, more complex system than one that lacks malls, and it has a different dynamical behavior and thus generates different spatial configurations. Although, at present, there is no evolutionary model of the retail system, the generic model of structural evolution in an economic system (Straatman, White, and Banzhaf, 2008) could be adapted as the basis of such a model.

Looking at the central place model from a different viewpoint, we see that it explains the fundamental bifurcation in spatial structure in mathematical or algorithmic terms, and in particular in terms of the value of the distance-decay parameter. But why does spatial interaction generally obey an inverse power or negative exponential relationship? John Niedercorn and Burley Bechdoldt (1969) on the one hand and Roger White (1976) on the other addressed this question by applying microeconomic utility theory, but neither of their studies showed that the relationship must have one of these two forms. Using an entropy-maximizing approach, Wilson (1970) showed that if movements between possible origins and destinations were assumed to be completely random in the absence of constraints, then the imposition of time or cost constraints would result in a negative exponential trip distribution function. But because none of these studies gives any insight into why, or under what circumstances, the distance-decay parameter takes on the values it does, none throws any light on the origin of the bifurcation that depends on that parameter. Since it is individuals who are engaging in spatial interaction, the most appropriate deep explanation would be one developed in terms of the psychology of individuals—their interests and desires—and in terms of the income and time constraints they face when deciding whether or not to make a trip. Such an approach would require individual-based modeling similar to that undertaken by Juval Portugali, Itzhak Benenson, and Itzhak Omer (1994, 1997; Portugali, 2000) to understand the development of new social groups with new behaviors in Tel Aviv.

But even though the urban system is a human phenomenon, and thus one in which the bifurcation in spatial structure is ultimately to be explained in terms of individual psychology and economic behavior, it is also a physical system that is far from thermodynamic equilibrium. It should therefore be possible to enrich our understanding of the bifurcation by explaining its appearance also in terms of energy flows. A formal theory of this sort has not yet been developed; therefore, we can only sketch the outlines of such an explanation.

From the thermodynamics point of view, human history is essentially a history of increasing energy density. At subsistence levels of consumption, the density of human energy use as embodied in food and fuel is proportional to population density. Agriculture permits a denser population than hunting and gathering, and as agricultural techniques improve with better crop selections, animal husbandry, crop fertilization, and better tools and storage techniques, agricultural population densities are able to increase. Whether agricultural settlement is in the form of villages (the usual case) or dispersed dwellings, as densities increase, more people are able to interact with one another on a daily basis. This larger effective group size permits increased cultural complexity, including material or technological culture (Bettencourt et al., 2007; Derex et al., 2013). Whereas at low densities every family typically makes its own pots, tools, and other implements, at higher densities, division of labor appears, and some families specialize in making these goods. Division of labor increases efficiency, which, in turn, permits a higher density. When transportation is faster, as with travel by horse or camel, or more effective in terms of the load that can be carried, as with boats or pack animals, then even greater numbers can effectively interact, and that further increases the possibilities for specialization, with consequent gains in efficiency and then density. This positive feedback cycle (see figure 4.6) eventually permits the appearance of a city—a further densification of the system—and then, as the process continues, the appearance of more cities. Each step in the cycle involves a greater density of energy flows through the system. Where greater energy flows are not possible, however, the cycle ceases to operate;

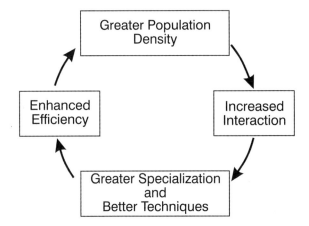

Figure 4.6
Feedback cycle of population density and economic efficiency.

that would be the case, for example, where natural environmental conditions are such that the population density and hence effective group size cannot reach the threshold necessary to generate a material culture that can overcome the immediate natural limitations. From a Prigogine-like perspective, then, the role of human culture is to increase the density of energy flows through the system and thus push it farther from thermodynamic equilibrium, with the consequence that the system becomes more highly organized.

One aspect of this ever more complex self-organization is an increase both in the number of products made and used in the system and in the variety of each type of product. When the density of the system and the number of products is low, every village will be similar in terms of the products available. But as density and the variety of products passes a threshold, due to an increase in energy density of the system, a bifurcation occurs in which some products continue to be offered in every village, but the provision of others becomes concentrated in just one, which is therefore differentiated from the other villages—it is now a true central place (figure 4.7). This bifurcation represents the splitting of a single spatial interaction parameter applying to all goods into two values—high and low, corresponding to low- and high-order goods. Or, to describe the same situation from another perspective, it represents the point at which the value of n, gradually declining as energy density increases, crosses the threshold to a functionally low value. In any case, the bifurcation leads to a change in the spatial structure of the system, from one where settlements are similar and regularly spaced, to one where one center is different because it is larger and more varied in its functions. The existence of activities characterized by a low distance-decay parameter depends on a sufficiently high energy

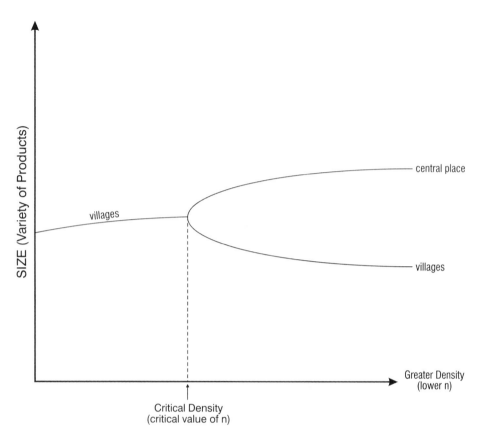

Figure 4.7
Bifurcation depending on energy input.

density—there is an inverse relationship between energy density and the value of the distance-decay parameter. The situation is shown in figure 4.7 and applies to the settlements in a system where at least one type of product has the potential for becoming a high-order good. When energy density is low, the effective distance-decay parameter is high, and only one settlement size is possible. Beyond the critical distance d_c, the value of the distance-decay parameter is low enough that two sizes are possible, but only one can be realized by any particular settlement. Whether this settlement follows the upper branch, and becomes a higher-order central place that is the major supplier of the product to the region, or follows the lower branch and remains a village, offering only minimal amounts of the good, depends on the settlement's spatial competition with the others. But at least one, and possibly several, settlements will move onto the upper branch of the bifurcation.

In the search for sustainable cities, a theory of urban form and development based on energy flows could have much to offer. As Ilya Prigogine points out, self-organization reduces the local entropy of the system by exporting entropy—that is, waste or pollution—from the organizing structure. The thermodynamics approach thus covers the two key concerns of sustainability—energy use and waste. But the processes of self-organization in human systems are much more complex, with many more degrees of freedom than is the case in simple physical and chemical systems. Energy use in human systems is mediated by technology, and the growing multiplicity of technological possibilities increases the variety of possible outcomes of the process of self-organization. Indeed, the system is now intentionally designed to increase the technological possibilities by diverting some energy use from production to research and development, thus, in effect, intentionally expanding the bifurcation tree and introducing new possibilities for structural evolution. In a general sense, an increase in energy efficiency increases the degree of self-organization that is possible by the same amount as an equivalent increase in total energy use. However, the increase in energy efficiency can only occur through changes in technology, whereas in the simplest case, an increase in total energy use could represent simply more of the same—that is, no qualitative change in the technology or the structure of the system. Furthermore, because of the cascading nature of the bifurcations that characterize any process of self-organization, the number of possibilities that exists at any particular level of energy use is very large. As a consequence of these complexities, it is likely to be difficult, at least initially, to make progress in developing an energy flow theory of cities.

Conclusions

The model presented in this chapter was an early attempt to reformulate location theory in a system dynamics framework. It performs well, both as a general theory of such systems and as a model that can be applied to a particular central place system or system of urban retail centers. It is complementary to the CA-based urban land use models presented in later chapters in that it gives an economic explanation of the commercial component of urban spatial structure.

The most powerful theoretical result of this model is the identification of a basic bifurcation that determines whether the spatial structure will evolve toward concentration or dispersal of activity. However, the success of the model in explaining one phenomenon raises other questions. What explains the range of values taken on by the distance-decay parameter? How do innovations in the form of new retail structures like malls arise to subvert the dynamics represented by the model? These questions can only be addressed by new models, operating at other levels, based in other knowledge domains, and using other techniques. For example, we have seen that the distance-decay parameter can, in principle, be explained by both an individual-based psychological model and an energy-flow model. These approaches are complementary; each covers aspects of the problem that are invisible to the other. This is the nature of explanation in the realm of complex human systems: one model, one theory is not enough. Understanding comes from a collection of complementary models.

5
The Fractal Forms of Urban Land Use Patterns

Every city has a unique spatial structure, and that structure evolves over the years. The unique form is due in part to the particular characteristics of the site, such as the configuration of the coastline or the location of hills and valleys. But, primarily, it reflects the particular historical path followed by the city as it grows and organizes itself. In other words, it expresses the fact that self-organizing systems generate complexity, and that a particular observed outcome, however complex, is only one of many that could have been generated. On the other hand, cities all seem to have much in common with one another in terms of the general characteristics of their form. These similarities of form reflect the fact that cities have many functions in common: for example, they must all produce and import goods and services and distribute them both locally and farther afield. But these generic features are also a result of the process of self-organization itself. Far-from-equilibrium self-organizing systems, whether physical, biological, or human, have a particular formal signature: they are complex and yet ordered. In particular, they almost always have a fractal structure. The fractal form is a sign, as we saw in chapter 2, that they are maintaining themselves far from equilibrium, poised between order and chaos, actively generating and regenerating themselves, and acting within their larger environment.

A city is fractal in several respects. The edge of the built-up area, the spatial distribution of land uses, the size distribution of internal clusters, the transportation networks, and various local features are all fractal. Because the fractal qualities of cities represent generic features of urban structure, fractal measures are important both for a theoretical understanding of urban processes and for calibrating and validating models of those processes; they may also turn out to be important in planning and policy formulation. For these reasons, we will examine them more closely in this chapter. Our treatment will focus, however, on aspects directly relevant to modeling cities—to calibrating, validating, and evaluating the models and understanding their implications. In particular, we will focus on the radial dimension and the cluster size–frequency dimension.

Cities were, in effect, recognized intuitively as fractal forms by architects, planners, and others who studied urban form long before the formal concept of the fractal was developed. Indeed, the expression "organic form" in the urban literature more often than not can be understood as referring to fractal form when it points to the typical forms generated by processes of self-organization, in contrast to those which result from conscious planning or design. And, once Benoit Mandelbrot (1975, 1982) extended Fry Richardson's unpublished work on borders (published posthumously as Richardson, 1961) by developing a mathematical treatment of fractals and citing many examples of fractals in natural and human systems, "organic" forms began to be widely treated as fractals. Although they are mathematically well defined, when it comes to adapting fractals to real-world applications, complications arise. Most notably, mathematical fractals deal with infinities, with infinite recursion generating infinite detail, whereas both real phenomena and our measurements of them are finite. For example, a fractal boundary generated mathematically has a well-defined dimension, D_b with $1 < D_b < 2$. But if we ask, as Michael Batty and Paul Longley (1994) did, what the dimension of the boundary of an urban area like Cardiff is, then, to find D_b, we must estimate it by measuring the length of the boundary at increasingly fine resolutions in order to extract the relationship between the resolution of the measurement procedure and the measured length. And because the measurement may be implemented in a variety of ways, all giving slightly different results, the translation of the mathematical concept of fractals to urban applications is always somewhat messy, although, ultimately, this does not present a serious practical problem. The important question is, how can fractals help us to understand cities? The answer is, by providing useful new measures of urban form and function.

Fractal analysis allows us to see and measure aspects of urban form that would otherwise be essentially invisible. Batty and Longley (1994) used the word *picturescape* in this context. To generate "realistic"—that is, fractal—images of urban structure, they took several different approaches, among them a recursive fragmentation process to generate land use patterns, and a diffusion-limited aggregation (DLA) model (see box 2.3) to generate a global urban form. *Picturescape* is an appropriate term for these images because the models that generated them do not represent actual urban processes and therefore they tell us little about how cities actually go about structuring themselves. Subsequently, however, Batty and Longley did undertake extensive empirical investigations of the fractal nature of cities. They focused on the urban perimeter, estimating its fractal dimension for a number of cities, but they also examined the radial dimension and discussed its relationship to traditional measures of the urban density profile (Batty and Longley, 1994; summarized and evaluated in Batty, 2013).

The *radial dimension* (see box 5.1) describes the relationship between the built-up area of a city and the distance (radius) from the city center. If the entire area of the city were built up, then this area would increase with the square of the distance from the center, but since, in general, the built-up area becomes less dense as the distance from the city center grows, it will increase only with a power $D_r < 2$ of distance from the center, where D_r is the radial dimension. The *correlation dimension* (box 5.1), though similar to the radial dimension, is calculated without reference to the center of the city. It is derived by treating *every* pixel of the built-up area as the

Box 5.1
The Radial and Correlation Dimensions

The radial dimension of a city describes the rate at which the built-up area, or the area of a particular land use, increases as the radius of the circle within which it is being measured increases; the circle is centered on the center of the city. The radial dimension thus represents a radial density gradient. It is an appropriate measure when the city grew from the center, as is usually the case; it is less appropriate when the urban area grew from several centers, as in the case of a conurbation like the Ruhr region (Ruhrgebiet). In the simplest case, the relationship is described by the equation

$$A(\varepsilon) = \varepsilon^D \text{ or } \log A(\varepsilon) = D \log \varepsilon$$

where $A(\varepsilon)$ is the area of the urban object within distance ε from the center and the exponent D is the radial dimension. Pierre Frankhauser (1994) suggests including a prefactor or coefficient, k, in the relationship to account for various phenomena:

$$A(\varepsilon) = k\varepsilon^D \text{ or } \log A(\varepsilon) = \log k + D \log \varepsilon$$

If $D < 2$, the urban object occupies progressively *less* of the available land as distance from the center increases. If, however, $D > 2$, as it is for some land uses like detached housing, the land use occupies progressively *more* of the available land as distance from the center increases; in this case, the prefactor $k < 1$.

In empirical applications, the radial dimension is determined by calculating the area occupied by the urban object as the distance ε from the center is incremented. D is then the slope of the plot of $\log A(\varepsilon)$ against $\log \varepsilon$. The plot itself is referred to as the "radial analysis."

The *correlation dimension* is a generalization of the radial dimension, in which each pixel or cell occupied by the urban object is taken as the center from which the distance ε is incrementally increased. If the urban object consists of N cells, for each increment of ε, there are N values of $A(\varepsilon)$, from which the mean value $\langle A(\varepsilon) \rangle$ is calculated. The correlation dimension is then the slope of the plot of $\log \langle A(\varepsilon) \rangle$ against $\log \varepsilon$. To determine whether the fractal dimension varies from one neighborhood to another, the mean can be taken over subareas of the city. This approach can also be used to calculate the correlation dimension of the perimeter of an urban object by restricting the operations to cells that lie on the boundary.

center and accumulating the area around each one as distance is incremented; the correlation dimension is then derived from the combined areas around *all* pixels. In other words, the correlation dimension is a kind of mean of all the radial dimensions that can be calculated by taking each occupied pixel in turn as the center.

Frankhauser (1988, 1990, 1994, 2008) was the first to undertake an extensive investigation of the fractal nature of cities. He has developed an extensive mathematical treatment of the radial and correlation dimensions and related it to empirical estimation methods that can be used in applications to actual cities. Based on this work, a European network of collaborators that includes Frankhauser, Isabelle Thomas, Cécile Tannier, and others has undertaken a series of studies of both the urban form of a number of cities and the settlement pattern of larger areas such as the Wallonia Region of Belgium. Although these studies rely primarily on the correlation dimension of the built-up area, they also use the correlation dimension of the perimeter, as well as the dilation dimension. The work is particularly interesting because the dimensions are calculated separately for individual subareas of cities, for example, twenty-six communes in the Brussels area. In this way, local variations in urban morphology are being discovered.

Once a city or region has been decomposed into a patchwork of local areas, each characterized by a particular value of a fractal dimension, it is possible to correlate the local dimensions to other urban characteristics. For example, Marie-Laurence de Keersmaecker, Frankhauser, and Thomas (2003) have correlated local values of the correlation dimension with the type of housing (detached, terraced, flats, etc.), the age of the housing stock, average rent, median income, and the population density. Local values of the correlation dimension have also been correlated with household evaluations of the quality of the immediate neighborhood—whether it is unpleasant, satisfactory, or very pleasant (Thomas, Frankhauser, and Biernacki 2008; Thomas, Tannier, and Frankhauser, 2008). Thomas and colleagues (2010) have used the scaling relationship underlying the correlation dimension to categorize the morphology of cities and neighborhoods. And Alex Anas, Richard Arnot, and Kenneth Small (1998) have shown that a fractal urban form reduces mean travel costs to green spaces as well as to some other kinds of destinations.

This work, though interesting in itself, is also important because it points to the possibility of finding local, intraurban measures of urban form that can be related not only to other local characteristics such as income or housing type, but also to local functional characteristics of the sort thought to be important for quality of life. For the calibration and validation of urban models, measures that represent functionally important features of the morphology are preferable to arbitrary ones. Such measures would also be valuable in assessing alternatives generated in applications of the models to planning problems. Unfortunately, as we will see in chapter 9, because most currently used measures of urban morphology have little to do with the way a city functions, they probably do not capture the significant aspects of urban form.

In contrast, the models described in this book are designed to capture the processes that generate the urban structure, and thus to be capable of replicating them. Their underlying assumption is that, since the basic processes apply to all cities, one model should be applicable to any city. Of course, the model should be able to replicate the particularities of the city being modeled, but those particularities emerge through the interaction of the generic urban self-organization process captured in the model with the specific local conditions specified in the model's initialization data—for example, site characteristics, initial land use and transportation network, and expected population growth. In calibrating and validating a model, it is customary to seek the best fit between the model output and the actual data. But the best fit almost always represents a case of overcalibration, which suppresses the expression of the generic, universal characteristics of the model. To avoid overcalibration, it is desirable to calibrate not just to the data for a specific city (for which the local correlation dimensions could be useful), but also to generic properties. Two fractal dimensions that seem to represent stable generic properties of cities—the radial dimension and the cluster size–frequency dimension—can thus provide calibration targets that are complementary to city-specific data. Because they are used in the calibration and validation of all the applications discussed in the following chapters, we will examine them more closely here.

The Radial Dimension

Frankhauser (1994) graphed the area-radius relationship for a number of cities around the world in order to calculate their radial dimensions. He found that with very few exceptions the value of this dimension fell between 1.9 and 2.0 (table 5.1). Radial analysis revealed another striking regularity, however, one that Frankhauser noted but did not analyze: toward the periphery of a city there was a kink in the area-radius relationship, which he called the "rayon de segregation" or "separation distance." Coincidentally, the first version of the land use model discussed in chapter 6 was also generating abstract cities with a kink in the area-radius relationship. This kink separated the inner part of the city where the process of urbanization was essentially complete from an outer zone where the city was still developing, converting rural land to urban. The model results taken together with Frankhauser's data suggested that cities are actually *bi*fractal in terms of their radial structure. In other words, it takes two values of the radial dimension to characterize a city. The inner area has a relatively high radial dimension, reflecting the fully developed status of this zone, but the outer zone, beyond the kink, has a much lower radial dimension because the area is still in the process of urbanizing (figure 5.1; see also tables 5.3

Table 5.1
Radial dimensions of selected world cities

	City	D_r
Europe	Berlin	1.95
	Dortmund	1.97
	Essen	1.97
	Stuttgart	1.94
	Paris	1.99
	Moscow	1.96
	Budapest	1.97
	London	1.99
North America	Boston	1.96
	Pittsburgh	1.91
	Los Angeles	1.99
	Mexico City	1.97
Asia	Taipei	1.97
	Beijing	1.98
Australia	Melbourne	1.99
	Sydney	1.95

Source: Frankhauser, 1994
Note: Lower D_r values are given for these cities in Frankhauser and Sadler, 1991, with typical values being in the neighborhood of 1.92.

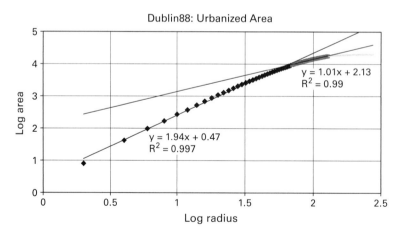

Figure 5.1
Area-radius plots of the Dublin urbanized area in 1988, showing the kink between the inner, developed (diamonds) and the outer, developing (triangles) zones. (Source: Calculated from maps supplied by the Joint Research Centre of the European Commission)

and 5.4). Since this bifractal structure of the urbanized area seems to be nearly universal, any model generating a map of an urban area must be able to reproduce it, or be judged inadequate.

The radial dimension is particularly reliable for this purpose because it is less sensitive to the scale of the map from which it is derived than the correlation or grid dimensions (Frankhauser, 1994, pp. 130–132, 140) and, by implication, because it should also be less sensitive to errors in the land use map as long as they are not correlated with distance from the urban center. This is important because land use maps are rarely strictly comparable from one city to another, or from one year to another: the data sources, definitions, methods, and criteria used depend on who is making the map, and even objective methods applied to many cities, especially those based on remote sensing imagery, depend on classification algorithms that are updated—i.e. changed—frequently, so that the results are not strictly comparable.

Nevertheless, the fact that most cities around the world have similar radial dimension values, especially for the inner zone, despite their different growth histories suggests that the radial dimension tends to be stable through time, although this is difficult to establish conclusively. As we have just noted, temporal comparisons are suspect because land use maps are almost never comparable from one year to another. Furthermore, while Frankhauser (1994) showed that the radial dimension is largely insensitive to changes in cartographic representation, in the case of Berlin, he has published three different sets of radial dimensions for the city over the years, all apparently based on the same series of maps. One shows radial dimension values for 1875, 1910, 1920, and 1945 as essentially stable, ranging from 1.71 to 1.77 (Frankhauser, 1990); another shows values for the same years that are also stable, but with a range of 1.94–1.97 (Frankhauser, 1994); and the third shows values increasing from 1.36 in 1875 to 1.81 in 1945 (Frankhauser and Sadler, 1991). Differences in the way the data were handled may account for the discrepancies among these three sets of results. Results from the cellular automaton–based model discussed in chapter 6 suggest that, in the earlier stages of urban growth, the radial dimension of the inner zone tends to grow over time toward a limiting value of between 1.9 and 2.0 and then to stabilize. If real cities behave similarly, that would resolve the issue of growth versus stability of the radial dimension, though not the discrepancy in the results presented for Berlin.

In contrast with the likely relative stability of the inner-zone radial dimension, the radial dimension of the outer zone should grow over time, at least up to some relatively low value, since this is the zone where the process of urbanization is most active, as rural land is converted to urban uses. Data for Dublin for the period 1956–1998 are consistent with the stability of the inner-zone radial dimension and the growth of the outer-zone radial dimension (table 5.3, col. 5). Logic suggests that the outer boundaries of the two zones defined by the radial dimensions of the bifractal

Table 5.2
Radial dimension of individual land uses in four U.S. cities, 1960

City	Commerce	Industry	Housing	Other
Atlanta	1.00	1.97	2.12	2.52
Cincinnati	1.10	2.11	2.51	3.42
Houston	1.24	1.51	2.76	2.77
Milwaukee	1.27	1.83	2.38	2.17

Source: Dimension values calculated from maps in Passonneau and Wurman, 1966.

city should also move outward as the city grows, and, indeed, the single empirical radial analysis available, for the metropolitan area of Dublin, suggests that this is in fact the case (table 5.4, col. 5). It is the outward shift of the outer zone that constrains the growth of the radial dimension of this zone since, as the city grows, the inner part of the outer zone becomes fully developed and thus part of the inner zone, whereas the outer edge progressively engulfs rural land as urbanization moves outward.

Individual land uses can also be characterized by the radial dimension. Table 5.2 shows the values for four land uses in four U.S. cities. The data used for the radial analysis come from a set of standardized land use maps produced by Joseph Passonneau and Richard Wurman (1966) for the year 1960.

The bifractal structure that characterizes urbanized areas also seems to be typical of individual land uses, although, with a few exceptions, it does not show up in the radial analysis used to determine the dimensions shown for the U.S. cities because the maps do not include the fringe of the urbanized areas. Evidence from other sources is limited because most radial analyses, like those of Frankhauser and of Batty and Longley, use a single aggregate "urban" or "built-up" category. However, we have calculated bifractal dimensions for individual land uses for three cities (table 5.3).

For individual land uses, the inner-zone radial dimension values seem to be less stable than those for all urban land uses taken together (table 5.3). For example, although the inner-zone dimension values for discontinuous sparse residential land use (col. 1) do seem stable, those for industry and services increase over the period, representing a relative shift of these activities away from the center. Over the same period, the dimension values calculated for commerce decline, indicating increasing concentration at the center. The outer-zone dimension values for all four land uses increase, as would be expected as urbanization proceeds. On the other hand, by 1998, a *third* zone of urbanization appears for industry and commerce. This anomalous situation, already visible for industry in 1988 (figure 5.2b), represents peripheral growth beyond what should have been the normal expansion zone for these activities—specifically, the appearance of large industrial zones and shopping malls

Table 5.3
Inner- and outer-zone radial dimensions for individual land uses: Dublin, Milan, and St. John's

	(1) Residential	(2) Industry	(3) Commerce	(4) Services	(5) Total urban
Dublin					
Inner zone					
1956	3.29	1.85	2.05	1.87	1.92
1968	3.12	1.94	1.98	1.92	1.87
1988	3.14	2.64	1.80	2.05	1.94
1998	3.27	2.67	1.59	2.06	2.00
Outer zone					
1956	0.65	0.81	0.25*	0.78	0.56
1968	0.72	1.12	0.33*	1.01	0.58
1988	1.05	1.27*	0.39	0.92	0.94
1998	1.21	1.05	0.24*	0.92	1.25
Third zone					
1998	—	1.63*	0.86*	—	—
Milan					
Inner zone					
1955	2.09	4.83	0.70	1.73	2.11
Outer zone					
1955	0.67	1.58	—	0.79*	0.85
St. John's					
Inner zone					
1977	2.48	—	—	—	1.74
1983	2.48	—	—	—	1.85
Outer zone					
1977	1.03	—	—	—	0.95
1983	1.13	—	—	—	0.75

*$R^2 < 0.98$ for the radial analysis.
Source: Values for Dublin and Milan calculated from maps supplied by the Joint Research Centre of the European Commission.
Note: For Dublin, "residential" is discontinuous sparse residential, the dominant residential land use class; for Milan and St. John's, "residential" is the total of all residential land use classes. The "total urban" column shows the radial dimension of the urbanized area, including all urban land uses.

Table 5.4
Dublin: Outer limit of zones in kilometers from the city center

	(1) Residential	(2) Industry	(3) Commerce	(4) Services	(5) Total urban
Inner zone					
1956	6.2	3.2	1.8	3.4	6.6
1968	7.8	1.8	1.8	3.4	7.6
1988	7.8	2.6	1.8	3.4	6.8
1998	7.8	2.6	2.4	3.6	10.0
Outer zone					
1988	13.8	6.0	6.8	10.8	14.6
Third zone					
1998	—	10.0	11.6	—	—

Source: Calculated from maps supplied by the Joint Research Centre of the European Commission.

on the fringe of the city. This development represents a rupture in what had been normal city growth, and means that, as far as these two activities are concerned, the city is not just extending its normal structure, but also beginning again on the periphery. In other words, for these two activities, the normal urbanization process that was underway in the second or outer zone during the 1956–1988 period seems to have come to a halt, leaving that zone with relatively little in the way of industrial and commercial activity. Instead, industrial and commercial expansion jumped to the periphery. This phenomenon perhaps reflects a lag in the expansion of these activities relative to that for residential development, so that they were left with no room to expand in what had been their outer zone and were then forced to leapfrog to the periphery to continue their growth. The appearance of this third zone also explains the apparent anomaly that, in 1998, the outer edge of the inner zone of the urbanized area was at a much greater distance than the outer edge of any of the individual land uses. In sum, the temporal evolution of the radial dimensions corresponding to individual land uses can tell us much about the restructuring of a city.

The Cluster Size–Frequency Dimension

Sometimes referred to as "$1/f$ noise," the *cluster size–frequency dimension* is common in the natural sciences but almost unknown in urban and regional studies, except for its applications in connection with the models described in this book. Yet it is an extremely useful measure of spatial structure, one that should be more widely used in the modeling community because it provides a partial answer to some calibration

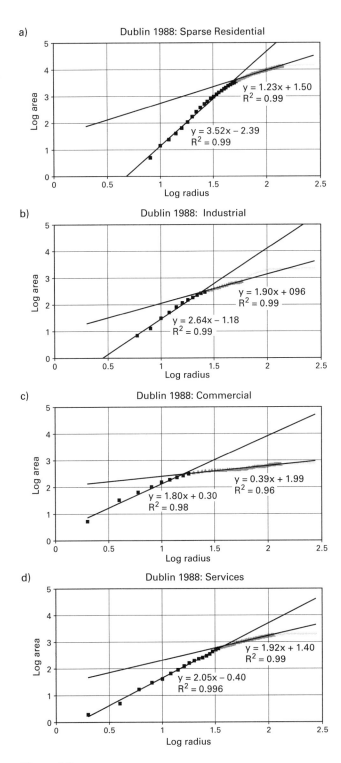

Figure 5.2
Area-radius plots for inner (squares) and outer (triangles) zones of Dublin, 1988: (a) low-density sparse residential; (b) industrial; (c) commercial; (d) services. (Source: Calculated from maps supplied by the Joint Research Centre of the European Commission)

problems that are otherwise completely intractable. The cluster size–frequency dimension (see box 5.2) represents the size spectrum of land use clusters; it is highly complementary to the family of fractal measures based on radial analysis that we have just discussed because it describes the relationship between the size of a cluster and the number of clusters of that size, regardless of the location pattern of the

Box 5.2
The Cluster Size–Frequency Dimension

Sometimes referred to as "1/f noise," the *cluster size–frequency dimension* describes the relationship between the size of a cluster and the number of clusters of that size that are found in a system. It can be used to characterize the size distribution of urban clusters in a region or of clusters of a particular land use in a city. The relationship is found by plotting the log of the number (frequency) of clusters of a particular size against the log of cluster size. If the plot is linear, then the relationship can be described by the equation

$N(s) = ks^{-D}$ or $\log N(s) = \log k - D \log s$

where $N(s)$ is number of clusters of size s, and D is the cluster size–frequency dimension. If the relationship is not linear, then the system is not a fractal in this respect.

The values of $\log k$ and D can be found by a regression analysis performed on the data in the plot. For geographical applications, however, although the plot is usually highly linear with very little scatter for most frequencies, when frequency numbers are small (e.g., $N(s) \leq 3$), the distribution flares out to become a highly scattered one. In other words, for the largest clusters, there is typically only one of a given size, and thus at a frequency of 1, there will be a number of clusters, each of a different size, some much larger than others. At frequencies of 2 and 3, there will be a similar but smaller scatter in the size of clusters. Several methods are available for dealing with this phenomenon in order to get a better estimate of D; for example, clusters of similar size can be represented by their mean size and the frequency adjusted accordingly. Clusters of cells can be defined either by horizontal and vertical adjacencies only or by also including diagonal adjacencies. The most common approach is to use only the horizontal and vertical adjacencies, and clusters defined in this way usually give higher R^2 values for the cluster size–frequency plot, at least in land use applications. All the results shown in this book use the rook (horizontal and vertical only) adjacency criterion for cluster definition.

Per Bak (1994, 1996) has developed an entire approach to understanding complex systems based on the idea of *self-organized criticality*, where a system moves toward a limiting or critical state. The system is unable to move beyond that state because it becomes unstable and collapses back to the vicinity of the critical configuration. A literal example is a sand pile built by continuously dropping grains of sand from above—a kind of input of energy. The pile becomes steeper as it becomes larger, up to the point where the slope reaches a critical angle. Beyond that point, as the sand grains continue to fall, avalanches of sand of various sizes occur at random intervals, so that the pile approximately maintains its shape as it continues to grow. The avalanches have a fractal distribution: their size–frequency distribution is log linear.

clusters. In that sense, unlike the correlation and radial dimensions, it is a nonspatial measure, much like the rank-size distribution.

Almost every land use map analyzed, whether of an urban area, region, or country—and including even a rural land cover map—has shown a linear cluster size–frequency relationship. In the single exception that has been found, the clusters of urbanized land in Flanders, the relationship is somewhat convex, implying that there are too few small clusters, probably because in that very densely settled region of Belgium what would otherwise be many small independent urban clusters have merged in a ribbon pattern of development.

Figure 5.3 shows cluster size–frequency graphs for the four U.S. cities whose radial dimensions for various sectors are given in table 5.2. It was only possible to analyze the land use corresponding to commerce because the other three land uses had too few clusters to give meaningful results, as did even commerce in the case of Atlanta.

Table 5.5 shows the cluster size–frequency dimensions for four land uses in the immediate Dublin area over several years, together with the R^2 values of the

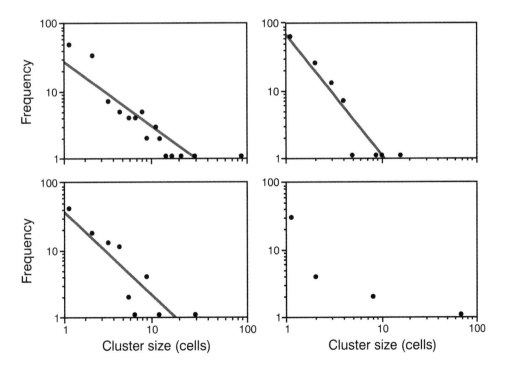

Figure 5.3
Cluster size–frequency plots for four U.S. cities, 1960: (*top left*) Houston; (*top right*) Milwaukee; (*bottom left*) Cincinnati; (*bottom right*) Atlanta. (Source: Calculated from maps in Passonneau and Wurman, 1966)

Table 5.5
Cluster size–frequency dimensions

	Residential	Industry	Commerce	Services
Dublin				
1956 D_c	0.52	0.99	1.13	1.50
R^2	0.62	0.76	0.95	0.92
1968 D_c	0.94	0.98	1.16	1.40
R^2	0.80	0.78	0.94	0.85
1988 D_c	1.01	0.77	1.20	1.60
R^2	0.93	0.87	0.88	0.89
1998 D_c	1.00	0.74	1.21	1.47
R^2	0.86	0.87	0.88	0.89
Greater Dublin				
1990 D_c	2.07	—	—	—
R^2	0.99	—	—	—
St. John's				
1961 D_c	0.85	—	—	—
R^2	0.72	—	—	—
1977 D_c	0.62	—	—	—
R^2	0.59	—	—	—
1983 D_c	0.67	—	—	—
R^2	0.67	—	—	—
Cincinnati				
1961 D_c	—	—	1.28	—
R^2	—	—	—	—
Houston				
1961 D_c	—	—	1.01	—
R^2	—	—	—	—
Milwaukee				
1961 D_c	—	—	1.75	—
R^2	—	—	—	—

	Residential (low density)	Residential (combined)	Industry	Total urban
Netherlands				
1990 D_c	1.87	1.58	1.81	1.91
R^2	0.99	0.99	0.98	0.99

Source: Values for Dublin and Greater Dublin calculated from maps supplied by the Joint Research Centre of the European Commission; values for Cincinnati, Houston and Milwaukee calculated from maps in Passonneau and Wurman, 1966; values for the Netherlands calculated from maps made available by the Research Institute for Knowledge Systems, Maastricht.

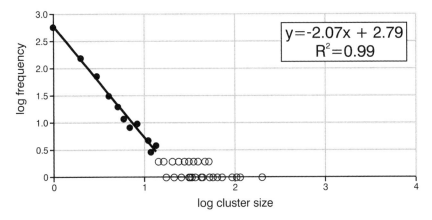

Figure 5.4
Cluster size–frequency plot for discontinuous sparse residential land use, Dublin, 1990. Data points shown as empty circles were not included in the regression. (Source: Calculated from maps supplied by the Joint Research Centre of the European Commission)

regressions used to determine them, as an indication of the scatter in the plots. In addition, the table shows results of an analysis of residential land use in the five-county Greater Dublin Region in 1990 at a resolution of 500 meters (see also figure 5.4). In this analysis of the GDR, all residential categories were combined, whereas the results for the immediate Dublin area are for discontinuous sparse residential land use, the largest of four residential land use classes. In addition, the 500-meter resolution of the GDR contrasts with the 100-meter resolution of the data underlying the other Dublin results. All relationships, for Dublin as well as for the Greater Dublin Region, are linear. Table 5.5 also shows the cluster size–frequency dimensions calculated for residential land use in St. John's, three U.S. cities, and the Netherlands. Again, all relationships were linear. The results for the Netherlands are for the entire country and are calculated excluding clusters with sizes greater than twenty in order to avoid the problem of the flared tail of the distribution. An analysis of the entire set of clusters of residential land use is shown in figure 5.5.

The salient characteristic of these results is that they are all linear. The actual values of the dimensions vary over time and from one city or region to another, and different land uses have different values. These variations may prove to be useful in understanding certain characteristics of the self-organizing city or region, much as is the case with other fractal dimensions. But, at present, the interest of the cluster size–frequency dimension lies primarily in the very linearity that permits the dimension to be defined, because that linearity seems to be a nearly universal feature of land use patterns characterized by clusters. The existence of a universal gives us a standard against which to measure the performance of our models, one which is independent

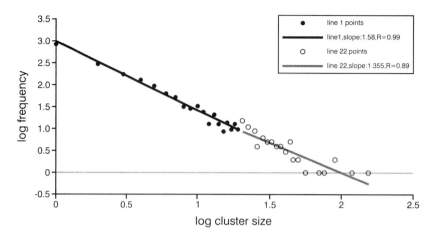

Figure 5.5
Cluster size–frequency plot for Netherlands, 1994. (Source: Calculated from maps made available by the Research Institute for Knowledge Systems, Maastricht)

of any particular application. This enables us to weed out some erroneously formulated models and some overcalibrations. If a model cannot be calibrated to maintain a linear distribution over the long run, then, more likely than not, it is incorrectly formulated. And if an apparently optimal calibration, based on a relatively short period of five or ten years, does not maintain a linear distribution over a much longer period when the model is run into the future, then, more likely than not, the model is badly calibrated. Of course, because there are many land use patterns that can give rise to a linear distribution, there can be many poorly formulated or badly calibrated models that will be able to pass this linearity test. In practice, however, it is surprising how frequently models and calibrations cannot pass the test and must therefore be modified. In other words, the linearity test is in fact useful in the daily practice of modeling. A model that fails to maintain an essential property such as the linear cluster size–frequency relationship is said to exhibit "drift." Drift is a notorious problem in simulation models; it has received much attention in the case of climate models, but very little in the case of models of socioeconomic phenomena.

6

Urban and Regional Land Use Dynamics: Understanding the Process by Means of Cellular Automaton–Based Models

Cities and regions are highly organized systems but, at the same time, extremely complex. This dual quality is expressed in a general way by the fractal dimensions discussed in chapter 5. But, because complexity is an essential characteristic of these systems, to understand them, we need to retain and work with that complexity, rather than abstract from it, as the fractal measures do. Whether we look at the daily movements of individuals, the spatial distribution of the various activities carried out in a city, or the land use patterns that reflect those activities, we see that the system is complex but organized, and hence functional. How do cities and regions generate such a structure? In this chapter, we will address the question by means of a cellular automaton (CA)–based model of land use. In chapters 7 and 8, we will extend the model so that it also captures the locational dynamics of population and economic activity, and we will begin to include daily movement patterns in these models.

To address the issue of complexity in all its spatial intricacies, we must have high-resolution data, for it is only at high resolution that the complexity appears. Administrative or statistical regions, for example, are typically too large to capture the details of spatial patterns. We must also have data for more than one urban land use. If we have only two classes, urban and rural, or developed and undeveloped, then land use data will show us nothing of the internal structure of the city. Because most CA-based urban models use only these two land use classes, they are only able to model the overall shape of the urban area. If those models are good, they are able to predict a fractal form of the sort we have discussed in chapter 5, and, in this sense, they capture one aspect of urban complexity. But knowing the radial dimension of the urbanized area or the dimension of the urban boundary, for example, will tell us nothing about the internal structure of the city. Yet, because most of the formal information about urban processes is coded in the internal organization of the city, it is important to model the internal structure. Only models that do so will offer significant theoretical insights and provide a foundation for the development of serious policy and planning tools.

A good CA-based model of urban land use dynamics should include not only the most important individual land uses, but also the major factors that together determine the land use. What are those factors? Common knowledge is a good guide here. First, the size of the city will approximately determine *how much* land will be occupied by each land use type; as the city grows, the areas devoted to the individual land uses will grow roughly in proportion. On the other hand, the *location* of the land occupied by each land use class will depend on several other factors, and, together, these other factors will determine the evolution of the land use pattern as the city grows. Because land uses represent activities that interact with one another, some land uses will be attracted to one another (or to themselves), while others will tend to repel one another. For example, residential land use will tend to be attracted to parks, but repelled by heavy industry. The location of various land uses will also depend on intrinsic qualities of the land itself. For example, land that is on a steep slope may be difficult or expensive to build on, and thus less likely to be developed for urban purposes. Some activities require better access than others to infrastructure networks like the highway system, and this can affect their location and hence the land use pattern. And some land may be subject to legal restrictions that prevent its development for certain purposes. Finally, location decisions are made by individual people and organizations, all with differing tastes and needs. For example, the land use class *commercial* represents a wide variety of businesses, from fast food restaurants to financial institutions, and each will have its own locational requirements in terms of the factors just mentioned.

The Basic CA-Based Land Use Model

The CA-based model described here is more complicated than most CA-based models, because it is designed to represent the processes that generate the evolving urban or regional land use pattern as realistically as possible while remaining computationally efficient. It includes all of the factors we have just mentioned. Together, those factors allow us to calculate a *transition potential* for each possible land use for each cell, which represents in a general way the value of the cell for each particular land use. Transition potentials are used to determine which land use the cells will actually receive at each time step. The characteristics of the CA are as follows.

The Time Step
Time is treated as discrete steps, and all cells are updated simultaneously. In most applications, one time step represents one year, although it can equally well represent any appropriate period.

The Cell Space

Consisting of a finite Euclidian space divided into an array of square cells, the cell space conforms to the shape of the application area. It is often rectangular, but sometimes not, as when the area to be modeled is defined by administrative regions. The size of each cell depends on the resolution of the land use map used; for the applications described here and in chapters 7 and 8, the resolution ranges from 100 meters to 1kilometer. Of course, the size of the cell space, and therefore the run time of the model, grows with the square of the resolution.

Most important, and in contrast to most other CA-based land use models, the cell space in this model is inhomogeneous. Each cell i has associated with it three vectors of values that represent the site-specific factors that affect land use. First, each cell is characterized by a vector of *suitabilities*—one value for each active land use j—representing the intrinsic quality of that cell for each of the land uses (figure 6.1). These suitabilities, S_{ij}, are typically the weighted sum of various physical and environmental attributes of the cell site, such as slope, aspect, soil type, and substrate. They are normalized to values in a range of $0 \le S_{ij} \le 1$, with 0 representing conditions that are completely unsuitable for the particular land use and 1 representing completely suitable conditions. Although these values are normally calculated before the initialization of a simulation and remain constant throughout the run, in a few variants of the model, they are actively updated during a simulation, for example, to reflect the impact of a drying climate.

Second, each cell has an associated vector of *accessibility* factors, again one for each active land use (figure 6.2), which represent the relative need for access to the several infrastructure networks; some land uses, such as commerce, are more strongly tied to the networks than others. The networks are represented in a vector format superimposed on the cell space. The networks can be updated as the model runs, with new versions read in at the appropriate times. This not only keeps the networks up to date by reflecting new links and upgrades of existing ones; it also permits users to test the effects of proposed additions or modifications by means of "what if" experiments. The accessibility factor of cell i for land use j, A_{ij}, is measured as a function of distance from the cell to the network:

$$A_{ij} = \left(1 + \frac{d_i}{a_j}\right)^{-1} = \frac{a_j}{(a_j + d_i)}, \text{ with } 0 \le A_{ij} \le 1 \text{ and } a_j > 0; \quad (6.1a)$$

If there is a repulsion effect between the network and a land use, then $a_j < 0$, and the accessibility factor is calculated as

$$A_{ij} = \frac{d_i}{(|a_j| + d_i)} \quad (6.1b)$$

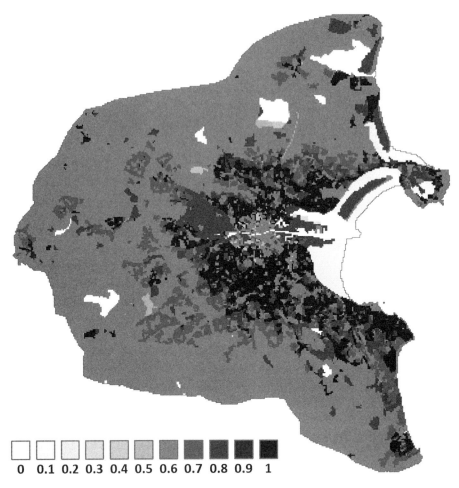

Figure 6.1
Suitability for discontinuous sparse residential land use, Dublin, ranging from 0 (completely unsuitable) to 1 (completely suitable).

where

d_i = the Euclidian distance from cell i to the network, with the distance measured either to a link (e.g., in the case of a road) or a node (e.g., a train station) as appropriate

a_j = a parameter representing the importance for land use j of accessibility to the network; this represents a distance-decay effect.

Third, each cell i has associated with it one or more vectors of legal restriction or *zoning* factors, Z_{ij}, for the active land uses (figure 6.3). When there is more than one

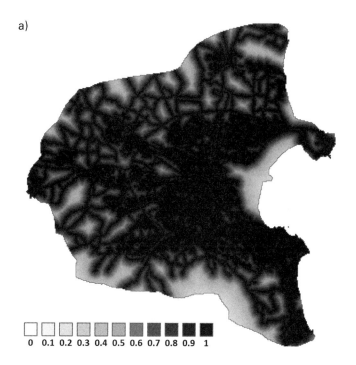

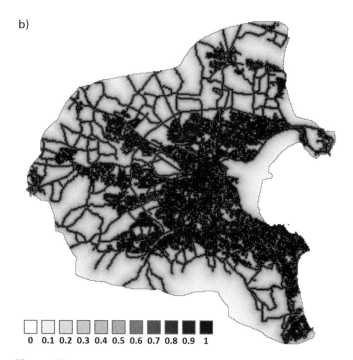

Figure 6.2
Accessibility to the transport network, Dublin, 1998, ranging from 0 (completely inaccessible) to 1 (completely accessible): (a) discontinuous sparse residential; (b) industry.

108   Chapter 6

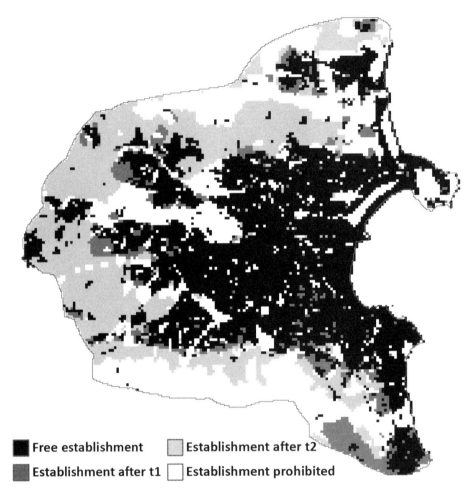

Figure 6.3
Zoning for residential, Dublin, 1998. t1 is the date of the initial zoning map and t2 is the date of a map that is introduced later, during the simulation run.

vector, each one is associated with a date that determines the iteration when it is to be fed into the simulation. Values of Z_{ij} are binary, indicating that the land use is prohibited (0) or permitted (1) on the cell.

Finally, a digital elevation model (DEM) is included among the inputs of each application. This, of course, expresses a particular spatial heterogeneity of the modeled area. The DEM is required in applications where the natural system model generates changing sea levels in order for the model to determine when a sea cell becomes dry land, or when a land cell is submerged and therefore converted to a sea cell. In all applications, the DEM can also be used to display the various maps (land use, accessibility, transition potential, etc.) draped over the relief surface. The digital elevation model is also used in preprocessing to compute slope and aspect if these are required as inputs to suitability calculations.

The Cell Neighborhood

Defined as the approximately circular region around the cell out to a radius of eight cells (although some early applications used a radius of six cells), the cell neighborhood contains 197 cells including the central cell itself. Because of the geometry of the grid, these cells fall into thirty discrete distance zones ($1, \sqrt{2}, 2, \sqrt{5}, \sqrt{8}, 3,...$; see figure 6.4). At the commonly used resolutions of 100 to 200 meters, the eight-cell

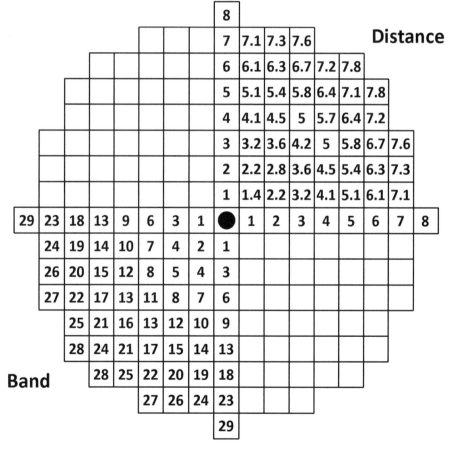

Figure 6.4
Cell neighborhood template, showing distance bands (*lower left*) and cell distances (*upper right*).

radius represents a neighborhood with a radius of 0.8–1.6 kilometers (~0.5–1.0 mile), which is assumed to be approximately the size of area that people would consider their local neighborhood. Recently, empirical support for this assumption has emerged, as will be discussed in chapter 8. In order to minimize the boundary problem, where land use data are available, a buffer eight cells wide is added to the cell space of the application proper in order to give cells near the edge of the modeled area a full neighborhood. Cells in the buffer zone thus affect the land use dynamics of cells within the modeled region, but they do not themselves change state.

The Cell States
Cell states represent individual land uses. Land uses are assigned to one of three categories depending on how they are to be handled in the CA: active, passive, and fixed. Most urban land uses will typically be designated as active land uses: participating fully in the dynamics, they can take over other active or passive land uses, and be taken over by other active land uses. Passive land uses normally change state only if they are replaced by an active land use, but if an active land use abandons a cell and is not replaced by another active use, then the passive land use for which the cell has the highest suitability will replace the departing active use. Finally, fixed land uses, or features, are those like lakes or parks which do not change state. The reason for this categorization of land uses will be made clear shortly.

The Neighborhood Effect
The neighborhood effect represents the positive and negative interactions between the land use on cell i and the land uses of all the cells in its neighborhood. Because we do not yet know what land use a cell i not occupied by a fixed land use will have at the next time period, we must calculate, for each cell not occupied by a fixed land use, the neighborhood effect for each possible land use that the cell could have. The interaction effects between individual cells are represented by weights that depend on the land use of the two cells and the distance between them. Positive weights represent attraction effects and negative weights, repulsion. Normally, the absolute value of the weights becomes smaller as the distance between cells increases, to reflect the fact that distant cells are generally less important as a determinant of land use (see, for example, figure 6.11). We refer to the sets of weights used to calculate the neighborhood effect of a cell as "influence functions" since each individual set of weights shows the influence, as a function of distance, of one land use on the desirability of the cell for another (see, for example, table 6.1, where each row represents an influence function). An inertia effect is included in the neighborhood effect calculations to represent the fact that there are usually various costs, both psychic and monetary, associated with changing land use. The inertia parameter is represented as the weight given to the effect of a land use on itself at zero distance. Other

Table 6.1
Influence functions (sets of w_{khd}) used to calculate potential for residential land use in the homogeneous cell space application

Distance	Residential	Industry	Commerce
1.0	2.0	-10.0	-2.0
1.4	2.0	-10.0	-1.0
2.0	1.5	-5.0	2.0
2.2	1.5	-3.0	1.0
2.8	1.0	-1.0	1.0
3.0	1.0	0.0	1.0
3.2	1.0	0.0	0.5
3.6	1.0	0.0	0.5
4.0	0.5	0.0	0.4
4.1	0.5	0.0	0.3
4.2	0.5	0.0	0.2
4.5	0.5	0.0	0.1
5.0	0.5	0.0	0.1
5.1	0.1	0.0	0.1
5.4	0.1	0.0	0.0
5.7	0.1	0.0	0.0
5.8	0.1	0.0	0.0
6.0	0.1	0.0	0.0
6.1–8.0	0.0	0.0	0.0

zero-distance weights can be specified to represent the effect of one land use on the potential for another on the same cell; for example, a negative weight for the effect of commerce on the potential of the cell for low-density residential would represent the likely remediation costs to prepare the cell for single-family housing.

We calculate the neighborhood effect as

$$N_{ij} = \Sigma_h \Sigma_d w_{khd} \Delta_{hd} \qquad (6.2)$$

where

N_{ij} = the neighborhood effect calculated for land use j at cell i
w_{khd} = the weight applied to land use k on the hth cell in distance band d
Δ_{hd} = the delta function: $\Delta_{hd} = 1$ if the cell has land use k; otherwise, $\Delta_{hd} = 0$.

The neighborhood effect does not have to be completely recalculated for every cell at each iteration. It is only necessary to update the value for cells with a neighborhood in which one or more cells changed state, and, even then, the update only involves adjusting the weights corresponding to the cells that changed state; the other cells in the neighborhood can be ignored.

The Stochastic Perturbation

To represent the heterogeneity among the underlying agents in the system, which we are not modeling directly, the basic model includes a stochastic perturbation term. For example, in calculating how good a particular cell is for commercial land use, we perturb the deterministic calculation to represent the fact that we do not know what kind of commercial activity is involved—is it fast food or financial services?—and that the different types would make different calculations if we were modeling at that level of disaggregation. The perturbation is given by

$$r = 1 + [-ln(\text{rand})]^{\alpha} \tag{6.3}$$

where

α = a parameter that controls the size distribution of the perturbation
rand = a uniform random variable, with 0 < rand < 1.

The distribution of r is highly skewed, so that most deterministic calculations will receive only a small perturbation, which will not normally affect the land use decision, whereas a few will receive a perturbation large enough to alter the deterministic land use assignment.

The stochastic perturbation is the most important factor determining the spatial structure in terms of clusters. If the perturbation is too low, too few seeds of future clusters are generated, and thus with too few small clusters, the cluster size–frequency distribution becomes convex (figure 6.5). Seeds are single isolated cells of a particular land use, but not all single cells become the nuclei of clusters; many remain in

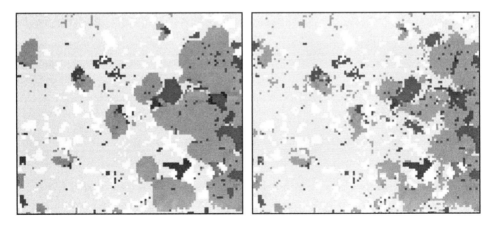

Figure 6.5
Effect of the stochastic perturbation on cluster seeding: (*left*) too little stochasticity results in too few small clusters; (*right*) correct level of stochasticity gives a realistic distribution of cluster sizes.

their isolated state. The stochastic perturbation, in effect, endows the model with stochastic resonance, which allows the model to explore the possibilities offered by the bifurcation tree. This will be treated further in the discussion of the transition rule below.

Land Use Demands

In the CA developed for this model, the dynamics are subject to an exogenous constraint. In conventional CA, the dynamics are completely endogenous: the number of cells in each state at each iteration is determined within the CA itself as an incidental outcome of the application of the transition rules. A real city or region, however, does not have purely endogenous dynamics. The amount of land required for each use is determined not by the local competition for land, but rather by the size of the city's population and economy, and the city's size, as well as its growth or decline over the years, depends on its role in the regional, national, and global system of cities and regions—in other words, it depends on the dynamics of the larger system in which it is embedded. In the simplest version of this model, the number of cells of each active land use type at each time step is specified exogenously, and the CA then determines, endogenously, their location. In more advanced versions, the numbers of cells are determined by exogenous models linked to the CA; for example, demographic and economic models generate demands for residential, industrial, and commercial cells, and these demands in turn drive the CA dynamics.

The Transition Potential

We calculate a vector of *potentials*—one for each active land use—for each cell:

$$V_{ij} = rS_{ij}A_{ij}Z_{ij}N_{ij} \tag{6.4a}$$

where

V_{ij} = the potential of cell i for land use j
r = the random perturbation
S_{ij} = the suitability of cell i for land use j
A_{ij} = the accessibility measure of cell i for land use j
Z_{ij} = the zoning status of cell i with respect to land use j
N_{ij} = the neighborhood effect on cell i for land use j.

If the neighborhood effect is negative (this happens only in the rare case where repulsion effects dominate), then we calculate the transition potential as

$$V_{ij} = r(2 - S_{ij}A_{ij}Z_{ij})N_{ij} \tag{6.4b}$$

Once the model is calibrated, the transition potentials for the various land uses that could occupy the cell effectively represent the value of the cell for each of those uses, or in other words, the willingness of potential users to pay to occupy the site, at least up to a monotonic transformation. Therefore, the potential surfaces over the area being modeled, one surface for each land use class, correspond to the bid rent curves in the Alonso-Muth land use model (Alonso, 1964; Muth, 1969). Of course, Alonso-Muth bid rent surfaces are smooth and deterministic, whereas here they are somewhat rough because they are altered cell by cell by the stochastic perturbation term $r \geq 0$, and also because the suitabilities and zoning may introduce local discontinuities.

The Transition Rule
The transition rule is straightforward:

Assign to each cell the state (land use) for which it has the highest potential as calculated by equation 6.4, until all land use demands have been met.

In order to implement the rule, it is necessary to rank the potentials for each cell, and then to rank the cells by their highest potential. Beginning with the top-ranked cell and proceeding to the next-ranked one, and so on, each cell is assigned the state for which it has the highest potential and is then removed from the list. But as cells are assigned land uses, a running count is kept of the number of cells assigned to each active land use, and when the exogenous cell demand for a land use is met, the potentials for that particular land use are removed from the ranked lists of the individual cells, the cells are reranked by their highest potential, and thus no more cells are assigned that land use.

This transition rule, the heart of the model's CA, is actually only the third in a hierarchy of transition rules. The rule with the highest priority, allowing the user to intervene exogenously, is to change the cell to a state specified by the user. This rule is used, for example, to introduce a planned development at a certain location in a certain year. The rule with the second highest priority is to change cells to the fixed-state sea if the natural system module raises the sea level above the elevation of the cell as given by the digital elevation model (DEM). Essentially all applications include a DEM among their input data.

Note that, in most cases, a cell is assigned the state it already has—that is, there is no change. This is partly due to the inertia factor, but also to the fact that potentials tend not to change rapidly, so that what was a good location for a particular land use tends to remain a good location. Nevertheless, at each iteration, every cell is in play. Also, it is often the case that a cell does not end up with the land use for which it has the highest potential because a sufficient number of other cells have higher potentials for that land use to satisfy the demand. Similarly, it may happen that none of the cells with the highest potentials for a particular land use end up with that use. This situation arises frequently in the case of land uses that have lower market value: what would be their best locations are preempted by land uses that have more market power. A well-known example is the preemption of the best agricultural lands by urban land uses.

Although these phenomena do not depend on the presence of a stochastic perturbation and will occur even in a deterministic system, the stochastic perturbation ensures that, occasionally, a cell will be converted to a land use that does not have the highest deterministic potential. When that happens, the cell may remain as a single isolated case of that land use. On the other hand, if the deterministic potential is just a little lower than the highest or dominant potential on that cell, then the presence of the new land use, through a positive neighborhood effect, may raise the potentials on nearby cells enough that what had been a lower, or hidden, potential becomes the dominant one locally, and a growing cluster of cells with the new land use is established. An example from the Dublin simulation discussed below is shown in figure 6.6. Of course, because the cluster would never have appeared had the original perturbation been smaller, this is a case of the system exploiting a bifurcation, and that may be enough to alter the spatial dynamics of the system beyond the local area. Exploiting a hidden potential by means of a stochastic perturbation is an example of stochastic resonance, the phenomenon whereby adding noise (a random signal) to a signal that is too weak to be detected (the inferior potential hidden under the dominant one) makes the composite signal (and hence the original weak signal) strong enough to be detected. Of course, here, because a random signal is being added to all potentials, we are only detecting a small sample of the hidden potentials.

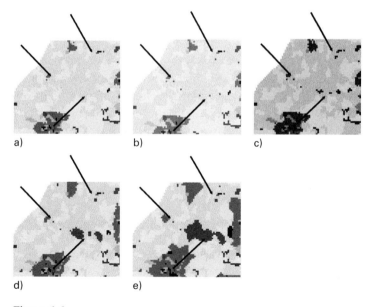

Figure 6.6
Stochastic resonance in Dublin simulation: industrial seeds (indicated by arrows) and cluster growth, 1988 (a); 1989 (b); 1991 (c); 1998 (d); 2008 (e).

Nevertheless, the sample, even if small, may still reveal something of the shape of the hidden potential. For example, most of the isolated industrial land uses that pop up in the simulation shown in figure 6.6 are near rail lines. Although we have been speaking of the stochastic perturbation in terms of system dynamics and stochastic resonance, it is important to remember that this perturbation represents actual heterogeneity among the individual actors: the people, corporations, and other organizations that are making the locational decisions.

Interventions

It is possible to interrupt a simulation at any iteration in order to intervene in the application and alter it in some way. For example, a simulation may be paused at a certain year so that the user can alter the suitability and land use maps in such a way as to represent the draining and infill of a wetland area to make it available for industrial and commercial uses; the simulation run is then resumed and works with the modified maps. Interventions can also target the land use, the infrastructure networks, the zoning and other legal restrictions, and certain parameters. Because interventions take priority over endogenous changes due to the model dynamics, the system must adapt to them.

Output

The primary output of the model is a land use map for each year of the simulation, as well as an animation of the series of maps if desired. Depending on the version and application, the model also generates various indicators from the annual land use maps, which are presented in the form of maps, tables, or graphs, as appropriate. Finally, some versions can be run in Monte Carlo mode, so that the model automatically runs a specified number of times and accumulates the results to produce probability maps of each land use for each year. Because of the stochastic perturbation, each time the model is run, a somewhat different series of land use maps results. From the ensemble of maps for each year, the probability of each cell being occupied by a particular land use is calculated to produce the probability map for that land use for that year. An example is shown in figure 6.7 (plate 1).

A Simulation for Generic Results

Before turning to more advanced versions or specific applications of the model, it will be useful to examine its generic behavior. Most conventional CA are defined on a homogeneous cell space, whereas the basic urban land use model just described runs on a highly heterogeneous cell space. It is primarily this heterogeneity that tailors an application to a specific city or region. If we begin a simulation with an urban seed consisting of a few commercial, industrial, and residential cells

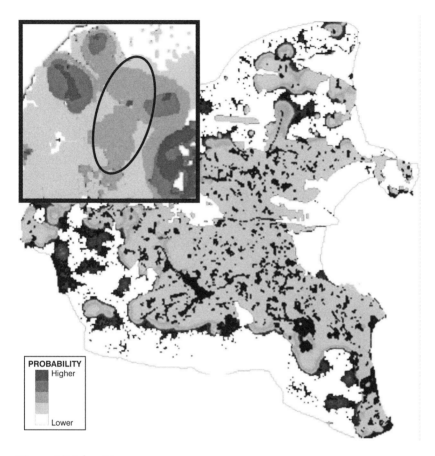

Figure 6.7 (plate 1)
Probability that a cell will be converted to an urban land use in Dublin simulation for 2008. Note the relatively large areas of intermediate probability in northwestern Dublin, shown in the inset enlargement of this area.

surrounded by rural cells covering the rest of the area to be modeled, but then include suitability, transportation, and zoning maps representing the Dublin area, then any city we generate will more or less resemble Dublin, because the growing simulated city will not be able to occupy the sea, will avoid the rugged terrain of the Wicklow Mountains to the south, and will tend to follow the main transportation routes, which in one form or another have been in place for centuries. In other words, if we use the full model, it will be difficult to discover the generic properties of the output, except by making many applications and analyzing the output for commonalities, like fractal dimensions. Therefore, we begin by running the model without suitabilities, accessibilities, or zoning, so that the cell space is homogeneous (see also White and Engelen, 1993). On this isotropic plane, we can generate generic cities, cities that owe their form entirely to the randomly perturbed neighborhood effect. Of course, it can be argued that the sets of weighting factors, or influence functions, used to calculate the neighborhood effect are city specific, and, to some extent, that is undoubtedly true, but applications to various cities and regions collectively suggest that the influence functions are broadly similar regardless of the application. This issue will be discussed further in chapter 10.

The simplest application uses three active land uses—commerce, industry, and residential—and one rural or vacant land use. The influence functions are specified for various pairs of active land uses; the passive land use—vacant—is assumed in this application not to influence the location of other land uses. Also, commerce is assumed to have no influence on industry. An example of the influence functions used is provided in table 6.1, which shows the three sets of weighting factors used to calculate the neighborhood effect, and hence the potential, for residential land use. In general, it is good practice to define influence functions for only the most important land use interactions because, with more land uses, the number of possible influence functions that can be specified grows rapidly; including all land uses makes the model difficult to calibrate and slow to execute. Since the application is hypothetical and generic, the weights are not calibrated; rather, they reflect common assumptions about the attraction and repulsion effects of land uses on one another. For example, commerce is shown as repelling residential use if it is located immediately adjacent to the cell in question; otherwise, it is attractive, though that effect becomes less at greater distances and disappears beyond a distance of 5.1 units of cell space. On the other hand, residential use is attracted by the presence of residential land use at all distances out to 6.0 units. The stochastic perturbation term is tuned so that the model produces fractal urban structures in terms of both the cluster size–frequency and radial dimensions.

An example of the output is given in figure 6.8, which shows the initial seed of the city and the land use maps generated at iterations 10, 20, 30, and 40. Because of the random perturbation, every run will produce a different city, and because the land use patterns are not constrained by preexisting suitabilities, zoning, or infrastructure networks, the configuration of land uses will be quite different in the different cities. On the other hand, the cities will be similar in terms of their fractal dimensions. The cluster size–frequency plot for commerce for these cities is linear (figure 6.9), and the radial analysis displays the characteristic kink in the area-radius relationship that defines the two zones with different radial dimensions (figure 6.10). The outer zone is the urbanizing area, and it is in this area that the cities generate their individual land use patterns.

This generic application, where the emerging land use pattern results entirely from the randomly perturbed neighborhood effect, shows most clearly the spatial

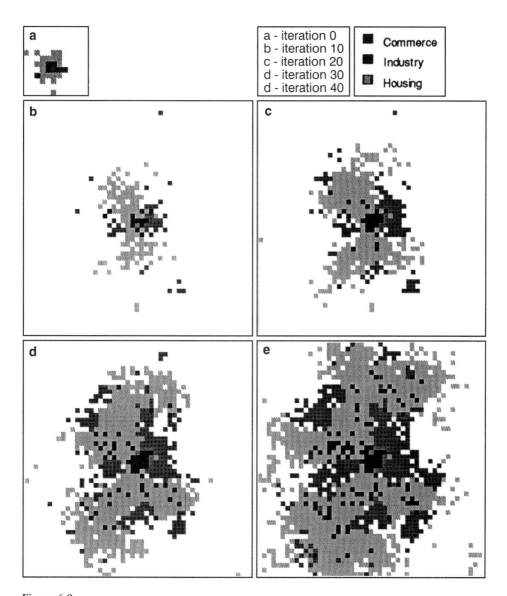

Figure 6.8
Iterations 0 (a); 10 (b); 20 (c); 30 (d); and 40 (e) of a simulation run on a homogeneous cell space and without a transport network.

120   Chapter 6

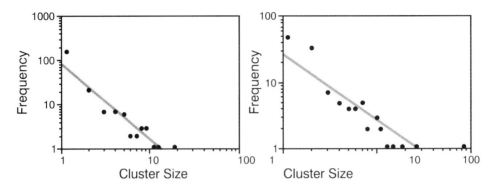

Figure 6.9
Cluster size–frequency distribution of commerce: (*left*) composite of iteration 40 of four simulations differing stochastically; (*right*) actual distribution for Houston, 1960.

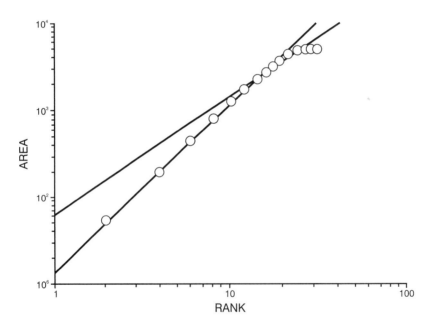

Figure 6.10
Area-radius relationship of the urbanized area, composite of four simulations, iteration 40. Slopes are 1.96 for the inner zone (*lower plot*) and 1.38 for the outer zone (*upper plot*).

consequences of the endogenous dynamics. As the city grows, single isolated cells of various land uses appear in this zone as a result of the random perturbation; some of them remain isolated, but others, again partly by chance, grow into larger clusters. The size distribution of the clusters is similar among the cities, but the actual location of the clusters, especially the larger ones that dominate the land use pattern, is completely different. Thus it is in the early stages of development of the zone that the future spatial structure is seeded. One implication is that a small planning intervention in this zone, to establish the seed of a cluster in a certain part of the zone or to prevent one from appearing there, will have a major impact on the future land use pattern of the city. In contrast, planning interventions in parts of the city where the spatial structure is already largely established will have only minor effects.

Applications of the Full Model

The full model, including suitabilities, zoning, and accessibility to one or more transportation networks, was tested with an application to Cincinnati (White, Engelen, and Uljee, 1997). Since land use data were only available for 1960, from Passonneau and Wurman (1966) the city was generated from a hypothetical protocity as it was assumed to exist in 1840, with the model calibrated to give a good approximation to the actual 1960 land use map. Suitabilities were based on steepness of slope since the topography of the Cincinnati area is characterized by valleys with steep walls cut into a relatively level plateau, so that both valley floors and uplands are easy to develop, but the valley walls are not. Both the railroads and the major highways follow the valleys. As a result, the land use patterns of both Cincinnati and its simulations reflect the topography: industry, having a greater need for accessibility to the transport networks, especially rail, is concentrated in the valleys; commerce, requiring good access to the highway network, is concentrated in the central business district and along major roads, and residential land use is mostly relegated to the plateau. The application is interesting because, so far, it is the only application where the model has been used to simulate the growth of an actual city almost from its initial settlement, and the result was reasonably successful. Calibration was by trial and error, and the quality of the match between the actual and simulated maps was judged visually. Validation relied on the same data set as the one used for calibration. Since this application, substantial progress has been made in both calibration and validation techniques appropriate to high-resolution models of complex systems, but calibration, validation, and map comparison remain important issues, which will be discussed more thoroughly in chapter 9.

Following the Cincinnati application, the model was applied to several European cities and regions in the context of the MURBANDY Project of the Joint Research Centre of the European Commission (JRC), developed within the Space Applications

Institute (now the Land Management Unit) of the JRC. Aimed, in part, at demonstrating the usefulness of remotely sensed data for urban planning, the project had three phased objectives. The first was to derive a set of land use maps for a representative sample of European cities, showing land use at intervals of approximately ten years over a forty-year period. The second was to develop a number of indicators of urban environmental conditions relevant to sustainability. And the third was to develop and implement a generic model of urban land use dynamics that would support a realistic exploration of urban futures under a variety of planning and policy scenarios. The CA-based land use model was adopted to achieve the project's third objective, and it was in this context that applications were made to several European cities, as well as one African city.

The project was designed to make use of land use and land cover data from CORINE, a standardized land use map covering member countries of the European Union derived from satellite imagery, with a minimum polygon size of 25 hectares (~62 acres). The MURBANDY Project added a fourth level to the standard CORINE classification, bringing the resolution to one hectare (~2.5 acres). At the time the modeling project began, the number of urban land use classes in the CORINE data set had recently been extended, thus increasing the usefulness of the data set. On the other hand, due to the inherent limitations of remotely sensed data, it was not possible to distinguish some important urban land use classes. For example, it is often impossible to discriminate between industrial and commercial land uses, or even, in the dense urban development typical of European cities, residential from commercial: a roof may shelter either retail shops or residential apartments, or frequently both. Because of these limitations, the remotely sensed data were supplemented with historical land use data from other sources collected by local research teams in each of the cities making up the MURBANDY sample. The resulting maps were just what was needed to support high-resolution modeling of urban land use. Once certain rural land uses were aggregated, the maps included twenty-three land uses; of these, ten were urban, eight of which could be treated as active urban land use classes. Furthermore, the availability of comparable data for several time periods facilitated calibration and validation of the model.

Of course, some of the data sets were better than others, and in several respects—accuracy, consistency, and area covered—the data for Dublin were the best. For that reason, we used Dublin as the test city for adapting the model to the MURBANDY data sets and output requirements, and we will focus here on the Dublin application. It was the first realistic application of the model, that is, the first one using a high-resolution multi-year data set with a large number of land uses, so that a proper calibration and validation could be carried out. Furthermore, as newer versions of the model were developed, Dublin was used as a test bed, both because of the quality of the data and because of the possibility of comparing new versions with previous ones in terms of performance. For this reason, Dublin applications will make frequent appearances in later chapters. Researchers at the Joint Research Centre made their own application of the model to Dublin, simulating over a longer period, specifically 1968–1998 (Barredo et al., 2003). They subsequently applied the model to several other European areas, including Madrid (Barredo and Gómez Delgado, 2008), the Friuli region in northeast Italy (Barredo et al., 2005), the Algarve in Portugal (Petrov, Lavalle, and Kasanko, 2009) as well as to Lagos, Nigeria (Barredo et al., 2004). Other versions of the model, developed for other clients or projects, were applied to Vitoria-Gasteiz (van Delden, Uljee, and Dominguez, 2006) and the Madrid region (Hahn et al., 2006), both in Spain.

The Dublin simulation uses the eight active urban land use classes shown in table 6.2, as well as eight agricultural and natural classes, which are passive—that is, they can be taken over by any one of the active land uses. The suitabilities (see, for example, figure 6.1) are primarily a function of elevation, so the Wicklow Mountains on the southern edge of the modeled area show up as being of low suitability, but the presence of wetlands also lowers suitability values. For ports, only cells that are close to the sea have high suitabilities. As for accessibilities, the transportation infrastructure consists of the city's road and rail networks. In this model, unlike the models discussed in the chapters 7 and 8, no distinction is made among links: a local street has the same significance as a superhighway when calculating accessibilities. Maps of the accessibility values for industry and discontinuous sparse residential are shown in figure 6.2. Zoning is minimal: protected natural areas are zoned to exclude all land uses; otherwise, active land uses are unrestricted as to location (figure 6.3). This simplified approach reflects both the difficulty of acquiring reliable zoning data and the relatively lax enforcement of most zoning at the time in the Dublin area.

Table 6.2
Urban land use classes used in the Dublin simulation

Active	Fixed
Residential continuous dense urban fabric	Construction sites
Residential continuous medium dense urban fabric	Road and rail networks and associated land
Residential discontinuous urban fabric	Airport
Residential discontinuous sparse urban fabric	Mineral extraction sites
Industrial areas	Dump sites
Commercial areas	Artificial nonagricultural vegetated areas (e.g., parks)
Public and private services	
Port areas	

Note: Rural land use classes were treated as passive land uses.

The main influence functions for the four most important active land uses are shown in figure 6.11. They reflect varying attraction and repulsion effects. For example, discontinuous sparse residential land use anywhere in the neighborhood makes the location more attractive (positive w_{khd}), whereas industry within the neighborhood makes the location less attractive (negative w_{khd}). On the other hand, in some applications, at greater distances industry enhances the attractiveness of the location, presumably because it represents conveniently located employment opportunities that are nevertheless far enough away so that the land use is not considered a disamenity. Commerce is strongly attracted to discontinuous sparse residential land use because it represents customers (the weights, though positive, are relatively small because there are many cells of this land use, so the cumulative effect is large). The effect of commerce on itself is strongly positive at short distances because a larger cluster size attracts more customers, whereas, at greater distances, the effect is negative because commerce located farther away represents a competing destination. The influence functions were calibrated over the period 1988–1998. The initial shapes of the functions either were established on the basis of common perceptions about attraction and repulsion effects among land uses or were borrowed from the Cincinnati calibration in cases where the land uses were roughly equivalent. The individual values making up the influence functions were then adjusted to improve the fit between the 1998 land use map generated by the model and the actual 1998 land use map. This process usually resulted in relatively minor changes in the shapes of the functions. Much more important is the relative height of the influence functions, which determines the relative dominance of the various land uses: commerce should normally be able to displace discontinuous sparse residential, for example, but the opposite should rarely happen. In effect, once influence functions are calibrated and the values of the neighborhood effect calculated, the transition potentials calculated from neighborhood effects by equation 6.4 represent the relative willingness of the various activities to pay to occupy the site.

The land use dynamics are forced by the growth of the city. In this application, as well as other MURBANDY applications, growth is represented by a file containing the total number of cells required for each active land use for each year of the simulation. Here the numbers were taken from the 1988 and 1998 land use maps and interpolated for the years between those dates. The trends were then extrapolated to 2008, the end date for the simulation, to establish a "business as usual" scenario; other cell demand trends for 1998–2008 represent high-and low-growth scenarios. With city growth specified by the yearly cell counts for the various land uses, the urban form emerges in a process of self-organization. Figure 6.12 (plate 2) shows the actual and simulated land use maps for 1998. By comparing them, we can see how the form that emerged in one particular simulation run compares to the form that emerged in reality. Other runs produced other, but similar, land use maps. The fully

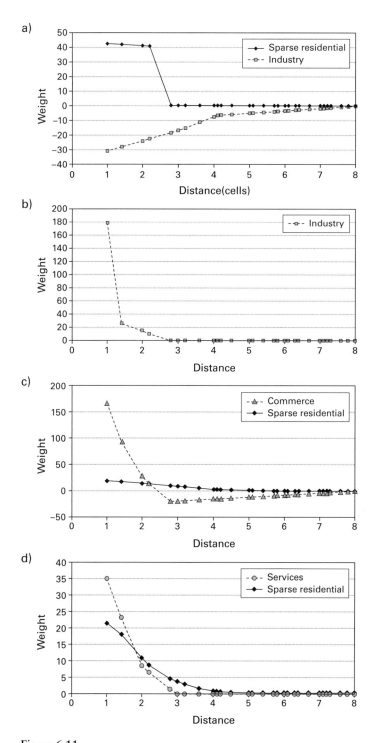

Figure 6.11
Influence functions used in Dublin simulation: (a) discontinuous sparse residential; (b) industry; (c) commerce; (d) services. Each curve within a panel shows the effect of a particular land use on the potential of the land use to which the panel applies.

126   Chapter 6

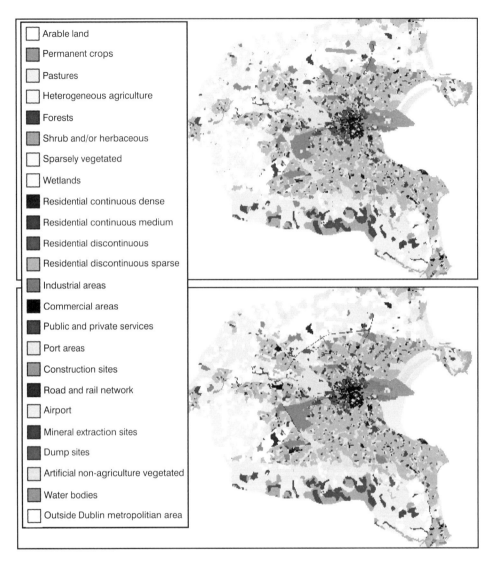

Figure 6.12 (plate 2)
Dublin application for 1998: (*top*) simulated land use; (*bottom*) actual land use.

developed inner zone of the city changes very little, whether in simulation or in reality. It is in the outer, urbanizing zone that we see most of the new urban structure emerging. In figure 6.6, we can follow local self-organization in detail. In 1988, there were no industrial cells in the three areas indicated by the arrows; in 1989, by a process of stochastic resonance, six new industrial cells appeared, one indicated by the top arrow, two by the arrow to the left, and three by the bottom arrow. Over the following years, some of these clusters grew and others did not; in other words, the system adopted some locations as good for industry, but rejected others. By 2008, the three most successful clusters had merged to make one large industrial area. In many runs of the model, industrial clusters appeared in this part of Dublin, although the actual location, size, and number of clusters varied from one run to another. The area thus seems to be a good one for that land use, partly because of good access to the rail and motorway (superhighway) networks.

Because, at the time of the application, land use data were not available for any year beyond 1998, the calibration could not be validated using the standard approach of running the model beyond the calibration period of 1988–1998 and comparing the results with a map of the actual land use. A comparison of the actual and simulated land use maps for 1998, however, permits a weaker, implicit validation. Since the model was calibrated on the basis of the same comparison, the validation is in a sense an assessment of the quality of the calibration. If it is not possible to get a good calibration, then the model has, in effect, failed an implicit validation test. Figure 6.12 (plate 2) shows the actual and simulated land use maps for 1998. Because the two maps appear to be similar, at least in a general way, we might judge the calibration to be good. But it is useful to make more specific comparisons. In figure 6.13, we see a comparison of the location of industry on the two maps. Since the model has a stochastic component and is subject to bifurcations, the specific locations generated are not significant; they will vary from one run of the model to another. What is important is the *pattern* of locations. Is the pattern generated by the model similar to the pattern on the actual land use map? To answer this question, it is helpful to look at the areas where the two maps disagree. Are the industrial areas found only on the simulated map in the same *kinds* of locations as the industrial areas found only on the actual map? Are they close to one another? Is the distribution of cluster sizes similar? It is not so helpful to concentrate on the areas where the two maps agree, even though these areas might be thought to represent the successes of the model. The first reason is that most of the cells in these areas were industry in the 1988 map and have simply remained in that state. Of course, the model could have changed the land use and did not, and that counts in its favor; but the inertia factor makes it unlikely that the model would have changed it. The second reason is that normally the maximum coincidence between maps represents an overcalibration of the model—that is, a bad calibration—and is therefore to be avoided.

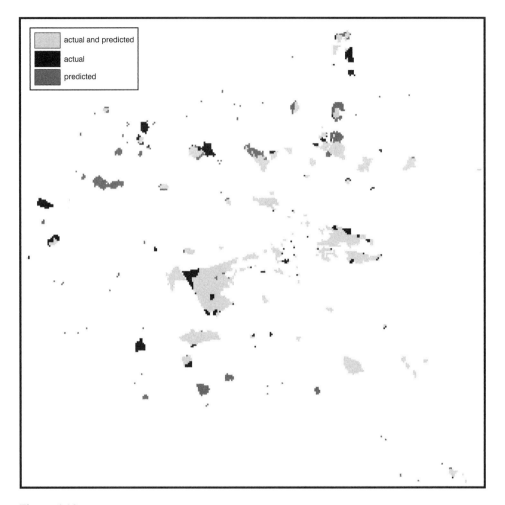

Figure 6.13
Comparison of simulated (predicted) and actual locations of industry, Dublin, 1998.

Making similar comparisons for the other active land uses permits us to make a global judgment about how good the calibration is and how well the model performs—or in which respects it performs well and in which not so well. Notice that we are making visual comparisons and judgments of quality, rather than relying on measurements and statistics. That is because, at present, the quantitative techniques available for making relevant comparisons of maps are either inadequate or completely inappropriate. For example, that the values of the Kappa statistics for these simulations of Dublin are generally above 0.80 largely reflects the fact that most cells do not change state. Furthermore, as a cell-by-cell comparison technique,

Kappa tells us nothing about the similarity of patterns between two maps. Yet it is the patterns that are important. When we are modeling complex systems, we can only hope to generate the correct patterns; we can never expect to model the details precisely. Nevertheless, it is very desirable to make quantified comparisons. Consequently, we have been developing appropriate techniques in parallel with model development (see chapter 9), although we are still a long way from having all the measures we need. In short, absolute, quantified validation is not possible for models of complex systems. These problems are difficult and messy ones, and therefore interesting. They will be taken up in chapter 9.

Integrated Models

The CA-based land use model described above is driven by a list of annual land use demands. Of course, those demands, if they are not for past periods for which data are available, can be generated by other models. For example, an economic model can generate estimates for future land use demands for various economic sectors by converting forecasts of output per sector into corresponding requirements for land; similarly, a demographic model can generate estimates of land needed for residential use. But such models can also be linked dynamically to the CA-based land use model, so that demands are generated as the integrated model runs. If the link is unidirectional, from the demand model to the CA-based model, then the advantage is largely one of convenience and flexibility. But if the link is bidirectional, then the CA-based model can influence the behavior of the demand model, and the performance of the integrated model should thereby be improved. Although it is commonly assumed that if two models are linked dynamically, the errors inherent in each one will be multiplied, the opposite is more often the case. Because the models are usually complementary, each one tends to constrain the errors that can be made by the other.

Given the fact that human and natural systems are intimately bound up with each other, it is surprising how infrequently models of the two domains are dynamically linked to each other. Even models of different human systems are rarely linked in this way. It is more common for models to be chained, so that one model can affect the next, but the second cannot affect the first; in other words, there is no possibility of dynamic feedback. Though in many cases this is a reasonable simplification, in others, it amounts to a serious misrepresentation of the system being modeled. In particular, the economy and land use are intimately intertwined. It is clear that various economic activities require land for their facilities. But it is also the case that land use patterns can affect the output of various economic sectors. For example, as good agricultural land is urbanized, output of the agricultural sector will tend to decline; this effect also illustrates why linking models may reduce their error levels:

an agricultural model that is unconstrained by the land use requirements of other sectors has more scope to predict output levels that are too high.

Because of the advantages of integrated modeling, it makes sense to link the basic CA-based land use model to other models. In particular, it has been linked to a nonspatial macro-scale model consisting of four linked submodels representing climate, demography, and the economy, as well as the land use intensities of the several sectors included in the economic model (Engelen, White, and Wargnies, 1996; Engelen et al., 2002; White and Engelen, 1997, 2000; White, Engelen, and Uljee, 2000). Dynamic feedback from the linked, inherently spatial CA-based model effectively introduces space into the essentially nonspatial macro-scale model, and thus strengthens its performance. Furthermore, the integrated model is not just a land use model like the stand-alone CA-based model; it also gives year-by-year scenario-specific demographic and economic forecasts—additional output that many users find desirable. The full integrated model was developed for the United Nations Environment Program to explore the possible effects of climate change on island states and was applied to the Caribbean island state of Saint Lucia as a test case. The macro-scale model is essentially generic, and has also been incorporated into the regionalized CA-based model described in chapter 7. The four integrated subsystems of the macro-scale model are linked as shown in figure 6.14. Although we will describe the subsystems separately, we will emphasize their links and the feedback effects that occur among them.

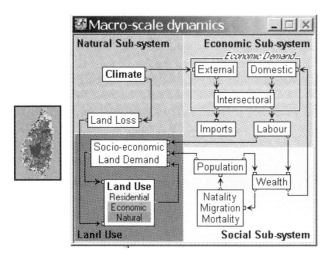

Figure 6.14
System diagram of the macro-scale model, which doubles as a graphical user interface (GUI).

Natural Subsystem

This subsystem is not a true model; rather it is a set of chained hypotheses that the user may easily change in order to define various scenarios. The first two represent the hypothesized trends in local temperature and sea level at yearly intervals over the simulation period. The next two represent hypothesized precipitation and storm frequency as functions of temperature. Finally, functional relationships between these four variables and demand in several economic sectors are specified; again, these are hypotheses that can be easily changed. For example, departures of temperature and precipitation from current mean values are assumed to affect agricultural output, and changes in storm frequency are assumed to impact tourism, which is part of the export sector of the economy. Thus these chained hypotheses lead from assumptions about the climate system to impacts on the economy (figure 6.15).

Economic Subsystem

The economy is represented by an input-output (I-O) model (see box 6.1). In the Saint Lucia application, there are five industry sectors: agriculture, industry, trade, services, and tourism. In addition there are two final demand sectors: external demand (exports) and domestic demand (consumption); the corresponding input sectors are imports and labor (see table 6.3). The I-O model calculates the total output of each sector of the economy for every year of the simulation on the basis of the values in the final demand columns. Those values are determined exogenously, on the basis of inputs from the natural system and demographic models. Given any particular values in the final demand columns, the model calculates the total output for each sector of the economy. Thus, if the volume of tourism goes up, as represented in the tourism cell of the external demand column, the model will calculate the final impact of that increase on all sectors of the economy. Similarly, if the population grows, various components of domestic consumption will increase, and that will have an impact on all sectors of the economy. Here we see the importance of a link with the demographic model, because demographic effects drive domestic consumption. The opposite is also the case. If the economy does well, there are demographic consequences: out-migration is slowed, and the death rate declines. All of these links are built into the macro-scale model. In short, the economic model is driven by exogenous changes in sectoral demands due to climate change and demographics. On the basis of these forcing factors, it generates new output levels for each sector of the economy. These are then translated into updated land use demands.

Using an input-output model to represent the economy has two major advantages. First, it captures multiplier effects by which change in one sector propagates throughout the economy. For example, an increase in tourism will benefit not just the tourism sector itself, but all other sectors, because it purchases inputs from them. Then, as each other sector expands, it also requires inputs from each sector, thus

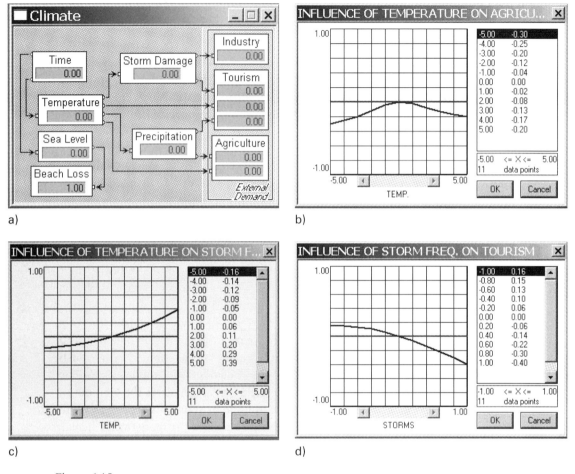

Figure 6.15
Inside the GUI of the macro-scale model: (a) climate module; (b) effect of temperature on agriculture; (c) effect of temperature on storm frequency; (d) effect of storm frequency on tourism. The agriculture, storm frequency, and tourism effects (b–d) are elements of the climate module GUI.

initiating a secondary expansionary round, and so on. Since the final result is that all sectors experience a change in output, all corresponding land use demands will be affected, not just the demand for land for tourism activities. The I-O model calculates the end result directly, so that land use demands can be updated. Second, because it amounts to a kind of accounting system, the I-O model ensures that the representation of the economy is always consistent. Some economic models that seem plausible in themselves are globally inconsistent. For example, the economic model used by Peter Allen (1997) inadvertently creates extra economic activity ex nihilo.

Table 6.3
Input-output table for Saint Lucia (millions of Eastern Caribbean $)

	Agriculture	Industry	Trade	Services	Tourism	External demand	Domestic demand
Agriculture	5.00	30.00	10.00	2.00	5.30	194.50	72.96
Industry	20.00	250.00	75.01	30.00	50.30	149.20	649.49
Trade	5.00	20.00	40.01	49.99	67.50	0.00	135.45
Services	6.00	30.00	30.01	20.00	46.00	22.30	370.14
Tourism	0.20	2.80	0.40	1.30	139.80	415.40	0.00
Imports	140.08	504.40	0.00	163.38	95.60	—	—
Labor	143.48	386.80	162.53	257.77	155.40	—	—

Box 6.1
The Economic Model

> The input-output model that is the basis of the economic subsystem is based on monetary flows, whereas the land use demands for each sector are calculated on the basis of employment in the sector. Therefore, it is necessary to first calculate the relevant sectoral outputs each year using the I-O model and then convert them to estimates of sectoral employment.
>
> The input-output table (table 6.3) consists of an interindustry matrix representing the intersectoral flows of intermediate goods, augmented by columns representing flows to final demand sectors and rows representing labor inputs (measured as wages and salaries) and imports. All flows are represented in monetary terms. Underlying the table of intersectoral flows is a matrix of technical coefficients calculated from the flow data. The technical coefficients represent in proportional terms the inputs necessary to produce the output of each sector; the input coefficients for each sector therefore sum to one. We use the technical coefficients to calculate the change in output of each industry sector—agriculture, industry, trade, services, tourism—induced by changes in the two final demand sectors, i.e., external and domestic demand. External demand, or exports, for all years of the simulation is specified exogenously as a scenario. On the other hand, domestic demand (largely household demand) is assumed to depend on the size of the population and the relative demands for the goods of each sector, both of which, in turn, are assumed to depend on economic status as measured by the relative employment level:
>
> $\Delta X_{Di} = c_i \exp(n_i (u_t - u_{t=0})) \Delta X_{P,t}$
>
> where
>
> ΔX_{Di} = change in domestic demand for industry sector i
> c_i = domestic demand coefficient for sector i
> u_t = per capita employment, the employment participation index for the current year t
> n_i = a parameter relating employment to domestic consumption in sector i
> $\Delta X_{P,t}$ = change in population.

Box 6.1 (continued)

New values for final demand are given by

$$\Delta X_{F,t} = \Delta X_{E,t} + \Delta X_{D,t}$$
$$X_{F,t} = X_{F,t-1} + \Delta X_{F,t}\text{f}$$

where

$X_{F,t}$ = vector of final demands; the elements correspond to the industry sectors i
$X_{D,t}$ = vector of domestic demands (elements are X_{Di})
$X_{E,t}$ = vector of external demands (exports).

We next calculate total output of each sector, as well as updated imports:

$$\Delta X_t = A_{i,j} \Delta X_{F,t} + \Delta X_{F,t}$$
$$X_t = X_{t-1} + \Delta X_t$$
$$\Delta X_{M,t} = M \Delta X_t$$
$$X_{M,t} = X_{M,t-1} + \Delta X_{M,t}$$

where

X_t = vector of total outputs
$A_{i,j}$ = matrix of intersectoral technical coefficients
M = vector of technical coefficients for imports
$X_{Mi,t}$ = imports of sector i products.

X and $X_{Mi,t}$ together constitute the solution showing the ultimate impact of an exogenous change in final demand, taking all multiplier effects into account. The input-output model is solved for these values at each iteration of the simulation, which amounts to an assumption that the economy reaches a new equilibrium within a year. Although this is certainly not the case, it is a reasonable simplification compared to the alternative of using round-by-round solutions initiated (but not completed) each year and then summed cumulatively as the simulation proceeds. The round-by-round approach would also need to be run on a faster timescale (e.g., monthly) than the rest of the simulation. The instant equilibrium approach, though unrealistic in its assumption of instantaneous adjustments, does perform the two necessary functions of generating multiplier effects while keeping the economy consistent both internally and with the exogenous forcing of the demographic scenario; the latter role represents the accounting function of the model.

Finally, we convert the sectoral outputs to sectoral employment:

$$J_{i,t} = \frac{X_{i,t}}{\mathcal{E}_i}$$

where

$J_{i,t}$ = current employment in sector i
$\mathcal{E}_i$ = employment coefficient for sector i (output per employee, estimated from sectoral output and employment data).

The new employment values are used by the land use demand module to calculate new cell demands for the land uses corresponding to these economic sectors. In addition, the sectoral output values calculated in the I-O model are used by the demographic model to adjust death and net migration rates.

A disadvantage of the input-output model as it is currently formulated is that the technical coefficients are assumed to remain fixed. In the short run, this is generally not a bad assumption. But land use models are typically used to simulate for a period of at least ten years and often twenty or more, and, over such time spans, the technical coefficients will certainly experience major changes in their value for a variety of reasons, such as technological change, import substitution, or factor substitutions in response to price changes. Although most of the changes in technical coefficients cannot be anticipated, some can be caused by shifts in land use. For example, as we have already mentioned, a loss of rich agricultural land to urban sprawl or rising sea level will tend to displace agriculture to less productive land, which would raise the technical coefficient expressing the labor input required to produce one unit of agricultural output. Incorporating this effect in the model could give us additional insights into the relationship between the spatial dynamics of land use and the productivity of the economy. Allen's (1997) model, mentioned above, is in some ways more capable of handling the effects of changes in productivity.

Demographic Subsystem

The demographic model calculates the population for each year of the simulation on the basis of births, deaths, and net migration (box 6.2). It is not disaggregated by age or sex cohort. Although in that sense it is a rather minimal model, disaggregating by age or sex cohort would probably not significantly improve the performance of the macro-scale model in generating land use demands. Unlike most simple demographic models, however, it does incorporate economic influences dynamically: birth, death, and migration rates are all specified as secular trends. These trends are established empirically over the period for which data are available, usually the calibration period. Beyond that, they are specified by the user—effectively, as scenarios. For mortality and net migration, the structural trends are treated as functions of economic performance: as per capita income increases, both trends are lowered. Per capita income is calculated annually on the basis of values in the labor row of the input-output table and the current year population. The effect is particularly important for net migration because migration tends to respond quickly to changes in economic conditions. The population estimates produced by this module are used to generate yearly demands for residential land.

Land Use Demand Subsystem

As the link with the CA-based land use model, this module takes the sectoral outputs generated by the economic model and the population estimates from the demographic model and converts them to demands for the corresponding land uses (box 6.3). It also adjusts the supply of land to reflect losses due to rising sea levels, as determined by the CA in response to inputs from the natural system component. If the density or

Box 6.2
The Demographic Model

The demographic model calculates the population at yearly intervals on the basis of birth, death, and net migration rates. These rates are estimated on the basis of assumed trends in their values; these trends constitute the structural component of the rates. The death and net migration rates also depend on economic conditions as measured by per capita output; this effect is the variable component of the rate. The model is not disaggregated by age or sex cohort.

The birth, death, and net migration rates are calculated as follows:

$$b_t = f_b(t)$$
$$d_t = 0.5 f_d(t)[1 + \exp(-r_2(u_t - u_{t=0}))]$$
$$m_t = r_3 + \frac{[1 - r_4 \exp(u_t - u_{t=0})]}{[1 - r_4]} - 1$$
$$\Delta X_{P,t} = X_{P,t}(b_t - d_t - m_t)$$
$$X_{P,t+1} = P_t + \Delta P_t$$

where

$X_{P,t}$ = population at time t
b_t = birth rate at time t
d_t = death rate at time t
m_t = net migration rate at time t
$u_t = \sum_i \frac{X_{i,t}}{X_{P,t}}$ = output per capita; i ranges over all intermediate and final demand sectors
$f_b(t)$ = structural birth rate
$f_d(t)$ = structural death rate
r_2 = variable death rate
r_3 = structural migration rate
r_4 = variable migration rate.

The birth, death, and net migration rates are the actual empirical rates for the years of a simulation for which data are available. For future years, the structural rate is estimated from past data or supplied by the user as a scenario.

Box 6.3
The Land Use Demand Model

Changes in the amount of economic activity and population alter the amount of land required for the corresponding land uses. The land use demand module converts changes in activity and population levels to numbers of cells required for them. The approach takes into account the tendency toward increasing density of occupation both as available land becomes scarcer and when its suitability is greater. The effect of scarcity depends on the amount of land currently occupied by the activity relative to the amount still available, which is taken to be the total area occupied by passive land uses—that is, the cells that could be converted to the land use in question, and which are not currently occupied by an active land use. The suitability effect depends on the mean suitability of cells occupied by the land use. Note that this changes over time—not because the suitability of individual cells is changing, but because additional cells, with suitabilities not equal to the current mean suitability, are taken in by the land use.

We first calculate the densities that will apply to newly converted cells:

$$W_{i,t=0} = \frac{J_{i,t=0}}{NC_{i,t=0}}$$

$$W_{i,t} = W_{i,t=0} \left(\frac{S_{it} S_{Ai,t=0}}{S_{Ai,t} S_{it=0}} \right)^{\delta_i} \left(\frac{S_{i,t} NC_{i,t=0}}{S_{i,t=0} NC_{i,t}} \right)^{\lambda_i}$$

where

$W_{i,t}$ = density of activity i (jobs / cell) at time t
$J_{i,t=0}$ = initial sectoral employment
$NC_{i,t}$ = total cells occupied by activity i
$S_{i,t}$ = suitabilities for activity i summed over cells occupied by the activity
$S_{Ai,t}$ = suitabilities for i summed over all cells with a passive land use (i.e., available for i)
δ_i = sectoral sensitivity to land pressure
λ = sectoral sensitivity to land quality as measured by mean suitability.

And for brevity we let the subscript i index not only the economic (jobs) sectors, but also population; J then represents population as well as jobs.

We then use the densities to calculate the number of cells required for each activity:

$$NC_{i,t+1} = \frac{J_{i,t}}{W_{i,t}}$$

$$NC_{P,t+1} = \frac{X_{P,t}}{W_{P,t}}$$

The required cell numbers are passed to the CA-based model, which determines their actual locations and thus updates the land use map.

A complication in many applications is that there is not a one-to-one correspondence between activity sectors, whether economic or demographic, and land uses. Thus it is necessary to establish a correspondence by conflating or expanding categories. In the Saint Lucia application, there are five productive sectors, but only four economic land uses. The problem is solved by combining the *trade* and *services* sectors into a single *commerce* sector, which can then be mapped to the commercial land use. In other applications, like those to Dublin, there may be more than one residential land use class corresponding to the single activity category *population*, in which case it is necessary to introduce a submodel to split population into subgroups that correspond to the various residential classes.

productivity of land could be assumed constant for each land use class, then the conversion of sectoral outputs to demands for land use would be straightforward. As land becomes scarcer, however, densities rise. Also, densities tend to be higher on land that is better suited. Both of these effects are reflected in the conversion formula, which includes both an estimate of the number of cells potentially available for each activity and a measure of the suitability of the available cells relative to the suitability of cells originally occupied by the activity. Notice that both effects require, as input, data that come from the CA-based model. Thus, although the purpose of the land use demand module is to supply cell demands to the CA at each time step, to do so requires a link in the other direction. In other words, the macro-scale model and the CA-based land use model are linked reciprocally and dynamically.

Linking them requires that a correspondence be established between land uses, on the one hand, and both population and individual economic sectors, on the other. Although the simplest scheme establishes a one-to-one correspondence, in some applications, it is necessary to work with many-to-one or one-to-many relationships. For example, population may have to be translated into demand for several housing sectors defined on the basis of housing type or proportion of sealed surface. In this one-to-many situation, the most common problem is that the conversion may be unstable: small changes in class definitions or in certain parameters in the conversion algorithm may lead to large swings in the proportion of land use assigned to the different categories. In the case of a many-to-one correspondence, the problems are usually less serious; however, the calibration of the neighborhood functions of a land use, like commerce, which corresponds to a diverse group of activities characterized by very different behaviors, may be more difficult.

Output
Although the primary function of the macro-scale model is to provide the cell demands to the CA-based model, it also generates predictions of population, sectoral employment and output, domestic or household demand, per capita output, and birth, death, and net migration rates, and does so for each year of the simulation. These predictions can be displayed as tables or graphs.

Variations on the Macro-Scale Model
As described here, the macro-scale model has been linked to several versions of the CA-based model and used in a number of applications, especially in the context of the regionalized model discussed in chapter 7. But because each application must to some extent take into account particular constraints in terms of data availability, and because each has its own special requirements that follow from the goals of the modeling exercise, the macro model is frequently modified to suit the requirements of the particular application. Although the most common modification is to replace the natural systems module with a regional growth scenario, occasionally, more

substantial changes are made. For example, in an application to the southwestern region of the Indonesian island of Sulawesi, the purpose of the modeling exercise was to assess the performance of an impoundment reservoir as a means of reducing flooding in the city of Makassar (de Kok et al., 2001; Uljee, Engelen, and White, 1996). The watershed feeding the reservoir was subject to severe erosion, which had the potential to fill the reservoir with silt and thus severely reduce its storage capacity, and hence its ability to minimize flooding. In this application, the natural system module was replaced with a series of appropriate physical models—for example, a rainfall event simulator and a soil loss model using as inputs both slope and land use, as some land uses leave the soil much more exposed to erosion than others. In addition, the natural system model ran on a time step of one month to take into account the seasonality of precipitation and flooding, whereas the rest of the model ran on the usual yearly time step. Also, at the request of the users, the input-output model was replaced by another economic model. In other respects, the simulation model (in particular, the CA) was the same.

Conclusions

The CA-based land use model described in this chapter differs from other such models in three respects. First, it works with a relatively large cell neighborhood. Second, the neighborhood effect is modified both by the properties of the heterogeneous cell space, as represented in maps of suitability, accessibility, and zoning, and by a stochastic perturbation term representing heterogeneity among implicit agents. Third, it works with a relatively large number of urban land use classes, so that it is able to model the internal structure of the city. The MURBANDY applications among others demonstrate that it gives very good predictions of land use patterns.

Linking the CA-based model to a macro-scale model increases the range of phenomena that can be modeled, and thus the model's usefulness. The macro model may in some cases improve the quality of the land use predictions through the feedback effects that it mediates, although any such improvement is probably small. It is more likely that feedback effects from the CA significantly improve the predictions of the linked models, as when land use changes alter the rates of soil erosion, sedimentation, and flooding.

In one respect, it is surprising that the CA performs as well as it does. In reality, land use patterns reflect and are the result of spatial interactions occurring on all distance scales. But the CA only reflects very local interactions, those at the scale of the cell neighborhood. Even the accessibility factor is a local one because it represents interactions from a cell *to* the network, not interactions *through* the network. Long-distance interaction effects are not modeled explicitly, yet they must play an important role in shaping the spatial structure. In chapters 7 and 8, we look at models that include long-distance interactions explicitly.

7

The Bigger Picture: Integrated Multiscale Models

Cities and regions are organized by processes operating at all spatial scales. They are linked into a national and global system, and their success depends on their role, both synergetic and competitive, within that system. The region itself is integrated functionally by the complex but highly structured daily flow of people, goods, and information. Although the pattern of these movements reflects the land use pattern, over longer time periods, land use itself evolves in response to the flows and to the growth induced by being part of the national and global system. It seems obvious that a realistic model of land use should take into account these multiscale spatial interactions, yet the CA-based model ignores all but the most local of them, those occurring within the cell neighborhood. From this perspective, it is surprising that the CA approach performs as well as it does.

A macro-scale model like the one described in chapter 6 takes care of the relationship between the land use model and the wider system of which it is a part. In the application to Saint Lucia (White, Engelen, and Uljee, 2000), for example, scenarios involving climate change, exports, and trends in demographic parameters represent links with the wider world that affect the island; these scenarios provide input to the macro-scale model's dynamically linked natural, economic, and demographic submodels, which together predict the impact of the external events on the island as a whole. But, once the impacts are converted to land use demands, the CA-based model locates the required land use without reference to any spatial processes operating beyond the scale of the cell neighborhood. Thus, for example, competition for growth between the two major cities at opposite ends of the island is only implicit in the CA-based model since the model includes no interactions over distances long enough to encompass both of them. At this point, then, what we have is an integrated simulation model for cities or regions that covers the two extremes of scale in the modeled area. What we need, however, is a model that will fill the gap and handle spatial processes operating at intermediate scales. This chapter describes a regional-level model inserted between the global and local levels. Another approach, one without regions, in which the CA itself handles interactions at all distance scales, is described in chapter 8.

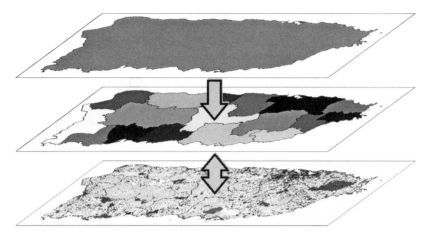

Figure 7.1
Three levels of the regionalized model: global (*top*), regional (*middle*), and local or cellular (*bottom*). Example is from the Puerto Rico application Xplorah. (Source: Maps produced by the Graduate School for Planning, University of Puerto Rico)

The simulation model incorporating long-distance spatial interaction operates at three levels, as shown in figure 7.1. The global level represents the dynamics of the modeled area as a whole; the regional level handles interactions among the regions; and the local level models the land use dynamics on the basis of the very short range spatial interactions captured in the neighborhood effect of the CA. The regional level, described in the next section, mediates between the global and local levels, so that estimates of various quantities such as total output by sector or total population are allocated and reallocated among regions on the basis of spatial interaction–based dynamics, and the regional totals are then passed down to the local-level CA-based model to be expressed as land use. The three levels are linked upwardly as well, with the cellular automaton passing information on land availability and other local characteristics to the regional model to be taken into account in the regional allocations; in some versions, the regional model in turn modifies certain parameters controlling the global-level dynamics. The regional model somewhat resembles a repurposed transportation model, one that deals with relocations of activity rather than traffic flows.

The Regional Model

Spatial interaction models of the sort mentioned in chapter 3 have been widely used for many years, mostly to model movements of people, especially frequent or repetitive movements like work or shopping trips, but only occasionally to model permanent relocations like migration. In our case, however, we are interested in permanent moves: land becomes residential when people move there to stay, not just to visit, and it becomes commercial when a shopping mall or big-box outlet is built: pop-up businesses do not affect the land use map. The dynamic central place model of chapter 4 represents an intermediate case, where a classical spatial interaction equation is used to model the flows of customers (or their money) to various competing commercial centers. But those flows, converted to estimates of profit, then become the basis for relocating commercial activity from one center to another, a permanent relocation. In fact, that dynamic model was incorporated in one version of the regionalized model discussed here to handle relocations of commercial activity; it was eventually removed, however, in order to avoid the complications of having two different submodels of activity migration in the same model.

Formally, the regional model works much like classical spatial interaction–based potential models, such as those introduced into theoretical geography by William Warntz (1965) or those discussed by Michael Batty (1976). Each region competes with all the others to attract population and economic activity; its success depends primarily on how attractive it is as measured by its current size in terms of population and economic activity and by its location with respect to the other regions. In this respect, the regional model is structurally very similar to most transportation models in use today. In addition, however, it measures a region's attractiveness in terms of the specific qualities of the land in the region as described at the cellular level by suitabilities, accessibilities, and the neighborhood effect. The regional model acquires summary measures of these land attributes from the CA-based model at each iteration. In return, it converts the updated regional values for population and economic activity into regional cell demands and provides these to the cellular automaton.

In this section, we describe the generic regional model (for a complete description, see Engelen et al., 2005). With particular applications, however, it is occasionally necessary to make minor modifications because of the nature of the available data or because the user desires a particular output.

The Regions
The regions may be either statistical divisions, such as census tracts, or administrative regions, such as municipalities or counties, which in any case almost always double as statistical units. When the regional model is being used not just to drive the CA-based land use model, but also to provide output at the regional level for the user, administrative regions are often the most appropriate from the user's point of view since such areas tend to be the ones that are relevant for planning and policy purposes. On the other hand, if the model is being used primarily to translate economic and demographic projections provided by the macro-scale model into regional

land use demands, then statistical divisions may be more appropriate. In either case, wherever possible, the regions should have some functional coherence in terms of the economic and demographic dynamics that will be modeled. For example, in a national application, a set of urban-centered regions, in which each region consists of a city together with its hinterland, would be very appropriate, whereas regions that were larger and thus typically contained more than one urban center would not. This is because the model will represent each region as being located at a single point. If the region is relatively homogeneous, then it can reasonably be represented by its centroid, or if it is urban centered, then the location of the city center is appropriate as the representative point. If, on the other hand, it is polycentric, then no point is sufficiently representative. We will see examples of both these situations in the applications described later in this chapter.

Interregional Distances
Because of the distance-decay effect, distance is one of the most important factors in the competition among regions to attract activity. As part of the initialization procedure, the model creates a matrix of interregional distances. Depending on the application and the data available, these may be either Euclidean or network distances, and network distances may be measured either as miles or kilometers or as travel times or costs. Some versions of the model, for example the one used in the Dutch application described below, are dynamically integrated with a four-stage transportation model. The Dutch application measures distances in terms of cost per kilometer, implicit travel time cost, and parking cost; the transportation model is solved at each iteration of the simulation to reflect changes in land use and the spatial distribution of economic activities and population. Although distances calculated by the transport model can be used for the interregional distances, that does not solve the problem of regions that are poorly defined or too large. This problem is negligible in the Dutch case (Engelen et al., 2005), but substantial in the Dublin application (Shahumyan et al., 2009, 2011). If the regions are not spatially coherent, that is, if they do not have a natural center, then no matter how sophisticated the representation of the transportation network, the calculated distances will be only rough approximations because the locations of the regions are poorly defined. This can be a major problem because calibration experiments show that the locations chosen to represent the regions are one of the most powerful determinants of the simulation results, especially when there are relatively few regions.

Another problem is the definition of the *self-distance*—the distance from a region to itself. The solution used in most applications is to calculate the self-distances as

$$d_{ii} = \sqrt{\frac{A_i}{k\pi}} \qquad (7.1)$$

where A_i is the area of the region in square miles or square kilometers and k is a calibrated parameter that accounts for the concentration of activity toward the center of the region. In applications where the regions have no single dominant concentration of activity, $k \approx 1$.

Finally, because transportation models generally work with zones that are much smaller and more numerous than the regions used in the simulation model, they can be used to improve the measure of accessibility in the CA-based model. For example, the Netherlands is divided into 345 zones for the national transportation model, but just forty urban-centered regions (COROPs) for modeling the spatial dynamics of population and economic activity. The accessibility measure as defined in chapter 6 represents only distance from a cell to the appropriate element of the infrastructure network. When a transport model has been integrated into the simulation program, however, the local accessibility measure can be integrated with a measure of global accessibility calculated for each of the transport regions.

Regional Attractivity

At each iteration, a certain number of people and a certain amount of economic activity move out of each region and into the other regions. The size of the flows going to each destination region depends on the relative attractivities of the regions with respect to one another. The absolute attractivity of a destination region is a function of its distance from the origin region, its size as measured by population and economic activity, and the quantity and quality of its land. (Because of the distance-decay effect, this is technically the *distance-discounted* absolute attractivity.) Note that only distances are derived within the regional model; information on size is ultimately derived from the global-level model or scenario, while the land characteristics are input from the CA-based land use model.

The regional model uses several measures of size because some activities may be attracted not only by population but also by the presence or absence of certain economic activities, as well as by other factors. For example, retail activity may be more attracted to a region with a larger population but a paucity of retail activity, whereas industrial activity may be attracted by both population (indicating the local availability of labor) and the presence of other industrial activity in the region (indicating availability of suppliers and customers, or just generally favorable conditions). Economic sectors may be measured in monetary terms or in terms of employment, depending on data availability.

Attractivity also depends on several aggregate cellular level measures of the quality and availability of land in the region—specifically, the density of the activity, the neighborhood effect, the suitability, and the accessibility. In each case, the measures are calculated as the mean value of the cells occupied by the activity. Zoning is also included, but is measured as the proportion of land zoned for the activity that is not yet occupied by it. The effect of density is inhibitory: the higher the density, the lower the attractivity. The effect of the other factors is generally positive.

The absolute attractivity of region I as seen from region j is calculated as

$$AT_{Ki} = (d_{ji})^{-nK} (X_{Pi,t-1})^{\beta_{1K}} (J_{i,t-1})^{\beta_{2K}} (X_{Ki,t-1})^{\beta_{3K}} (W_{Ki,t-1})^{\beta_{4K}} (\langle N_{Ki,t-1} \rangle)^{\beta_{5K}} (\langle S_{Ki,t-1} \rangle)^{\beta_{6K}}$$
$$(\langle A_{Ki,t-1} \rangle)^{\beta_{7K}} (Zr_{Ki,t-1} + 1)^{\beta_{8K}}$$

(7.2)

where

AT_{Ki} = absolute distance-discounted attractivity of region j
d_{ji} = distance from region j to region i
$X_{Pi,t-1}$ = population of region i
$J_{i,t-1}$ = total jobs (all sectors) in region i
$X_{Ki,t-1}$ = activity in sector K in region i
$W_{Ki,t-1}$ = density per cell of activity K in region i
$\langle N_{Ki,t-1} \rangle$ = mean neighborhood effect of cells occupied by activity K in region i
$\langle S_{Ki,t-1} \rangle$ = mean suitability of cells occupied by activity K in region i
$\langle A_{Ki,t-1} \rangle$ = mean accessibility of cells occupied by activity K in region i
$Zr_{Ki,t-1}$ = cells in region i occupied by passive land uses, zoned for activity K but not occupied by it
$\beta_1 \ldots \beta_8$ = influence parameters.

Note that population is treated as one of the activities K. Therefore, when $K = P$, either β_1 or β_3 must be set to zero in order to avoid including population twice in the equation. Some variables are subscripted $t - 1$ because the values are calculated in the previous iteration.

The logic of attractivity is that the factors included in equation 7.2 determine the *absolute* attractivity of a destination region i as seen from an origin region j, although the *relative* attractivity of the destination region depends on the alternatives available to the origin region. If the origin has a number of other attractive regions close by, the relative attractivity of the destination region will be less than if there are few other attractive destinations nearby; in other words, region i is competing with all the other regions to attract activity from region j. The collective attractivity for activity K of all regions as seen from origin region j is the potential, V_{Kj}, at j:

$$V_{Kj} = \sum_i AT_{Ki}$$

(7.3)

and the relative attractivity of destination region i is then given by $\dfrac{AT_{Ki}}{V_{Kj}}$.

Note that because the origin region is included among the destination regions, some of the activity relocated by equation 7.4 moves to the region it is coming from—that is, it does not move at all, or it may be moving internally.

Activity Migration

The amount of activity migrating to region i depends both on its relative attractivity and on the amount of activity present in the origin region j and thus potentially available to move. But, owing to an inertia effect, not all activity is available to move: in any given year, most business and institutional establishments, and most people, will not move at all (the actual proportions are often available in national statistics). Therefore, to calculate the migration of activity, whether of population or economic activities, only the proportion that will move has to be considered. That quantity is then allocated among the various destination regions according to the relative attractivities:

$$X_{OKji} = (1 - \varphi_K) X_{Kj,t-1} \left(\frac{AT_{Ki}}{V_{Kj}} \right) \quad (7.4)$$

where

X_{OKji} = the outflow of activity K from region j to region i
φ_K = the inertia factor (the proportion that will not move in any one year) for activity K
$X_{Kj,t-1}$ = amount of activity K in region j.

The total amount of activity K migrating into region i, X_{IKi}, is then

$$X_{IKi} = \sum_{j \neq i} X_{OKji} \quad (7.5)$$

where

X_{Iki} = the total inflow of activity K to region i.

Because inflows to one region represent outflows from another, the total outflow of K from region i, X_{OKi}, is given by

$$X_{OKi} = \sum_{j \neq i} X_{OKij} \quad (7.6)$$

Equations 7.5 and 7.6 together represent the competitive reallocation of activity among the regions. But regional activity levels are also affected by the acquisition of activity new to the system.

Allocation of New Activity

In most applications, the modeled area is growing, and the actual amount of growth of each activity, including population, is determined in the macro-scale model. At each iteration, these amounts are sent to the regional model to be allocated among the regions. The basis for the allocation is both the relative size of the region and its relative competitiveness. Size is measured as the amount of the activity in question, with the amount of new activity allocated to the region dependent on the amount of the activity already there: regions with a large amount of an activity get a larger share of new activity. Competitiveness is measured as the ratio of inflows to outflows of migrating activity, and the higher this ratio, the more competitive the region is assumed to be. The ratios are adjusted according to the relevance of competitiveness to the location of new activity; they are then rescaled so that, over all regions, they sum to one. Specifically, the allocation of new activity to a region is given by

$$X_{EKi} = E_K \left\{ \frac{\left[(X_{Ki,t-1})^{\beta_{9K}} \left(\frac{X_{IKi}}{X_{OKi}} \right)^{\beta_{10K}} \right]}{\sum_j (X_{Kj,t-1})^{\beta_{9K}} \left(\frac{X_{IKj}}{X_{OKj}} \right)^{\beta_{10K}}} \right\} \quad (7.7)$$

where

X_{EKi} = amount of new (exogenous) activity K allocated to region i
E_K = total amount of additional activity K
β_{9K} and β_{10K} = influence parameters
and in Σ_i, j includes i.

Finally, the regional activity levels for the current year t, X_{Ki}, are calculated:

$$X_{Ki,t} = X_{Ki,t-1} + X_{IKi} - X_{OKi} + X_{EKi} \quad (7.8)$$

Generating Regional Cell Demands from New Activity Levels
Because the new regional activity levels will require additional land, new regional cell requirements for the various activities must be calculated and passed to the CA-based land use model, where they will force changes in the land use map. The procedure is apparently simple:

$$NC_{Ki,t} = \frac{X_{Ki,t}}{W_{Ki,t}} \quad (7.9)$$

where

NC_{Ki} = the number of cells required for activity K in region i
$X_{Ki,t}$ = the new activity level of sector K in region i
$W_{Ki,t}$ = the new cell density of sector K in region i.

The devil is in the denominator, however. As population and economic activity grow, they require more land. But as they occupy more land, less is available; some regions may even run out of sufficient land for the various activities. Consequently, it is necessary to increase densities for each activity on the basis of the relative amount of land still available, the growth rate of the activity, and the changes in mean values of the neighborhood effect, suitability, and accessibility. But the procedure must also take into account the total amount of land being claimed by all activities. The details are given in box 7.1.

Box 7.1
Calculating Cell Densities

During initialization, we calculate densities as

$$W_{Ki,t=0} = \frac{X_{Ki,t=0}}{NC_{Ki,t=0}}$$

where

$W_{Ki,t=0}$ = initial density of activity K in region i
$X_{Ki,t=0}$ = initial amount of activity in region i
$NC_{Ki,t=0}$ = initial number of cells of land use K corresponding to activity K in region i.

For all iterations after initialization, however, we must recalculate densities to reflect the increased number of cells required as the modeled system grows, and we must also increase densities to reflect the decreasing amounts of land unused by, but available for, the activities and to ensure that sufficient cells are available for all active land uses. First, we calculate cell requirements using the currently available densities, that is, those available from the previous iteration. Then we find the total number of cells, $NC_{i,t}$, required for all activities at these density levels:

$$NC_{i,t} = \sum_K \left(\frac{X_{Ki,t}}{W_{Ki,t-1}} \right)$$

Next, we compare the required number of cells with the total number of cells potentially available for all activities, including cells already occupied:

$$L_{i,t} = \frac{NC_{i,t}}{\left[\sum_K NC_{Ki,t-1} + \sum_R NC_{Ri,t-1} \right]}$$

where

$L_{i,t}$ = the ratio of cells required for all activities in region i relative to the number available, based on current density levels
$NC_{Ri,t}$ = the number of cells currently occupied by passive (mostly rural) land uses.

If $L_{i,t} > 1$, then there are not enough cells available at the current density to meet the cell demand as currently estimated.

Now we calculate the new densities for each activity:

$$W_{Ki,t} = \delta(t)_{1K} W_{Ki,t-1} \text{Wcor}_{Ki,t} \text{Wcel}_{Ki,t}$$

where δ_{1K} = a trend parameter to adjust the effect of the increasing activity level on changes in density. Values of Wcor and Wcel are determined as follows.

$$\text{Wcor}_{Ki,t} = \left(\frac{X_{Ki,t}}{X_{Ki,t-1}} \right)^{\delta_{2K}} [\max(1, L_{i,t})]^{\delta_{3K}}$$

Box 7.1 (continued)

Wcor thus adjusts the density on the basis of the rate of increase of the activity, and, if there are not enough cells available in the region ($L_{i,t} > 1$), also on the basis of the cell deficit. Note that $L_{i,t}$ can only have the effect of increasing the densities.

$$\text{Wcel}_{Ki,t} = \left[\frac{\langle N_{Ki,t}\rangle}{\langle N_{Ki,t-1}\rangle}\right]^{\delta_4} \left[\frac{\langle S_{Ki,t}\rangle}{\langle S_{Ki,t-1}\rangle}\right]^{\delta_5} \left[\frac{\langle A_{Ki,t}\rangle}{\langle A_{Ki,t-1}\rangle}\right]^{\delta_6} [Zr_K]^{\delta_7}$$

where

$\langle N_{Ki,t-1}\rangle$ = mean neighborhood effect of cells occupied by activity K in region i,
$\langle S_{Ki,t-1}\rangle$ = mean suitability of cells occupied by activity K in region i,
$\langle A_{Ki,t-1}\rangle$ = mean accessibility of cells occupied by activity K in region i,

and

$$Zr_K = \frac{\left[\left(\frac{Z_{RKi,t-1}}{Z_{Ki,t-1}}\right)+1\right]}{\left[\left(\frac{Z_{RKi,t}}{Z_{Ki,t}}\right)+1\right]}$$

where

Z_{RKi} = number of cells in region i occupied by passive land uses, zoned for activity K but not occupied by it
Z_{Ki} = total number of cells in region i zoned for activity K.

The effect of Wcel is to adjust densities on the basis of the change in the average quality of the land occupied by the activity in the region: decreasing quality has the effect of lowering densities, all other factors being the same.

Finally, we use the new densities to calculate the numbers of cells required for each activity in each region:

$$NC_{Ki,t} = \frac{X_{Ki,t}}{W_{Ki,t}}$$

Introducing an Activity to a Region That Has None

If, for some reason, a region lacks a particular activity, then equations 7.2–7.8 will ensure that it never gets any. Since this is not realistic, a stochastic procedure is included in the model to occasionally assign activity to regions that lack it. The ratio of regional potential for the activity to the mean potential for all regions is calculated and then compared to a number drawn from a suitably scaled random distribution. If it is larger than the random number, then an amount of activity proportional to the ratio of potentials is assigned to the region. Because this activity comes out of the current year's growth, it must be subtracted from E_K before equation 7.7 is evaluated. Cell numbers are calculated on the basis of a parameter representing the minimum allowed density.

Modifications to the CA-Based Model

When the simulation framework was augmented by including a regional-level model, improvements were made as well to the CA-based model—specifically, to the calculation of the accessibility factor. As described in chapter 6, accessibility was calculated simply as the shortest distance to the transportation network. But because some links or nodes are relatively more important than others, all levels of links and types of nodes of all transport networks are now included in the calculation of the accessibility measure. For example, the Dublin application includes one type of node and five levels for the road network: motorway (superhighway) junctions (node), and motorways, dual carriageways (divided highways), national routes, regional routes, and local roads (levels). Both superhighway junctions and superhighways are included because the presence of a superhighway is irrelevant for accessibility if it cannot be accessed, and access is only by means of the junction. On the other hand, a nearby superhighway can be a disamenity because of noise and fumes. Thus, for a land use such as discontinuous sparse residential, distance to the superhighway junction would be highly weighted, whereas distance to the superhighway itself would receive a zero or even a negative weighting. Now that there are several networks (road, rail, light rail, etc.), each with several nodes and levels, the original distance-decay parameters a_K, one for each land use K (described in chapter 6), must be redefined as a_{Kj}, so that, for each land use K, there is now a set of parameters containing a parameter for each level or node j of each network. Furthermore, since some elements of the networks are more important than others for particular land uses, we must introduce a second set of accessibility parameters, b_{Kj}, to represent the relative importance of the various elements of the several networks (see table 7.1 for an example). To calculate the overall accessibility to the network, the accessibilities to the individual elements and levels must be weighted by the parameters representing relative importance and then combined:

$$A_{NiK} = \frac{[1 - \Pi(1 - b_{Kj} A_{iKj})]}{[1 - \Pi(1 - b_{Kj})]} \tag{7.10}$$

where

A_{NiK} = overall accessibility to the network
b_{Kj} = relative importance of accessibility to element or level j of the network
A_{iKj} = accessibility to element or level j as calculated by equation 6.1.

The value of A_{NiK} increases as the number of network elements and levels increases, but the contribution of any single element or level decreases.

Finally, the road network used in applications typically does not include the lowest level of the network, the most local streets and roads. Yet this level is significant in that it ensures access to the rest of the network. But, even if it is included, as the model runs and land is converted to urban uses, the network will not be automatically extended by the model into those areas, and thus their accessibility will be underestimated. To handle this problem, an *implicit accessibility*, U_{KL}, is introduced, with two values, one for urban and the other for rural land uses: $U_{KL} = (U_{K-\text{urban}}, U_{K-\text{rural}})$. The user of the model specifies the land uses included in each category. In one recent version of the model a value of U_{KL} may be specified for each land use. Unlike the other components of accessibility, U_{KL} does not depend on location, only on land use. Generally, the value for urban land uses is higher than that for rural uses, but, in any case, $0 \leq U_K \leq 1$.

Including a transportation model in the integrated model makes it possible to define a measure of accessibility *through* the network to the rest of the urban or regional system. Since a transportation model works with traffic zones, accessibility to the system will be defined not for cells, but for zones—that is, *zonal accessibility*. The general equations to calculate movements over the network from origin to destination zones typically are distance-decay functions similar to equations 4.4 and 4.5, but more elaborate. In the Dutch application, for example, distance is measured as a generalized cost based on cost per kilometer, travel time, and parking costs, over three networks: road, rail, and waterways (de Nijs, 2009). Because both numbers of trips and modal split among the networks are determined by purpose of travel or type of trip—for example, recreation, shopping, journey to work, and so on (as well as by other factors), accessibility will vary according to the purpose of travel. A composite flow corresponding to zone i is given by the weighted sum of flows calculated for the individual trip types:

$$F_{zKi} = \sum_p (w_{pK} F_{zip}) \tag{7.11}$$

where

F_{zKi} = total weighted flows associated with zone i
F_{zip} = flows for trip purpose p associated with zone i
w_{pK} = weight specific to land use K applied to flows for purpose p.

Note that the weights are specific to land uses because the composite flows will be used to establish a zonal accessibility factor for each possible land use; the transportation model, as such, does not use land uses. To convert the weighted zonal flows to zonal accessibility factors, A_{zKi}, they must be rescaled so that $0 \leq A_{zKi} \leq 1$:

$$A_{zKi} = v + (1-v) \frac{[F_{zKi} - \min(F_{zK})]}{[\max(F_{zk}) - \min(F_{zK})]} \tag{7.12}$$

where

υ = a parameter to be calibrated that sets a minimum value for A_{zKi}
$\min(F_{zK})$ = the lowest value of F_{zK} among all zones
$\max(F_{zK})$ = the highest value of F_{zK} among all zones

Finally, the composite accessibility factor for land use K on cell i is calculated as the product:

$$A_{Ki} = A_{NiK} U_K A_{zKi} \qquad (7.13)$$

where the value of A_{zKi}, that is, the value for cell i, is taken from the value of the zone in which it is located. Of course, if the integrated model does not include a transportation component capable of generating interzonal flows, the zonal accessibility term, A_{zKi}, is dropped from the equation.

Note that, because of the A_{zKi} term in equation 7.13, long-distance effects of the sort treated in the regional model are now included in the CA-level accessibility factors. Since they come from the transportation model, these long-distance effects do not mitigate any problems in the regional model caused by regions that are too large or poorly defined, but they may have a small effect on the regional-level dynamics through their contribution to regional attractivity as calculated in equation 7.2, which includes A_{Ki} as a factor.

Applications

Although the regional model just described could be used on a stand-alone basis by removing the links with the cellular automaton, it was developed to augment the CA-based land use model by introducing an explicitly spatial representation of the dynamics of the activities that find expression as land uses. To that end, it is always embedded in an integrated model, where it serves to link the top-level scenario or model to the CA-based land use model. Consequently, applications always make use of the complete integrated three-level model (Engelen et al., 2007). The model has seen a number of applications—to the Netherlands, Belgium, Flanders, Dublin, the Belfast–Newry corridor, the Côte d'Azur, Puerto Rico, and several areas in New Zealand, among others. Although these applications were carried out by various groups, each with its own institutional context, interests, and goals, all were nevertheless able to use essentially the same model, with only minor customization to accommodate particular project requirements. The most important differences occur only at the top level, which drives the regional and CA levels: some applications simply use a growth scenario, while others use various integrated models of the natural, economic, and demographic systems. In the following sections, we will examine some of the applications of this model, known variously as "MOLAND"

(JRC applications), "LOV" (LeefOmgevingsVerkenner) or "Environment Explorer" (Netherlands), "RuimteModel" (Flanders), "Xplorah" (Puerto Rico), and "WISE" for Waikato Integrated Scenario Explorer (New Zealand); we will use *MOLAND* to refer generically to all these versions. The application to Flanders will be described in chapter 11, where it will receive a more thorough treatment.

Applications: Dublin

The successor to the MURBANDY Project at the Joint Research Centre was the MOLAND Project, which replaced the model discussed in chapter 6 with the integrated regional CA-based model just described. The MOLAND model remains scenario driven, and its CA-based land use component is essentially the same, except for a more comprehensive treatment of accessibilities as described above. The major difference is that it includes a regional model. By agreement with the Joint Research Centre, the MOLAND model was adopted as the core of the Urban Environment Project (UEP), a joint project between the Urban Institute Ireland and the Irish Environmental Protection Agency whose twin goals were to acquire a greater understanding of sustainability issues in the urban context and to provide support for policy development and implementation. The model was the basis for a number of specific projects concerning urban sprawl, urban wildlife, traffic and emissions, transit use, wastewater treatment, and climate change impacts on the region.

As part of the Urban Environment Project, new land use maps were derived, and these meant that the simulation period could be extended to more recent years. Specifically, land use data were now available for 1990, 2000, and 2006, at a resolution of 200 meters. With data for three dates, it is possible to calibrate over the first period and validate the calibration over the second period, a procedure that was not possible in the earlier applications. The UEP also defined a much larger application area than had been used in the MURBANDY simulations. This Greater Dublin Region (GDR) consists of the former County Dublin (since divided into four smaller counties) and four surrounding counties. It is a large area, one that extends well beyond the urban fringe and satellite towns, and as far as the border with Northern Ireland (figure 7.2). Counties were chosen as the regional units because most of the data necessary to drive the regional model are available for them but not for smaller spatial subdivisions. Unfortunately, except for County Dublin itself, the units are not urban centered; some are largely rural, but contain several widely separated towns. Thus, except for County Dublin, it was difficult to choose an appropriate point as the representative center; consequently, the point chosen was inevitably somewhat arbitrary.

In applications involving the regional model, data is often a major problem, and Dublin was no exception. The regional model is driven by the global scenario for the five-county region, which supplies inputs to the regional model for each year of the

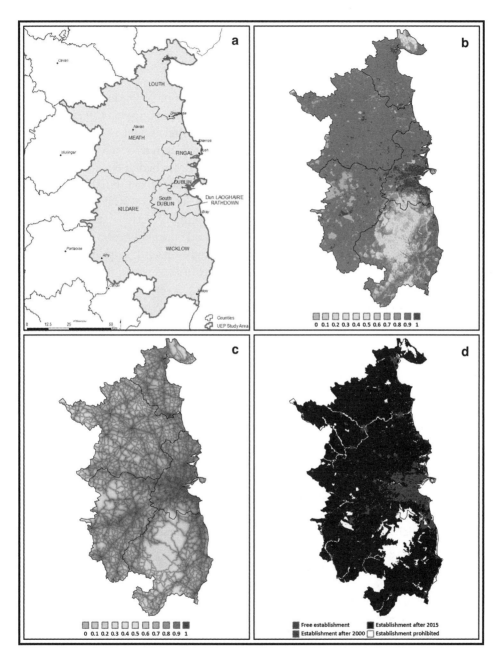

Figure 7.2
Greater Dublin Region (GDR): (a) UEP study area; (b) suitability; (c) accessibility; (d) zoning. (Source: Maps available from the Urban Environment Project)

simulation. For past years, the inputs are either actual data or interpolations between the years for which the data are available. For future years, they are either projections of past trends or more elaborate forecasts. In the Dublin application, for the years spanned by actual data, the global total is simply the sum of the data for the five counties or interpolations for years between data points; but, for future years, it is estimated from the output of national economic and demographic forecast models by downscaling to the five-county region. The regional model is initialized with county data, but, for all subsequent years, the county activity levels are calculated from the global totals received from the scenario, as described in equations 7.2–7.8. Even though the regional model uses only county data for the initial year, county data for as long a period as possible beyond that year are essential for calibration and validation. The model produces estimates of county activity data, and these must be compared with the actual figures both to guide the calibration and then validate the calibrated model. The procedure is straightforward in principle, but, in practice, difficulties abound because, for the procedure to work, the data must be comparable over the entire period, and that is almost never the case.

For population data, on the other hand, the problems are usually minor. In the case of Dublin, the fact that most of the census dates (1991, 1996, 2002, 2006) do not coincide with dates of the land use maps (1990, 2000, 2006) is only a minor annoyance since interpolations of activities to the years with land use maps introduce only very small errors. A more significant issue arises in converting the yearly population estimates to requirements for residential land use since the UEP MOLAND application uses four residential classes, as was the case in the MURBANDY application. The population must therefore be divided into four groups, with each group generating a corresponding land use demand. This was done by estimating the population density of each residential land use class using small area (electoral district) population data, and then multiplying by the number of cells of each class to get the corresponding population, with adjustments to keep the sum equal to the actual population. The procedure was carried out for each of the three years for which a land use map was available; that made it possible to estimate trends to be used in the simulation. For future years, the trends were continued as estimated or replaced by scenarios expressing other trends.

For the economic activities, however, the situation was much more difficult. Most of the necessary data are available from the Irish Central Statistical Office (CSO), and they are arranged in hierarchical classifications according to an industrial classification system broken down into highly specific industries. The initial difficulty is that the four active economic land use classes used in the simulation—industrial, commercial, public and private services, and ports—do not correspond to any of the major economic activity classes used by the CSO. Therefore it is necessary to go to highly disaggregated levels of the data to find very specific industry classes that clearly belong to one or the other of the land use classes, and then to aggregate these to build up a new set of four industry classes that correspond to the land use classes. The problem becomes much worse not only because it is necessary to do this for each of the years covering the simulation period, but also because the industry classification system is changed occasionally, with classes being split or combined, or simply redefined. If two industrial classes that are combined in a later year both previously corresponded to the same land use class, then there is no problem. But if they corresponded to different classes, then the new combined class must either be arbitrarily assigned to one or the other of the land uses or be subdivided on the basis of data for the two original classes. Many of these problems are due to the change, beginning with the 2002 census, from the Irish CSO classification system to the standardized NACE (Statistical Classification of Economic Activities in the European Community) system mandated by the EU.

Another problem is that census data on employment by industry are by place of residence, whereas the model should be using place of work data since the data are being used to drive the corresponding classes in the land use model. For some recent years, survey data of employment by place of work are available, and these were used to get some idea of the magnitude of the discrepancy between data by place of work and by place of residence. Of course, as long as place of residence and place of work are both in the same county, then there is no discrepancy. In the end, the only option was to use employment by place of residence and to assume that, because of the size of the counties, commuting between counties was not common enough to cause major discrepancies.

Data for the networks used to calculate accessibilities for the CA were much easier to come by. Two networks were used: road and rail, with rail including the metro system. The road network includes five levels, from superhighways to local roads, as well as superhighway junctions. The rail network has only one level, but includes stations. The network maps were prepared for the years 1990 and 2006, as well as several years beyond 2006, depending on the scenario. These are introduced automatically at the appropriate iterations as the simulation runs. With each new network, the accessibilities are recalculated immediately in order to reflect the new infrastructure. For future years, additional networks are supplied showing planned additions and modifications. In some applications, the point is to investigate the likely effect of alternate transport policies; in these cases, the alternative networks are tested against one another in "what if" simulations.

Suitabilities largely reflect the topography, with some contribution from a wetlands map. Zoning, which has been largely ineffective in the Dublin area, is essentially a map showing various protected areas, from city parks to natural areas and archaeological sites, where development is forbidden. This treatment also reflects the need for a business-as-usual baseline scenario simulation—one with no constraints

Table 7.1
Example of accessibility parameter values

Implicit accessibility		
Built-up area	1.0	
Non-built-up area	0.8	

	Accessibility	
Links and nodes	Relative importance	Distance decay
Superhighways	0.3	10
Superhighway junctions	0.3	10
Divided highways	0.3	10
National and primary roads	0.3	7
Regional roads	0.2	3
Local roads	0.1	1
Railroads	0.2	5
Railroad stations	0.0	0
Light rail	0.0	0

on urban development—for use in various UEP studies investigating the effect of various planning and policy initiatives. Accessibility, suitability, and zoning maps for discontinuous sparse residential land use are shown in figure 7.2; parameter values for calculating accessibility are listed in table 7.1.

For the Urban Environment Project, the regional model was calibrated separately over the periods 1990–2000, 1990–2006, and 2000–2006; all three calibrations were validated on the 2006 data as shown in table 7.2, although only the results for the 1990–2000 calibration period are, strictly speaking, a validation. As can be seen, the simulation results for the three economic sectors are very poor, except for the calibration over the 1990–2000 period. The large errors are due in part to the likelihood that the sectoral economic activity data are not entirely comparable for the three dates, especially since the switch to the NACE classification occurred in 2002. A more significant likely source of error is the use of place of residence rather than place of work data. Although the working assumption that this was not a serious problem may have been true in 1990, the rapid growth of the entire region, and especially of the counties surrounding County Dublin (see table 7.3), undoubtedly increased the amount of commuting between counties. The result would be a greater discrepancy between place of work and place of residence data, and thus greater apparent errors (figure 7.3). The results for the 1990–2006 calibration look much better than those for either of the two sub-periods. This counterintuitive situation is due to the reversal of the direction of the errors for most counties and industries between the earlier and later periods (table 7.2).

Table 7.2
Errors in simulated activity values for the Greater Dublin Region for three calibration periods

	Population			Industry			Commerce			Services		
Base year	1990	1990	2000	1990	1990	2000	1990	1990	2000	1990	1990	2000
End year	2000	2006	2006	2000	2006	2006	2000	2006	2006	2000	2006	2006
Louth	2.4%	2.4%	0.7%	20.1%	7.2%	-9.1%	16.4%	-0.8%	-9.8%	0.6%	-6.9%	-6.6%
Meath	8.2%	2.3%	-3.2%	24.9%	-4.8%	-18.0%	61.9%	-6.0%	-25.6%	57.0%	0.1%	-20.4%
Dublin	-0.6%	0.0%	0.2%	-7.2%	0.1%	7.4%	-8.6%	-0.2%	6.0%	-9.1%	-0.6%	6.1%
Kildare	-7.5%	-8.9%	-2.3%	3.4%	-10.0%	-13.4%	57.6%	6.1%	-12.2%	50.7%	6.8%	-11.1%
Wicklow	5.0%	7.7%	4.7%	26.3%	17.3%	0.4%	39.5%	1.5%	-15.3%	37.4%	1.1%	-14.9%
RMSE*	2.5%	2.5%	1.2%	13.0%	4.4%	11.9%	18.5%	1.6%	11.2%	19.1%	2.1%	10.7%

*Root mean square error

Table 7.3
Annual growth rates of counties in the Greater Dublin Region for two periods

	Growth: Annual Rates	
Base year:	1991	2002
End year:	2002	2006
Louth	1.05%	2.16%
Meath	2.21%	4.96%
Dublin	0.83%	1.38%
Kildare	2.67%	3.22%
Wicklow	1.51%	2.45%

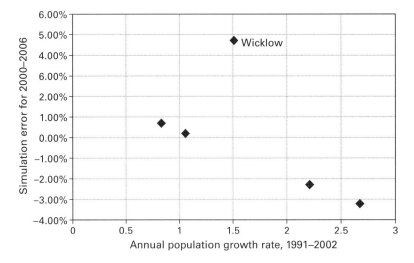

Figure 7.3
Error of simulated county populations in GDR, 2000–2006, as a function of annual growth rates, 1991–2002.

The calibration results for population are generally much better, although errors for Counties Meath, Kildare, and Wicklow are mostly high. The case of County Wicklow, located just to the south of Dublin, is particularly interesting: in all three calibrations, the regional model predicted it to grow much more than it actually does. This overprediction can be traced to the model's use of counties as the regions. All of the counties of the GDR are large, and mostly undeveloped; even County Dublin, which contains most of the population of the area being modeled, remains more than 50% rural. Because County Wicklow is essentially as close to Dublin as County Kildare or Meath, it should perform like those counties in the competition for population. In reality, however, County Wicklow is not able to receive as much of the urbanization radiating from Dublin as the other two counties because its northern part, the area immediately adjacent to the city of Dublin, is occupied by the Wicklow Mountains, a protected natural area not open to development; Dublin overspill development in the county is essentially limited to a narrow coastal strip. Because the regional model allocates to County Wicklow urban development comparable to what it gives Counties Kildare and Meath, it seriously overestimates development in that county in all three calibrations.

The dynamic feedback between the regional and CA-based models captured in equations 7.2 and 7.7 should, in principle, correct this problem. Although the data on accessibility, suitability, and availability of land that are passed from the CA to the regional level are designed to inform the regional model of the local limitations within the county that affect its attractivity, in this case, the signal is too weak to have a noticeable effect. That is partly due to the size of County Wicklow, much of which is not mountainous and not prohibited to development, with much land available relative to what has already been developed. Thus the indices of suitability and developable land have favorable values, values similar to those of the other two counties. Consequently, in the calibration of the regional model, most of the parameters scaling the feedback effects from the cellular automaton either disappear from the model ($\beta = 0$) or receive very low values, and the corresponding CA-level phenomena have very little effect on the regional dynamics. In sum, all three counties have very similar underlying conditions in terms of the CA-level measures. But most actual growth would come in the form of development adjacent to the urbanized area of Dublin, and this is precisely where it cannot occur in County Wicklow because of the Wicklow Mountains. The model discussed in the next chapter is designed in part to avoid this kind of problem.

Although our focus has been on the regional model, it is, after all, just one component of the larger integrated model. The output of the larger model includes not only predictions of regional activity levels but also a high-resolution land use map for each year of the simulation. One such land use map is shown in figure 7.4 (plate 3).

The MOLAND model was eventually integrated with a classical four-stage transportation model in order to examine in much greater detail the relationship between land use, traffic congestion, and public transport use under various growth and planning scenarios. The transport model uses land use data from the cellular automaton together with activity data from the regional model as input to the trip demand module, returning traffic volumes on individual links and nodes of the network to the CA to augment the calculation of local accessibilities. The model uses forty-four zones. It calculates trip production and attraction on the basis of population, jobs, and other factors such as recreational land use (which acts as a trip generator) for

162 Chapter 7

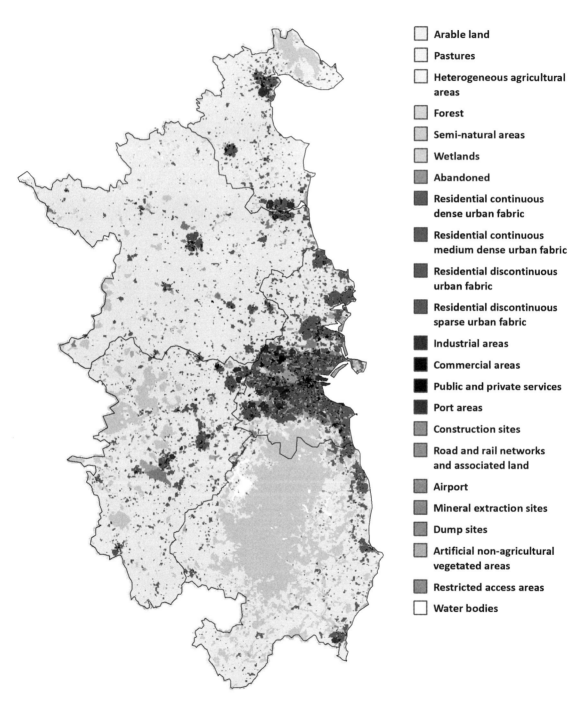

Figure 7.4 (plate 3)
Simulated land uses in GDR, 2026.

each zone. It then assigns trips to the transport network on the basis of travel demands and interzonal distances, with distances measured as a composite of physical distance, travel time, and costs. Capacities on network links permit congestion levels to be modeled as well (Shahumyan, Convery, and Casey, 2010; RIKS, 2007).

The integrated model was used to assess the impacts of a proposed rapid transit line, Metro North, running from the city center via Dublin Airport to Belinstown, on the northern fringe of the urbanized area. The model was run for the period 2006–2026 both with and without the new line. Although introduction of the Metro North line did not significantly affect land use patterns, it did have a major impact on the use of public transport in the six transport zones it traversed (figure 7.5), with the number of public transport trips being 20% greater in the Metro North than in the business-as-usual scenario (Shahumyan, Convery, and Casey, 2010).

Dublin: An Assessment of Wastewater Infrastructure
When the old County Dublin was dissolved and replaced by four counties covering the same area, the Dublin Regional Authority (DRA) was established to carry out a coordinating and planning role for the new counties. One of its responsibilities is the wastewater collection and treatment infrastructure, with a planning horizon of 2020 at the time of the Urban Environment Project. Past experience had shown that planning controls in the area were largely ineffective in guiding growth: residential development, in particular, frequently occurred in areas outside those zoned for it. Since current wastewater facilities had been planned and built on the assumption that development would largely take place in the areas zoned for it, the result was catchment areas that remained more rural than had been expected, so that treatment facilities operated well below capacity. At the same time, many newly developed areas were outside the catchment areas and therefore not serviced by the wastewater infrastructure.

The Dublin Regional Authority and the Urban Environment Project decided jointly to use the MOLAND modeling framework to evaluate planned extensions to the infrastructure (for a fuller treatment of this study, see Williams et al., 2012). Two key questions were to be examined: (1) whether the land most likely to be urbanized in the coming years was covered by the planned catchment areas; and (2) whether the planned treatment capacities were adequate for the expected volumes of wastewater. To answer these questions, the calibrated model of the Greater Dublin Region was run under three growth scenarios for the period 2006–2026. The Central Statistical Office's regional population projections for the period were used as the medium-growth scenario. The high-growth and low-growth scenarios were defined as the medium-growth projection plus 15% and minus 15%, respectively. The planned catchment areas (figure 7.6) were then overlaid on the 2026 land use maps generated by the model to determine (1) how well the catchment areas covered the developed

164   Chapter 7

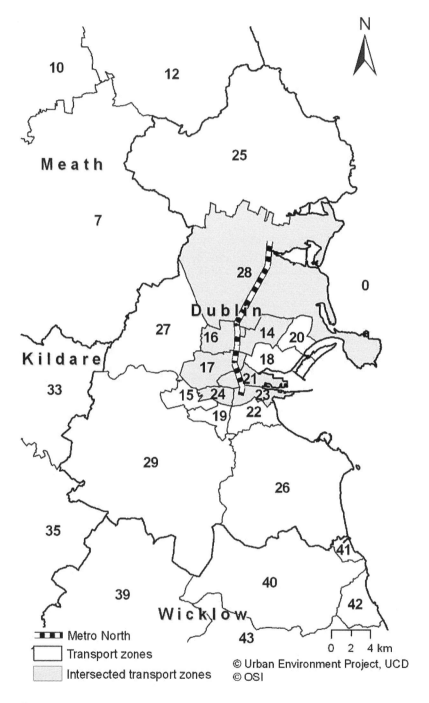

Figure 7.5
Planned route of Metro North and transport zones in GDR. (Source: Shahumyan, Convery, and Casey, 2010)

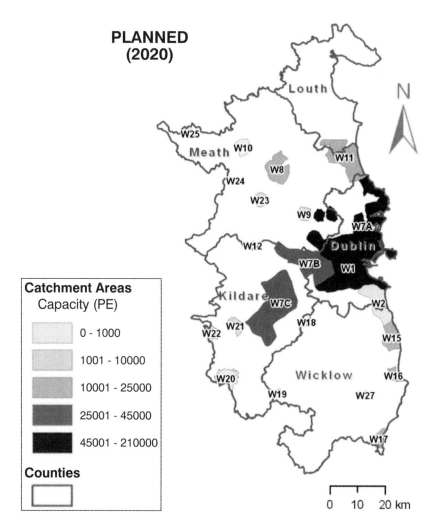

Figure 7.6
Planned wastewater catchment areas and treatment capacities, 2020, in the Dublin area. PE, population equivalents. (Source: Williams et al., 2012, fig. 9)

areas and (2) to what degree the planned treatment capacity for each catchment area matched the expected volumes of wastewater. The first question was answered immediately by the overlay. The second, however, required an estimate of wastewater volumes to be generated in each catchment area in 2026. This was made by using mean population densities per cell for the several residential land use classes to estimate the total 2026 population in each catchment area and then multiplying the estimated population by the expected 2026 per capita wastewater production. Notice that this application as described assumes that the presence of wastewater infrastructure does not influence the location of urban development. In the GDR, that is apparently more or less the case. But it is easy to include an influence if it is suspected that developers will prefer serviced areas. This can be done by including the catchment areas, suitably weighted to represent the degree of importance they are thought to have, in the calculation of suitabilities.

An example of the overlay is shown in figure 7.7. Under all three scenarios, a large amount of residential development occurs outside and to the north of the catchment area. The extent of such development depends on the growth scenario: the higher the regional growth rate, the greater the amount of development that occurs outside the catchment area in this small corner of the region, as we would expect. But, contrary to expectations, there is more residential development inside the catchment area under the medium-growth than under the high-growth scenario. The immediate reason provided by Brendan Williams and colleagues (2012) is that, under the high-growth scenario, a more than proportional amount of development occurs outside the catchment area, primarily because of a positive feedback effect due to the attraction of residential land use to existing residential land use as represented in the influence function. And that leaves the catchment area with fewer residential cells under the high-growth than under the medium-growth scenario. This sort of effect is common in complex self-organizing systems, and it represents a local spatial bifurcation that is a function of the growth rate.

The example involving a single land use map points to the hazard of relying on the output of one run of the model. If the model is run again, the effect could fail to appear due to the variation in output caused by the stochastic perturbation term. Even running all three scenarios with the same seed for the random number generator will not solve the problem because the differences in the numbers of cells to be located will mean that the identical sequences of random numbers will be out of phase in the three runs, and hence equivalent to sequences that are not identical. The lesson is this: never rely on the output of a single run of the model because the details of that output are arbitrary. The proper way to use a complex systems model is in Monte Carlo mode, where the output is expressed in proportions or probabilities—for example, the probability that a cell will receive residential development. In the case of the wastewater project, the aim is to know the *expected*

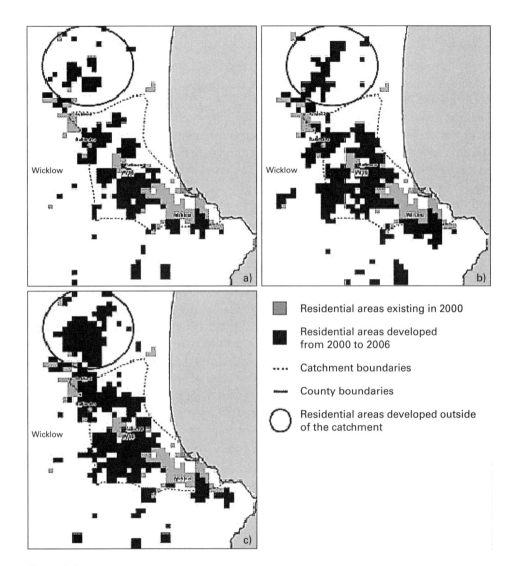

Figure 7.7
Residential development and the Wicklow catchment area, 2026. (Source: Williams et al., 2012)

amount of development both inside and outside the catchment areas, not the amounts generated by one arbitrary run of the model. In fact, in the actual study, the model was run a number of times, and the results described here are robust.

Applications: The Netherlands

The first major application of the dynamically integrated regional model was to the Netherlands. The model known as "Environment Explorer" or, in Dutch, "LeefOmgevingsVerkenner" (LOV) was adopted by the Netherlands National Institute for Public Health and the Environment (RIVM) as a tool to strengthen their understanding of spatial processes and the ways these processes affect the natural environment and the landscape. Natural areas in the Netherlands are small and therefore highly vulnerable to local changes in land use or activity location. Traditional human landscapes are also vulnerable to development in this small and densely populated country, and being highly valued, they are protected in various ways—most notably, through spatial planning. The model was used to evaluate the effects of alternative socioeconomic development scenarios on the sustainability of natural systems and cultural landscapes and, later, to evaluate the National Spatial Strategy to determine whether enough space would be available in designated areas of concentrated development to accommodate expected growth, or whether environmentally sensitive areas were likely to be threatened. The Environment Explorer was the first of the CA-based models to be fully integrated with a four-stage transportation model, and applications of this version were used to assess transportation and spatial planning policies (Geurs, 2006; Geurs and van Wee, 2006; see de Nijs, 2009, for the most comprehensive discussion of the Environment Explorer).

The model was implemented with a regional component running on forty urban-centered economic regions (COROPs; figure 7.8a), a transportation network including roads, rail, and waterways (figure 7.8b), and a CA-based land use model running at a resolution of 500 meters. At the CA level, eight land uses correspond to economic activities, of which only three—industry, services, and sociocultural—are primarily urban, the others (various agricultural sectors and recreation) being primarily rural. Two land uses correspond to population: low- and high-density residential. Finally, there are three natural land use classes. The model behavior is much more highly constrained than is the case with the MOLAND applications in Dublin because most land uses are forced by scenario trends; indeed, even some natural land covers are forced in simulations representing policies that call for an increase in natural areas. The model was modified to permit the user to specify minimum and maximum levels of activity in specified COROPs in order to give the model the capacity to represent development policies that were under consideration. In general, the model specifications were tailored to the requirements of the end user and, specifically, to the policy exercises carried out.

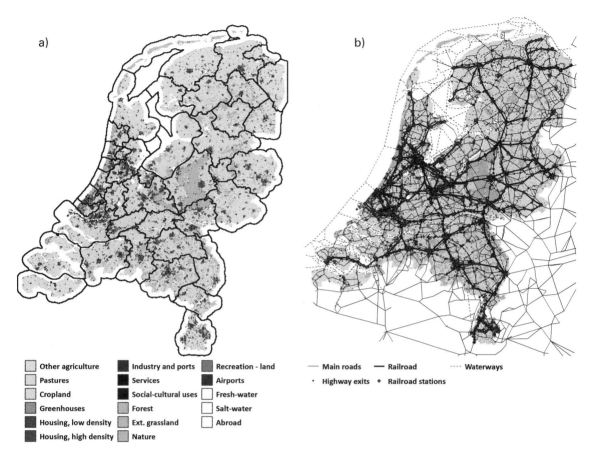

Figure 7.8
Netherlands: (a) forty urban-centered (COROP) regions; (b) transport infrastructure. (Source: Netherlands National Institute for Health and the Environment [RIVM])

The calibration period was 1989–1996, and the validation period, 1996–2000. Although calibration of the regional model was relatively successful, once the difficulties of constructing comparable data sets for the three years for the economic activities were overcome, calibration of the cellular automaton was less definitive. The problem was that there were very few changes in land uses over the six-year calibration period, or even over the whole eleven-year time span, and close examination of the three land use maps revealed that many of these changes were spurious, the result of classification errors in the maps. Therefore the calibration relied to a greater extent on measures such as maintaining the linear cluster size relationship and plausible general land use patterns over long time periods (figure 7.9; plate 4). It was also realized early on that, even though both calibration and validation of the CA-based

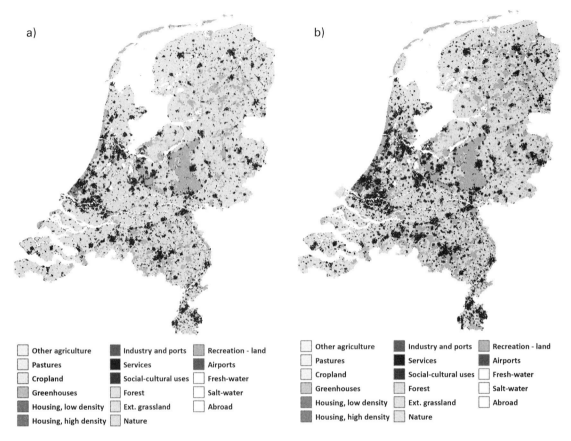

Figure 7.9 (plate 4)
Land use in Netherlands: (a) 2000 (actual); (b) 2030 (simulation). (Source: Netherlands National Institute for Health and the Environment [RIVM])

land use model require the comparison of a simulated map with the map of the actual situation, there were very few appropriate map comparison measures available. On the other hand, this problem had the fortunate effect of stimulating the development of new tools, some of which will be discussed in chapter 9.

In its final use for policy assessment, the model was run under various scenarios to 2030. In this phase the users relied heavily on a number of indicators, especially indicator maps, which collectively give a clearer picture of the implications in policy terms of the predicted land use patterns and activity levels. For example, in examining a 2030 land use map overlain by the transportation network, it is virtually impossible to get an idea of the degree of fragmentation of natural areas, even though the information is there, whereas an indicator map makes the picture immediately clear (figure 7.10). Furthermore, these indicator maps are dynamic, so that users can see changes from year to year and note threshold points.

A scaled-down version of the Environment Explorer or LeefOmgevingsVerkenner (LOV) model—BabyLOV—was provided with additional graphical user interface tools that made it possible to translate scenarios from storylines to numerical values and enter them quickly. This version was developed for the Visions Research Project of the European Union, which used public participation to develop integrated scenarios for a sustainable Europe for the years 2020 and 2050. These were developed for the European Union as a whole and for selected local regions, including the Green Heart area of the Netherlands. The main objective of the exercise with BabyLOV was to come up with representative scenarios that were internally consistent. Once a scenario was entered and run, the output showed, by means of land use maps and population and activity levels, what the scenario implied for the future. At this stage, it became clear that some scenarios were inconsistent. For example, maintenance of land use policies for nature and landscape would become impossible at some point under a high-growth scenario that also specified protection of rural areas. Although this example seems obvious, many seemingly logical qualitative scenarios are found to be inconsistent, either because they do not take into account the effects of secondary interactions among phenomena, many of which are not immediately apparent, or because they do not take into account the effects of detailed spatial constraints (White, Straatman, and Engelen, 2004).

Applications: New Zealand
New Zealand's unusual planning framework relies less on prescriptive regulation and more on a regulation of outcomes (Robert Makgill and Hamish Rennie, 2012; Rennie, 2011). It is also more strongly oriented toward environmental protection than is the case in other countries. Landcare Research, a Crown Research Institute owned by and accountable to the New Zealand government, took an early lead in advocating an integrated CA-based land use model as an aid in addressing planning policy issues (Price, 2007; Rutledge et al., 2007, 2008; Huser et al., 2009; van Delden et al., 2011). In this context, the Waikato region of New Zealand, on the North Island, has been using versions of the MOLAND model for a decade to explore environmental and land use issues, and as a spatial decision support tool to serve planning and policy ends. The current version, Waikato Integrated Scenario Explorer (WISE), has been used in several projects, to investigate, for example, the consequences of urban growth to the year 2050 in the area around Hamilton, Waikato's most populous city. The specific focus of interest was a proposed policy to protect areas of high-quality soils by means of zoning. The model used as inputs planned infrastructure improvements over the period and projected population growth, and it was run under two scenarios: zoning and no zoning.

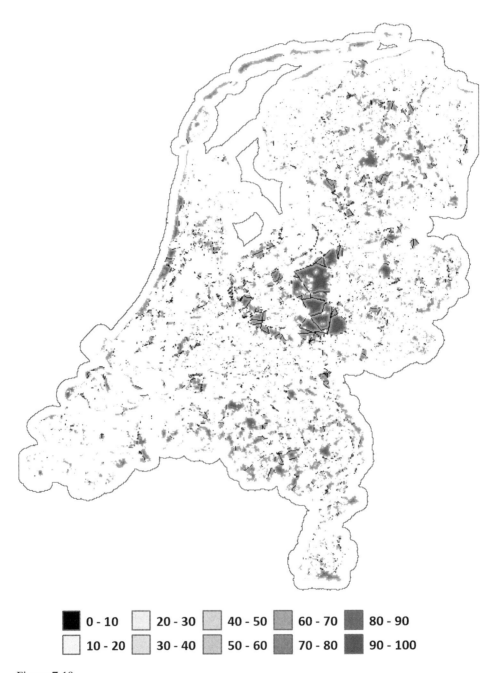

Figure 7.10
Fragmentation index (natural areas) for Netherlands, 2030. The index (the Kans op Voorkomen or KOV indicator) expresses potential biodiversity as a function of the size of an unfragmented natural area and distance from the edge of the area. Values are scaled from 0 to 100.

The WISE model has also been integrated with a terrestrial biodiversity model to forecast where native ecosystems are likely to become threatened as a result of future land use changes. Based on the likelihood of conversion to agricultural or urban uses or of other detrimental outcomes as shown by model runs to the year 2050, areas are classified into one of five levels of threat. With maps the model produces for each year of the simulation, users can visualize spatial and temporal trends in threats to native ecosystems. Although it has been run under a business-as-usual scenario, the model can also be used to help minimize the loss of local ecosystems by assessing the impact of various policies under consideration. Several other applications of the WISE MOLAND model are underway, and similar versions of the MOLAND model are being used in Auckland and Wellington.

Conclusion

A number of policy and planning organizations around the world have adopted, at least on an experimental basis, a three-level integrated model of the MOLAND class. They have done so because it provides a formal tool for investigating the impact of alternative plans and policies before they are implemented, one that integrates a number of different factors interrelated in complex ways that are difficult to understand without a computational model. When the full model includes, as its top-level driver, linked models of natural, economic, and demographic systems, it is one of the most comprehensive integrated models to date, and perhaps the only one that carries out the integration at medium and high spatial resolution. This is especially important in the context of research and policy development related to sustainability, because most interactions, and most environmental impacts, are localized. That space is important in dynamical systems can be seen in models such as those of predator-prey systems, which are unstable in non-spatial versions but behave realistically once their dynamics are constrained by space. Consequently, integrated, spatially embedded models are probably the only ones that have the potential to give usefully reliable, if only approximate, insights into urban and regional systems.

8

The Cellular Automaton Eats the Regions: Unified Modeling of Activities and Land Use in a Variable Grid Cellular Automaton

Cities are the home of diversity, interaction, and useful confusion. In the models we have discussed so far, we have attempted to capture some of the diversity and interaction that underlie their dynamics. But confusion, whether useful or not, is rarely welcomed by modelers. The MOLAND model described in chapter 7 handled the dynamics of population, economic activity, and land use by linking a regional model to a CA. In this chapter, we present an alternative approach to modeling these phenomena, and we will include a bit of useful confusion even as we simplify the model.

The *multiple activity variable grid cellular automaton* is based on the idea that, because the land use of a cell is an expression of the activities carried out there, both activities and land use should be modeled at the same time and by the same mechanism, specifically, a CA. The useful confusion is introduced by allowing multiple activities on a single cell, whatever its land use or land cover state. Thus, for example, a residential cell may have not only a population—in fact, it is residential *because* it has population—but also a certain amount of commercial and service activities, and even, perhaps, some agricultural activity. And finally, the CA should, just as the regional model did, handle spatial interactions at all distances.

It is easy enough to include activities along with land use in a CA: we simply define a complex cell state consisting of the land use as well as the various activities found on the cell, and make the activity levels a function of the transition potentials. But to do this without sacrificing the advantages that have been achieved using other modeling techniques is not so straightforward. The regional model linked to the CA was introduced to capture the effects of spatial interaction over the entire range of distances, not just the local distances of the cell neighborhood. In principle, we could treat each cell of the cell space as a region. Such an approach would avoid the problem of regions that are poorly defined or too large, and it would largely eliminate the artifacts in the dynamics due to the modifiable areal unit problem. But because the land use map of a typical application contains on the order of a half million cells, the run time would be excessive, and it is essential to keep run times low in order to be able to understand the behavior of the model, as we will see in chapter 9. To solve the run time problem while including long-distance spatial interactions, we use a *variable grid*, in which more distant cells are aggregated into larger supercells when calculating interaction effects, so that fewer cells are involved in the interaction calculations. The approach, borrowed from astrophysical simulations of gravitational collapse, was introduced into urban modeling by Claes Andersson and colleagues (Andersson, Rasmussen, and White, 2002; Andersson et al., 2002) and then adapted by Roger White (2005) for use in an activity-based approach.

The regional model described in chapter 7 is a *multiactivity* model because each region typically has all of the activities. A conventional CA-based model, on the other hand, is *not* a multiactivity model because it does not allow cells to have more than one state at a time and typically treats states as being qualitative and unitary—for example, "blue" or "dead" or "residential." We can easily generalize a CA, however, by defining cell states as vectors of values, and, once that is done, it is straightforward to model multiple activity cell states. Although this creates some modeling complications, allowing multiple activities on a cell is realistic, and it avoids several problems that would be encountered if the CA did not allow multiple activities. For example, even though, in most cities and regions, a significant proportion of the population resides in areas not shown on the land use map as residential, during initialization of the conventional CA, that part of the population would nevertheless be assigned to residential cells, thus misrepresenting the spatial distribution of the population and consequently biasing the dynamics. Permitting multiple activities also minimizes the arbitrary nature of assigning a single land use to a cell that may have several activities, as is typically done. A final advantage of the single model approach is that it significantly reduces the number of parameters. The half dozen or so additional parameters required in the CA are more than offset by the loss of all the parameters that disappear with the regional model, including those that were required to link it to the CA.

The Multiple Activity Variable Grid CA-Based Model

The multiple activity variable grid CA-based model is in many respects the same as the CA-based model already described. It still includes a top-level model or scenario that provides activity levels that must be accommodated by the CA. Cell state transitions still depend on a set of transition potentials calculated for each possible activity. The transition potentials are still a function of suitability, accessibility, zoning, and the neighborhood effect. And cells are still ranked by potentials and converted to the land use with the highest potential until the land use demands have been satisfied. But this common framework conceals several major differences. First, the neighborhood is now defined as the entire modeled area. In this way, interaction effects operating over all distances are automatically included in the calculation of the neighborhood effect. The calculations are made using a variable grid, that is, one in which more distant cells are aggregated into larger supercells. Second, a measure of negative externalities is introduced. Arising in denser and more centrally located areas due to factors such as greater congestion and higher land costs, these externalities are known to have an important influence on activity location in urban regions. The negative externality measure is used in combination with the neighborhood effect in calculating transition potentials. Finally, the cell state transition process assigns not only a land use, but also specific amounts of various activities (White, Shahumyan, and Uljee, 2011; White, Uljee, and Engelen, 2012; van Vliet, White, and Dragićević, 2009).

The Variable Grid
The use of a variable grid permits us to enlarge the cell neighborhood to include the entire modeled region—to reflect the reality that *all* the other cells of the region have an influence on a given cell's state—while keeping run times reasonable. Once it was demonstrated that a neighborhood could encompass all possible interactions in the modeled area, the possibility of replacing the spatial interaction–based regional model of activity location with a generalized CA became obvious. In other words, the locational dynamics of both activities and land uses could be modeled within a single CA.

The variable grid can be thought of as a moving template centered in turn on each cell of the basic cell space, for the purpose of calculating the neighborhood effect and negative externalities. The template (figure 8.1) has at its center the cell itself and the eight around it that constitute the Moore neighborhood. Individually, these nine cells belong to level 0 of the template cell hierarchy, level 0 being the level of the cell space itself. Collectively, the 3 × 3 square of nine cells constitutes a *supercell* of level 1, which together with its eight-cell Moore neighborhood forms a 9 × 9 cell supercell of level 2, and so on. Thus each grid cell of level L contains 3^2 cells of the level $L-1$ grid, or (3^{2L}) cells of the basic L_0 grid. Because the expanding rings are always Moore neighborhoods, all locations are in either rook or bishop directions with respect to the center cell; thus only a limited number of discrete distances are possible, as given by $\log_3(d) = \log_3(3^L)$ (rook) and by $\log_3(d) = \log_3(3^L) + \log_3(\sqrt{2})$ (bishop) or 0, 0.315, 1, 1.315, 2, 2.315….

Since the size of the supercells grows exponentially, a relatively small number of these cells can cover a very large area. For example, at a level 0 resolution of 200 meters, the 197 cells in the neighborhood used by the MOLAND cellular automaton together cover an area of only 1.93 square kilometers (~0.75 square mile), whereas, at the same resolution, the variable grid CA requires only 48 cells to cover the entire area of the Greater Dublin Region (7,812 square kilometers, or ~3,016 square miles).

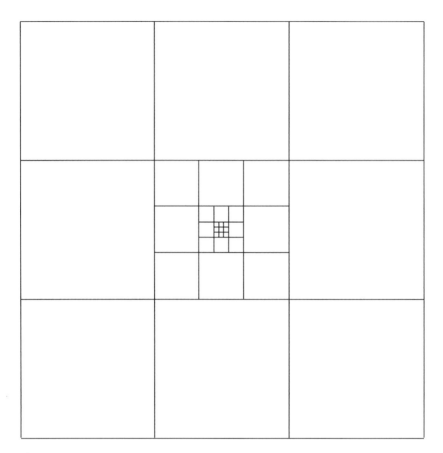

Figure 8.1
Variable grid template.

Cell States

Each level-0 cell has a state that consists of a land use together with a vector of activities. Each supercell has as its state the activity vector containing the sum of the activity vectors of the L_0 cells included in it; land use is not included in the supercell state vector. The land use of a cell corresponds to the dominant activity on the cell. In current applications, many land use classes are not associated with a modeled activity, in which case the activity level corresponding to the land use is set equal to one. But even these land uses will normally have nonzero levels of the modeled activities; for example, a forest cell may also have a few inhabitants and a small amount of commercial activity. On the other hand, the model structure permits any land use to be associated with an activity, and that opens up new possibilities for integrated modeling. Thus the forest cell in our example could be associated with the activity "biomass (trees)" and each year the volume would grow according to local suitabilities up to a biologically determined density limit.

As before, land uses fall into three categories—active, passive, and fixed (features)—depending on the way they interact in the dynamics. The number of cells required each year for each active land use is still determined by a density or productivity function that converts activity levels to cell demands. In the multiple use variable grid CA-based model, however, that conversion is carried out at the top level and then provided as total cell requirements for each land use along with the activity demands at each iteration. In most of the applications discussed below, cell and activity demands are determined exogenously and provided to the simulation model as top-level scenarios.

The activities in current applications include both population and several economic sectors. Each activity is divided into two components: primary and secondary. The primary part is that which is located on cells with the corresponding land use—for example, population located on residential cells. The secondary part is that located on cells with other land uses—for example, population on commercial cells. A set of parameters q_K, with $0 \leq q_K \leq 1$, specifies for each activity K the proportion that is to be located as primary activity, with the remainder to be located as secondary activity. Each cell may have several secondary activities, but some pairs of activities may be more compatible than others, and some may be incompatible. Consequently, another set of parameters, c_{KL}, with $0 \leq c_{KL} \leq 1$, specifies compatibility among the activities, with $c_{KL} = 0$ representing complete incompatibility. The total amount of primary and secondary activity in the system for each activity K is calculated as

$$XP_K = q_K X_K \qquad (8.1a)$$

$$XS_K = X_K - XP_K \qquad (8.1b)$$

where

XP_K = total primary amount of activity K
XS_K = total secondary amount of activity K
X_K = total amount of activity K
q_K = parameter specifying the proportion of activity K that is located as the primary activity.

Since all cells are the same size, cellular activity levels are also activity *densities*.

The suppleness of the variable grid approach in handling the spatial dynamics of activities comes from modeling the activities at the relatively high resolution of the basic cell space, rather than at the scale of regions. This often presents a problem, however, when setting up applications because the model must be initialized with activity data at the individual cell level, and such data are almost never available at that resolution. For population data, the challenge is usually manageable because the data are typically available for very small areas such as enumeration districts or census blocks, and they can then be interpolated to the cell level with some confidence, since the small size of the statistical regions limits the size of possible errors at the cell level. We have developed a procedure for doing this that distributes activity taking into account the same factors used in the model itself, so that the resulting distribution among cells in a region is relatively realistic, while minimizing discontinuities across regional boundaries (see box 8.1). For economic activities, the problem is much worse, because data are normally available only for relatively large regions (e.g., counties in the case of the Greater Dublin Region). Furthermore, there may be no reliable way to downscale to the cell level. At worst, all cells in a region corresponding to a particular activity can be assigned equal amounts of the activity, and, even in this case, the simulation results should be somewhat better than they would be for a regional model because, however arbitrary the individual activity levels may be, at least the distances are representative. Although techniques are being developed for estimating population on grid cells from satellite or land use data (see, for example, Gallego and Peedell, 2001; Harvey, 2002; Wu and Murray, 2007), these are likely to be less successful for economic activities. On the other hand, very detailed spatial data are becoming increasingly available that can be used

Box 8.1
Initialization Procedure for Activities

> Since activity data are normally available only for regions, but the model requires them to be available by cells, the initialization procedure distributes activities to cells in such a way as to arrive at a distribution as similar as possible to the (unknown) actual distribution while keeping the regional levels correct and minimizing density discontinuities across regional boundaries. Because the distribution mechanism allocates activity in proportion to the activity potential raised to a power m, the aim is to find the value of m that gives the lowest total of regional errors before cellular activity levels are adjusted to eliminate the errors so that discontinuities are minimized. The actual distribution is assumed to resemble the one that would result from the application of the model if the model were initialized and calibrated. Our procedure is thus an iterative bootstrapping one.
>
> First, we set the model up with best-guess values for the various parameters that will ultimately be calibrated, but with inertia factors and diseconomies eliminated by setting the relevant parameters appropriately. Then, for each activity K, the total activity X_K is divided into the amount to be allocated as a primary, XP_K, and secondary, XS_K, land uses. The total primary activity is distributed equally among all cells with the corresponding land use (i.e., we ignore regions) and the secondary activity is distributed equally among all other possible cells, but in accordance with the compatibility factors for each land use.

Box 8.1 (continued)

We now begin the iteration loop to find the value of the potential exponent, m, that gives the lowest total of regional errors. Using the current activity distribution, the activity potentials are calculated as

$$V_{Ki} = rS_{Ki}A_{Ki}Z_{Ki}N_{Ki} \qquad (8.1.1)$$

where

V_{Ki} = activity potential for activity K on cell i
S_{Ki} = suitability for activity K on cell i
A_{Ki} = accessibility for activity K on cell i
Z_{Ki} = zoning for activity K on cell i
N_{Ki} = neighborhood effect for activity K on cell i (see equation 8.2 in main text)
r = stochastic perturbation term.

Activities are assigned to cells in proportion to V_{Ki}^m, where $m = 0.1$ initially, with primary activities allocated to cells with the corresponding land use and secondary activity to all other cells. Once all activities are allocated to cells, activity levels are summed by regions to find regional totals, $X(\text{est})_{RK}$, and regional errors in allocated activity ($E_{RK} = X(\text{est})_{RK} - X_{RK}$) are calculated. Then the total relative error is

$$E_K = \frac{\left(\sum_R \text{abs}(E_{RK})\right)}{X_K} \qquad (8.1.2)$$

where

X_K = total amount of activity K
E_{RK} = error in predicted amount of activity K in region R
E_K = total relative error.

If this is the initial calculated value of E_K, then set $E_K^* = E_K$. Otherwise, if $E_K < E_K^*$, then $E_K^* = E_K$ and $m_K^* = m_K$.

Next calculate the relative error in activity levels in each region so that the cell values can be adjusted in order to eliminate the errors in regional activity levels:

$$r = \frac{X_{RK}}{X(\text{est})_{RK}} \qquad (8.1.3)$$

where

$X(\text{est})_{RK}$ = the estimated activity level in region R.

Then the corrected activity levels of the individual cells are given by

$$XP_{RKi} = rXP(\text{est})_{RKi} \qquad (8.1.4a)$$
$$XS_{RKi} = rXS(\text{est})_{RKi} \qquad (8.1.4b)$$

After making a final minor adjustment to correct the proportions of primary and secondary activity, increment m_K by 0.1 and return to equation 8.1.1. Continue in the loop until $m_K = 3.5$ and then assign the cells the activity values from equations 8.1.4a and 8.1.4b that correspond to m^*: that is, the activity values that give the lowest regional errors.

in a dasymetric mapping to produce reliable estimates of cell-level data for both population and economic activities. The problem of modeling at the level of the cell space is thus likely to become much less serious as we advance into the era of geo-referenced data.

The Neighborhood Effect

The impacts of both long-distance and local interactions are captured in the neighborhood effect. As before, the neighborhood effect is calculated as the weighted sum of the contents of the neighborhood, with weights being a function of distance. But now, because the neighborhood consists of the entire modeled area, the weights can reflect even long distances, and the content is characterized not just by various land uses, but by activity levels as well. In other words, the neighborhood effect now accounts for all land uses and activities—wherever they are located. Specifically,

$$N_{Ki} = \sum_J \sum_j w_{JKd(j)} \left(\frac{X_{Jj}}{X_J} \right) \tag{8.2}$$

where

N_{Ki} = neighborhood effect on cell i for activity K

X_{Jj} = amount of activity J (either primary or secondary) in supercell j (including the L_0 cells of the first ring)

X_J = total amount of activity J in the system

$w_{JKd(j)}$ = weight for the contribution of activity J, located at distance $d(j)$ from i, on the potential for activity K on cell i.

Since the different activities J may be measured in very different units—for example, economic activities could be measured in dollars, which would then be incommensurate with population—to standardize the measures of activity, we need to divide the activity level by the total amount of that activity in the system. Note that since the neighborhood effect at any cell i is a distance-discounted sum of the contents of all cells, it is in fact a potential, analogous to the potentials calculated in the regional model of chapter 7.

Each set of weights for a pair of activities represents a distance-decay function. An example of a calibrated set of weights is shown in table 8.1 and figure 8.2. Note that the distances are shown there as $\log_3(d)$, whereas the distances used in the neighborhood calculations are actual distances, whether in units of L_0 cells, kilometers, or minutes of travel time. The weights clearly fall into three groups depending on distance. The first group consists of a single weight—the inertia factor—at a $\log_3$ distance of -1. The value shown in table 8.1 may seem extremely high, but it applies to

Table 8.1
Influence functions used to calculate the neighborhood effect for population showing effect on population of population itself, industry, commerce, services and forests

Distance	Population	Industry	Commerce	Services	Forests
-1	500,000	0	0	0	0
0	600	0	70	50	50
0.315	400	0	25	35	30
1	100	5	—	5	15
1.315	60	—	10	3	—
2	5	0.5	3	0	5
2.315	4	0.3	—	0	—
3	2.5	0.2	0.2	0	0
4	1	0	0	0	0
5	0.42	0	0	0	0
6	0.41	0	0	0	0
7	0.41	0	0	0	0
8	0.4	0	0	0	0

Note: Each entry in the table is a particular value of w_{khd}; distances are cell distances in units of $\log_3(d)$. Each column represents a weighting function.

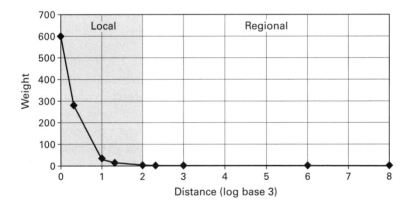

Figure 8.2
Influence weights.

only a single cell, whereas the other weights collectively apply to the 195,340 cells of the modeled area in this application. The second group has very high values, but the values decrease very rapidly with distance. In terms of the range of distances over which it applies, this group roughly corresponds to the local neighborhood as defined in the other CA-based models. Here the distance of the outer cells of the group is nine L_0 cells, or 1.8 kilometers (~1.1 miles), similar to the eight-cell radius (1.6 kilometers or ~1.0 mile) of the neighborhood in many MOLAND applications. The third group has much lower values, and they decline only slowly with distance. The curve here resembles a typical distance-decay function; in some applications, the values in this group were actually calculated with a negative exponential equation, thereby reducing the number of parameters directly involved in the calibration of the model. The sharp differentiation between a local and a long-distance set of weights that has emerged in all calibrations to date seems to reflect a real phenomenon. Specifically, people seem to judge their local neighborhood, roughly the area within a convenient walking distance, on one basis, and the area beyond it, where they are interested in accessibility to a wide range of opportunities in the region, on another. This behavior would also seem to justify the strategy followed in the models described in chapter 7 of using a CA to model the consequences of local interaction, and then linking it to a regional model to include the long-distance effects.

The use of the variable grid in neighborhood calculations means that the results are only an approximation of the true values because the L_0 cells within a supercell are treated collectively and are therefore, in effect, assumed to be at the same distance from the cell to which the template is being applied. But the resulting small deviations from the true values, visible as faint rectilinear patterns in the potential maps, do not noticeably affect the land use patterns. These artifacts are the price we pay for feasible, even good run times. It is a price well worth paying, however, because of the benefits gained in terms of better calibration and validation, more extensive sensitivity analysis, and a generally better understanding of the behavior of the model. The values for each supercell are updated efficiently by a cumulative process beginning at the individual cell level. The activity values of the L_1 supercell surrounding each L_0 cell are calculated, and then the activity levels of the L_2 supercell surrounding each L_1 cell are determined, and so on up the hierarchy. During the updating, at each level, cell counts for passive and feature land uses are also established, and these together with the activity levels are used to cumulatively calculate the neighborhood effect for all cells. This method has the advantage that location data attached to particular cells can be passed efficiently up the hierarchy, which is useful for determining the representative center of a supercell when the point to be treated as the center is not the geometric center but a location reflecting the concentration of activity. This is useful, as we shall see, in calculating network distances in the variable grid context.

Diseconomies of Agglomeration

As activities cluster at the most desirable locations—for example, places where accessibility to the region is high—the cost of land increases because of growing demand coming up against the limited availability of space. This cost is market mediated. But in addition, the growing number of people and increasing amounts of activity lead to other, implicit, costs that are *not* market mediated, such as more serious traffic congestion leading to longer delays; these are externalities. Nevertheless, because both types of costs are functions of accessibility to the system as a whole, the larger the agglomeration, and the more central the location within the agglomeration, the higher these costs. In other words, they are a function of activity potential. These *diseconomies of agglomeration* are calculated as follows:

$$D_{Ki} = \left\{ \max\left(\kappa_K, (1 + V_{\text{pop},i} - V_{\text{crit}})\right)^{\lambda_K} \right\}^{-1} \tag{8.3}$$

$$V_{\text{crit}} = \varepsilon \langle V_{\text{init}} \rangle$$

where

D_{Ki} = relative level of diseconomies of agglomeration for activity K at cell i
$V_{i,\text{pop}}$ = population potential at cell i,
V_{crit} = critical level of population potential at which diseconomies appear
$\langle V_{\text{init}} \rangle$ = mean value of initial population potentials
λ_K = relative importance of diseconomies for activity K
ε = parameter expressing the critical level for the appearance of diseconomies relative to the initial mean population potential
κ_K = parameter used to establish a ceiling on agglomeration *economies* for activity K ($\kappa_K > 0$).

$V_{i,\text{pop}}$ is essentially a neighborhood effect for population (pop). There are several options for calculating it. First, it can be calculated by letting K = pop in equation 8.2, in which case it is the full neighborhood effect for population. Or it can be calculated with equation 8.2 by letting $K = J$ = pop. In this case, it is in fact the neighborhood effect calculated on the basis of population only, without including the effect of other activities; it is thus equivalent to population potential as conventionally calculated. In addition, it is possible to exclude one or more of the inner bands of the neighborhood from the calculation. The rationale for doing this is that the inner bands have very high weights and thus exert a large influence, so that including them in the value of $V_{i,\text{pop}}$ would tend to be more a measure of the local neighborhood, whereas the potential is supposed to reflect accessibility to the entire region. In effect, in choosing to exclude the inner bands, we base the population potential on the long-distance rather than the local effects, which has the effect of encouraging contiguous urban development. Because, however, V_{crit} is always calculated *without* any band exclusions, $\langle V_{\text{init}} \rangle$ is normally greater than $\langle V_{i,\text{pop}} \rangle$ when one or more bands are excluded.

Although used to calculate *dis*economies of agglomeration, equation 8.3 will generally also yield economies in peripheral regions. This is realistic, but the effect may be minimized or eliminated depending on the value of κ_K. If $\kappa_K > 1$, then diseconomies are present everywhere. The diseconomies factor D_{Ki} is used only to calculate the activity potentials that determine land use transitions; it is not used in activity assignment.

Since both the diseconomies effect and the neighborhood effect are functions of the population potential, but the diseconomies effect is given by an inverse function, they tend to counteract each other. The neighborhood effect draws activities to the main clusters or agglomerations, where the advantages are greatest, whereas the diseconomies effect repels them from the same locations because the costs are highest there. In short, the best locations are also the worst locations. This situation is characteristic of self-organizing systems: positive feedback effects like the neighborhood effect eventually generate negative feedbacks like diseconomies of agglomeration.

Land Use Transition and Activity Assignment
For each year of the simulation, the top-level scenario supplies the CA with both the number of cells needed for each land use and the total amount of each activity required. The CA must then satisfy these land use and activity demands. The first step is to calculate activity potentials that include all the factors that together determine the quality of a cell for each of the activities. These activity potentials are essentially the same as the potentials used in the CA-based models of chapters 6 and 7 except for the calculation of the neighborhood effect:

$$V_{Ki} = rS_{Ki}A_{Ki}Z_{Ki}N_{Ki} \tag{8.4}$$

where

V_{Ki} = activity potential for activity K on cell i
S_{Ki} = suitability for activity K on cell i
A_{Ki} = accessibility for activity K on cell i
Z_{Ki} = zoning for activity K on cell i
N_{Ki} = neighborhood effect for activity K on cell i
r = stochastic perturbation term.

Note that S_{Ki}, A_{Ki}, and Z_{Ki} are calculated exactly as in the previous CA-based models. In particular, A_{Ki} represents *local* accessibility, that is, accessibility to the networks. Accessibility to the region—long-distance accessibility—is captured in the neighborhood effect.

The land use transition potential is given by

$$VT_{Ki} = D_{Ki}(V_{iK})^{m_K} + I_K \text{ (if } V_{Ki} < 0, \text{ set } m_K = 1) \tag{8.5}$$

where

VT_{Ki} = transition potential for land use K on cell i
D_{Ki} = diseconomies of agglomeration experienced by activity K on cell i
V_{Ki} = activity potential for activity K on cell i
$I_K = w_{K,d=-1}$ = inertia of activity K
m_K = a parameter to be calibrated.

The transition rule, as before, is to change each cell to the land use for which it has the highest potential as given by equation 8.5 until all cell demands have been met. The procedure is again to rank the transition potentials on each cell and to rank all cells by their highest transition potential. Then, starting with the highest-ranked cell, each cell is changed to its highest-ranked use. When the cell demands for a particular land use have been met, the corresponding transition potentials are ignored as the process continues. Under this procedure, each cell that ends up with an active land use will have undergone exactly *one* transition, though usually that transition will have left it with the same land use as before.

On the other hand, whenever there is an actual *change* of land use, if it is to an *active* land use, whether from another active use or from a passive one, a quantity of the corresponding activity is assigned to the cell, along with other, secondary activities:

$$XP_{Ki} = XP_K \left[\frac{(V_{Ki})^{\gamma_K}}{\sum_{i \in K}(V_{Ki})^{\gamma_K}} \right] \qquad (8.6a)$$

$$XS_{JKi} = XS_{JK} \left[\frac{(V_{Ji})^{\gamma_K}}{\sum_{i \in K}(V_{Ji})^{\gamma_J}} \right] \text{ for all } J \neq K \qquad (8.6b)$$

where

XP_{Ki} = amount of primary activity K on cell i
XP_K = total primary amount of activity K
XS_{JKi} = amount of secondary activity J on cell i with primary activity or land use K
XS_{JK} = total secondary amount of activity J
$\gamma_K, \gamma_J,$ = parameters to be calibrated
$\Sigma_{i \in K}$ indicates that the sum is taken over all cells i with land use K in the modeled area.

Notice that the activities assigned in equations 8.6a and 8.6b are a function of activity potentials rather than transition potentials. The reason is that the factors like high land costs that underlie the diseconomies effect and that tend to repel activities are also the ones that lead to higher densities when activities do move in despite the diseconomies. Thus equation 8.5, which includes the diseconomies effect, tends to spread activity, viewed as land use, more widely across the region; whereas equations 8.6a and 8.6b, which do not include diseconomies, lead to much higher activity densities in the central areas, the same ones with serious diseconomies.

As the system grows and changes, the relative desirability of various locations, as measured by the potentials, changes as well. The activities assigned to cells in equations 8.6a and 8.6b, both primary and secondary, reflect these changes since they are based on the current potentials. On the other hand, cells that did not experience a change of land use are left with their previous levels of activity. In reality, activity levels change to reflect changes in the quality of the location; for example, as a city grows, the potential of many areas increases, which leads to greater densities. Therefore (skipping some technical details), we adjust the activity levels (i.e., densities) of cells that did not change state to reflect the changing relative activity potentials:

$$XP_{Ki} = \left[\frac{\left(\frac{V_{Ki}^{m_K}}{\sum_i V_{Ki}^{m_K}} \right)}{\left(\frac{V_{(t-1)Ki}^{m_K}}{\sum_i V_{(t-1)Ki}^{m_K}} \right)} \right]^{\tau_K} XP_{Ki} \text{ for all } K \quad (8.7a)$$

$$XS_{KJi} = \left[\frac{\left(\frac{V_{Ji}^{m_J}}{\sum_i V_{Ji}^{m_J}} \right)}{\left(\frac{V_{(t-1)Ji}^{m_J}}{\sum_i V_{(t-1)Ji}^{m_J}} \right)} \right]^{\tau_J} XS_{Ji} \text{ for all } i \in K, J \neq K \quad (8.7b)$$

where the m_K are parameters to be calibrated and τ_K is a parameter that scales the effect; for $\tau_K = 0$, there is no adjustment of densities. As for equation 8.6, $i \in K$ indicates all cells i with land use K.

Due to this density response to changing potentials, as a simulation is executed, the population densities of rural cells (which have population as a secondary activity) change, with the densities of rural cells near large urban centers increasing significantly. As a result, in some simulations of the Dublin region, a few periurban rural cells eventually have larger populations than some more peripheral residential cells.

Network Distances

The key to the neighborhood effect on a cell is the set of weights applied to the various activities located at various distances from the cell. As figure 8.2 makes clear, each set of weights collectively represents a distance-decay function. Earlier versions of the variable grid approach used the Euclidian distances to supercells in the neighborhood to determine the weight to apply. Thus the only distances that occurred were the discrete set given by $\log_3(d) = \log_3(3^L)$ and by $\log_3(d) = \log_3(3^L) + \log_3(\sqrt{2})$. The current version of the model, however, uses network distances for cells beyond the local neighborhood (see box 8.2; Crols et al., submitted). These are weighted averages of travel times through the road and rail networks, with distances through the road network taking into account the different average speeds on different types of links (e.g., superhighway, highway, local road). These can be changed by the user to represent improvements or degradations in the network, or the difference in travel times between off-peak and peak periods. Because network distances can take on any value, to find the proper weight to apply at a certain network distance, the value must in general be interpolated between the discrete weight values shown in figure 8.2.

Box 8.2
Calculating Network Distances

> Local distances from a cell, that is, those to supercells of a level lower than L_E (where E is specified by the user) are calculated as Euclidian distances to the geometric center of the supercell. For example, in applications to Flanders, which is modeled at a resolution of 100 meters and with $E = 2$, distances out to points within the level-one supercells are Euclidian. The challenge is to calculate the distances to higher-level supercells in the neighborhood through the network, and to do so in a computationally efficient manner (Crols et al., 2015). Once we know the origin and destination nodes on the network, calculating the distances through the network is straightforward. Finding the origin and destination nodes is more difficult since it is rarely the case that a cell is also the location of a node, and a supercell may contain many nodes or none. Thus each cell and supercell must be associated with a network node.
>
> For the cell itself, the closest node is chosen. For the supercells, the node closest to the representative center of the supercell will become the associated node. The representative center is the cell that normally best represents the concentration of activity in the supercell; it is found as a by-product of the calculation of the aggregate activity levels that define the state vector of the supercell. This calculation proceeds in a cumulative fashion from the L_0 grid upward and can thus efficiently pass information on activity concentrations upward to higher-level supercells. Starting at level L_2 the activity levels of the nine subcells are compared, and, for the L_1 cell with the most activity, the L_0 cell with the most activity is taken as the representative center of the L_2 cell. At each level $L_n > L_2$, the activity levels of the nine L_{n-1} subcells are compared, and the representative center of the one with the greatest activity is chosen as the representative center of the cell. Thus the original L_1 centers are passed up the hierarchy, with the number of centers decreasing by a factor of 9 at each higher level. Because of this procedure, the centers do not have to be recalculated at each level. Although this approach may miss

Box 8.2 (continued)

the major concentrations of activity in some special cases, in general, it finds a representative center that reasonably approximates the concentration of activity in each supercell. It also avoids the boundary problem: the representative center will always lie within the modeled region, whereas some other methods, such as choosing the geometric center of the supercell as the representative center, may place the center outside the modeled area—for example, in the sea.

Using the Dijkstra algorithm, distances are calculated from each node to the node closest to the representative center of each supercell of level $L_n \geq L_E$ in the variable grid neighborhood of the level L_E supercell containing the origin node. Since, in general, neither the origin cell nor the representative center of a supercell coincides with a node, in both cases, the Euclidian distance to the nearest node is added to the network distance. Box 8.2, figure 8.2.1 shows schematically the route from an origin cell, O, to a destination cell, D. The link Oa is the Euclidian route to the associated node on the network, ab, bc, and cd are links on the network, and dD is the final Euclidian link. The distances are stored in memory so that they do not have to be recalculated with each iteration of the model. On the other hand, if the representative center of a supercell changes from one iteration to the next as a result of the changing location pattern of activities (which may also result in a different node being the closest one), then the distances to that supercell must be recalculated. As a further simplification for the sake of efficiency, we use a single grid, referred to as the "network grid," for level L_E, and define all cells of $L_n \geq L_E$ in terms of that grid. Therefore, the Euclidian add-on distance from the origin cell is to the closest node associated with this grid, which is not necessarily the closest node to the origin cell.

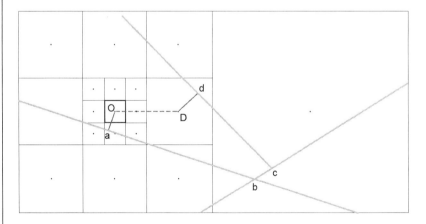

Figure 8.2.1
Diagram of a route through the network (from O to D).

Box 8.2 (continued)

To simplify the discussion of the geometry, we have spoken simply of "Euclidian" and "network" distances. But there may be several different kinds of networks involved (e.g., road and rail), and each network has several classes of links; for roads, these range from superhighways to local roads. These distinctions are necessary because we actually calculate distances as travel times, and, in order to do this, each class of network links, as well as the Euclidian links, must be associated with an average speed. For the road network, these speeds may come from traffic studies; rail travel times are taken from an origin-destination matrix based on the system timetable, and modified with an added constant that depends on service frequency (box 8.2, table 8.2.1). We can change these speeds to represent improvements or degradations in the network or the difference between travel during off-peak and peak periods. The shortest path is then determined as the one with the shortest travel time. These calculations are relatively straightforward for each travel mode, but when there is more than one mode available, the distance is treated as a weighted average of the travel times by the two modes.

Finally, although distances beyond L_E are calculated through the network, if the route is very circuitous, the low-speed Euclidian distance (e.g., from O to D in box 8.2, figure 8.2.1) may actually be faster than the higher-speed but longer trip through the network. We therefore calculate both trip times and store the faster time, using it as the distance from the cell to the supercell in calculating the neighborhood effect.

Table 8.2.1
Average speeds in kilometers per hour on link types in Flanders

Link type	Legal maximum speed (reality)	Average speed (model)
Superhighway	120	100
Express road	100	85
Major road	90	70
Secondary road	70	55
Local road	50	40
Urban low-speed zone	30	30
"Euclidian speed"	—	5

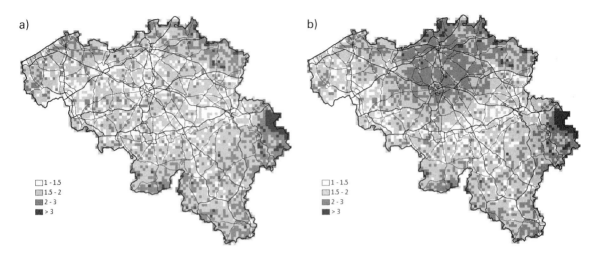

Figure 8.3
Accessibility by means of the road network, Belgium: (a) off-peak (no congestion); (b) peak periods (congestion). Values show aggregate travel time to all cells in Belgium, weighted by population, relative to the minimum value. 1 = maximum accessibility, >3 = least accessibility.

Figure 8.3 shows general accessibility maps corresponding to off-peak and peak travel times in Belgium. The part of the country containing Brussels and Antwerp is generally the most accessible, as would be expected since it is both most central and contains the greatest concentration of activity, and thus has shorter average distances to all activity. But this is only true in the absence of congestion (figure 8.3a). When the road network is congested, it has the *lowest* accessibility in the country (figure 8.3b). Thus the neighborhood effect calculated for commerce or industry in this area will be much lower if the peak period travel times are used to determine the values of the weights, and this is likely to have a noticeable impact on the evolution of the location patterns of these activities.

Regions

Although, in some applications, activity data by region may be used as input to an initialization procedure that distributes the activity to individual cells, the actual modeling is carried out entirely at the cellular level: regions are not involved. Nevertheless, in order to calibrate and validate the model, activity levels generated by a simulation must be compared to actual values, and these are available only by region. Furthermore, because most end users require predictions of activity levels for at least one set of regions, the model aggregates cellular activity levels to regions. In the Dublin application described below, results are aggregated to two sets of regions: the 629 electoral districts and the five counties. Since the calculations of the model do not make use of regions, which are simply a convenient way of presenting the model output, they can be changed at will without the need to recalibrate.

Output

At each iteration, the activity-based variable grid model produces not only a land use map, as the other models do, but also a density map for each activity, a transition potential map showing the values calculated in equation 8.5, and a population potential map showing the values used to calculate the diseconomies effect in equation 8.3. These can be saved both as animations and as log files for use in subsequent analysis. Finally, it produces a table of activity levels in each region.

Application to the Greater Dublin Region

The variable grid model was applied to the GDR using the same data as the UEP applications of the MURBANDY model described in chapter 7. This permits us to compare the two approaches and to evaluate their relative strength. There were, however, two notable differences in how the data were used in the variable grid model. First, the four residential land uses in the UEP application were combined into a single class. And, second, because activity data for the four economic sectors were only available at the county level, population was the only activity that was fully modeled. The economic activities were provided with zero-growth scenarios and effectively frozen. Since this treatment would affect the spatial behavior of population to some degree, the results for that sector would probably be somewhat better if the economic sectors had been fully modeled.

Population was initialized using data for the 629 electoral districts of the five-county region. The districts are small enough to provide a reasonable approximation to local densities, and since many of them cover areas that are largely nonresidential, they can also be used to estimate the density of population as a secondary activity on various land uses. The population of the electoral districts was distributed among the cells using a procedure developed for that purpose (box 8.1). It first divides the population of the GDR into primary and secondary components and then uses the variable grid model, running with its initialized parameter values and influence rules, to distribute it among the cells. The result is a smooth distribution of population over the region with no discontinuities at electoral district boundaries. But, because the distributed population summed within individual electoral districts does not match the actual value, densities are adjusted within each electoral district so that the population is correct. And, because this correction introduces discontinuities, the procedure generates a discontinuity index. The procedure is iterated until the discontinuities no longer decrease. Since results depend on the initial, assumed, values of parameters that are yet to be calibrated, the results can be improved by reinitializing the population distribution once the model has been calibrated.

The first versions of the variable grid model did not include network distances (White, Uljee, and Engelen, 2012). Here we present an application to Dublin of the version that does. The density and diseconomies parameters have been recalibrated, but, otherwise, the two versions are run with the same parameter values and the same data, so their results can usefully be compared. We will also compare output of both versions of the variable grid model with the results of a UEP MOLAND application.

Parameters

A few comments on the effect of various parameters, especially the density and diseconomies parameters, may be helpful. The influence functions (weights) on population are shown in table 8.1; these are identical in the applications with and without network distances. The values of the parameters controlling density, the diseconomies effect, and several other factors are given in table 8.2 for both versions. With the network distances version, because diseconomies begin at a lower potential level, as given by ε in equation 8.3, they are experienced over a larger proportion of the region, but because they also increase more moderately as the potential increases (lower values of λ), the extreme values are not as high. When population is assigned to a cell that has changed state, the density is much more responsive (higher γ) to the potential of the cell (V_{Ki} in equation 8.6a), and thus densities can become much higher. The lower value for m in equation 8.5 means that the transition potentials of cells are more similar to one another than they were in the Euclidian distances

Table 8.2
Values of key parameters used in simulations with activity-based model

Parameter	Network value	No-network value
Band	2.00	2.00
ε	1.07	1.35
λ	0.62	0.85
γ	2.00	1.00
τ	1.50	0.90
m	0.20	0.40
α	0.70	0.60
Q	0.82	0.85
Network speed (km/hr)	54.00	N/A
Euclidian factor	3.50	N/A

Note: Euclidian factor is equivalent to 15.4 kilometers per hour.

Table 8.3
Local accessibility parameters applying to population

Network element	Relative importance	Distance decay
Superhighway	0.00	0
Superhighway junction	0.90 (0.99)	9
Divided highway	0.70	9
National routes	0.70	4
Regional roads	0.60	2 (4)
Local roads	0.60 (0.5)	2 (4)
Railroads	0.00	0
Railroad stations	0.00	1
Light rail	0.99	2

Note: Values in parentheses are from the application without network distances.

version, which will tend to make the transitions more sensitive to the stochastic perturbation. Similarly, in equations 8.7a and 8.7b, the lower value of *m* would reduce the density adjustment in response to changing activity potentials, but this effect is counteracted by the higher value for τ. For calculating travel times through the network, we used a single speed (54 kilometers or ~34 miles per hour) because we lacked data for the average speeds on the five different road classes. The speed used for Euclidian distances (the distances to and from the network, or within the local area) was 15.4 kilometers (~10 miles) per hour, arrived at by calibration. Local accessibility calculations made use of essentially the same set of relative importance and distance-decay parameter values in both applications, though a few values did change marginally during calibration (table 8.3).

Results

The base year for the simulations was 1990, and the model was run forward to 2000 and 2006. Predicted and actual land uses in the year 2000 are shown in figure 8.4 (plate 5) for the network version. Figure 8.5 (plate 6) shows the differences between the predicted and actual locations of residential land use for both the version using Euclidian distances and the network version. A comparison of these two maps shows that the results are very similar for the two versions of the model, as indicated by both the detailed location of residential cells, although the prediction errors are somewhat less in the network version. Comparing the two versions on the basis of errors in the predicted amount of residential land use in each county confirms that there is little difference in their performance; note that the results shown in table 8.4 are averages over ten runs, which is necessary because of the stochastic variation from one run to another. When the model is run forward to 2006, however, it shows

196   Chapter 8

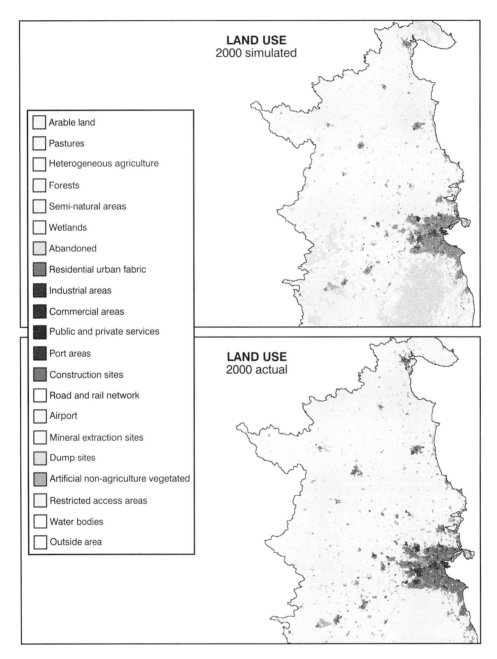

Figure 8.4 (plate 5)
Land use, Dublin, 2000: (*top*) simulated, using network distances; (*bottom*) actual.

The Cellular Automaton Eats the Regions 197

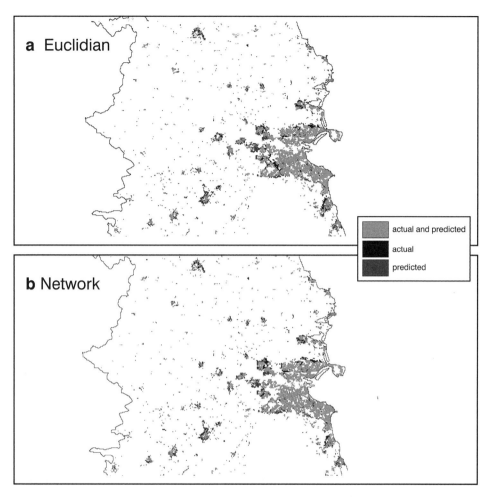

Figure 8.5 (plate 6)
Error in simulated residential land use, Dublin, 2000: (*top*) simulation using Euclidian distances; (*bottom*) simulation using network distances.

Table 8.4
Errors in predicted residential land use per county, 2000

County	Network		No network	
	Error (%)	SD (%)	Error (%)	SD (%)
Louth	−2.08	0.87	−6.61	0.77
Meath	5.22	1.17	0.79	0.86
Dublin	−0.34	0.39	0.61	0.20
Kildare	2.53	1.21	2.18	0.92
Wicklow	−4.16	0.84	−1.77	1.20

Note: Error values are the mean for ten model runs from 1990 to 2000; standard deviations are shown as a measure of variability among runs.

too much growth of residential land use in the towns surrounding Dublin (figure 8.6; plate 7), although the cluster size–frequency plot for 2056 remains linear and very similar in slope to the 1990 distribution (figure 8.7). The activity potential for population (figure 8.8; plate 8) and the predicted year 2000 population density (figure 8.9; plate 9) closely resemble each other, as is to be expected. Notice that the major transportation routes show up clearly on the potential map, but hardly at all on the population density map; this may be an artifact of the scale intervals.

Mixed land uses show up clearly in a comparison of land use and activity density maps. The green areas on the population density map (figure 8.9; plate 9) represent low-density rural population occupying agricultural, forest, or other natural land use classes as a secondary activity. The yellow areas also indicate population as a secondary activity on rural cells, but at much higher densities—up to 400 people per square kilometer (~1,040 per square mile)—in areas immediately peripheral to Dublin; they will in many cases be converted to residential land use at much higher densities as the model runs forward. Notice that most cells in the central core of Dublin also have very high densities even though many of these are not residential; their mixed commercial and residential use is typical of the dense core of large cities. At the other extreme, the areas with no population (white on the map) are either areas where zoning has prohibited residential development or the compatibility factor has excluded population as a secondary activity. Notice that Phoenix Park, the large park just to the northwest of central Dublin, is shown with a modest population density. This is because the compatibility factor of population on park cells is small but positive, with the result that parks receive some population as a secondary activity. Phoenix Park does in fact have a resident population: it is home to both the president of Ireland and the U.S. ambassador.

The population densities—that is, the cell populations—can be summed over the counties to get the predicted county populations. These can be compared with actual

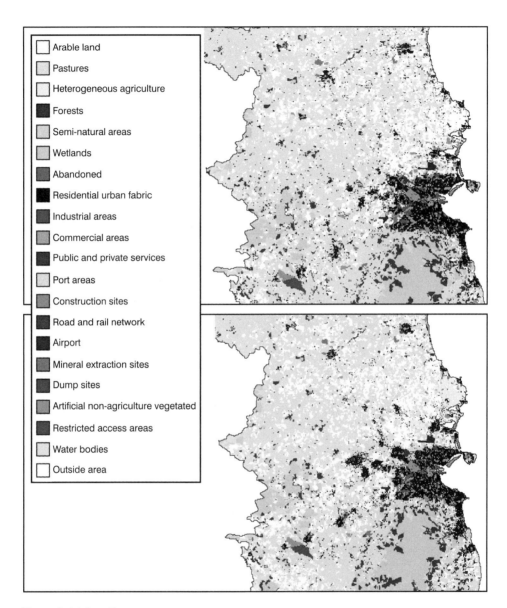

Figure 8.6 (plate 7)
Land use, Dublin, 2006: (*top*) actual; (*bottom*) simulated.

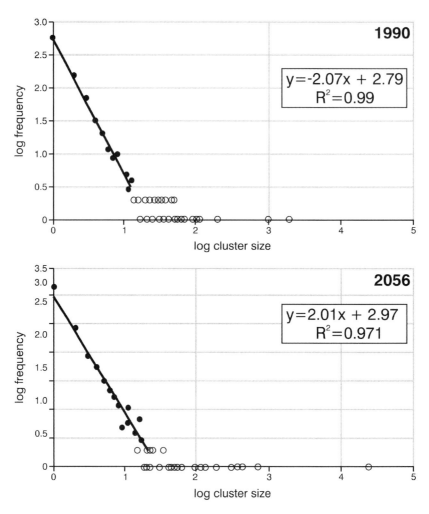

Figure 8.7
Cluster size–frequency relationship, Dublin: 1990 (*top*); 2056 (*bottom*).

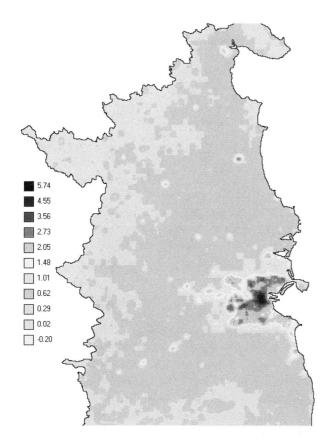

Figure 8.8 (plate 8)
Activity potential (population), Dublin, 2000, from simulation using network distances. Values are as calculated by equation 8.4.

populations for purposes of calibration and validation. The results for both versions of the multiple activity model, the UEP MOLAND model, and the "constant share" estimates—a "null" prediction where each county keeps a constant share of the growing population—are shown in table 8.5. It seems that it makes little difference overall whether distances are measured as travel times through the network or simply as Euclidian distances, but this may be due to the fact that the network links were all weighted with the same speed (54 kilometers per hour) and congestion was not taken into account. In an application to Belgium that makes use of better speed data, real differences emerge between the network and Euclidian distance versions of the model (figure 8.10; plate 10). Note that use of network distances favors residential development in the area between Antwerp and Brussels, whereas Euclidian distances favor the Liege area, although differences in population densities are less spatially

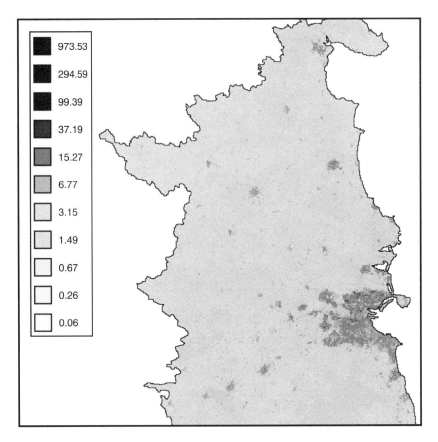

Figure 8.9 (plate 9)
Simulated population density, Dublin, 2000. Density is population per cell.

structured. Returning to the Dublin simulations, both versions of the activity-based model did give better predictions than the UEP MOLAND model, and all three models clearly outperformed the constant share estimates. Errors for 2006 predictions are shown in table 8.5, although the results for the two versions of the activity-based model are not strictly comparable to those for the UEP MOLAND because the former were produced by running the model as calibrated over the 1990–2000 period forward to 2006, whereas the UEP MOLAND results for 2006 were generated by a calibration over the entire 1990–2006 period. The calibration over the entire period of the run should produce better results than a 2006 prediction based on a 1990–2000 calibration, yet the activity-based approach clearly produces better county population predictions. This is important: one of the reasons for using an activity-based CA rather than linked regional and CA-based models is that it *should*

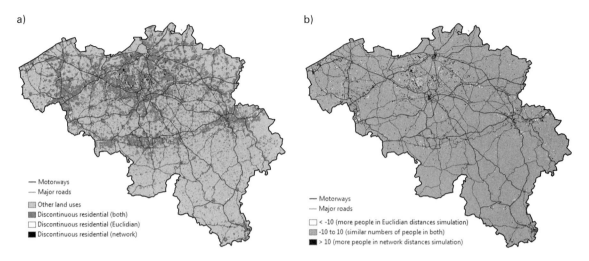

Figure 8.10 (plate 10)
Differences between Belgian simulations using network and Euclidian distances: (a) residential land use; (b) population density.

Table 8.5
Errors in predicted county populations for four models

	Error (%)					
	Activity Based Model 1990–2000		Moland Model	Constant share	Activity Based Model (Network)	Moland Model
County	Network	No Network	1990–2000	1990–2000	1990–2006	1990–2006
Louth	5.67	4.38	2.4	1.98	2.63	2.4
Meath	0.01	–4.21	8.2	–7.73	–11.67	2.3
Dublin	–0.14	0.03	–0.6	2.27	0.87	–0.0
Kildare	–0.18	0.51	–7.5	–13.02	3.96	–8.9
Wicklow	–3.37	0.69	5.0	–3.37	–1.33	7.7

Note: Both activity based models were calibrated over 1990–2000; results for 1990–2006 are for 1990–2000 calibrations run forward to 2006. MOLAND model was calibrated over 1990–2000 and 1990–2006; it was not run forward beyond the calibration period. Constant share results were calculated on assumption that each county maintained its initial share of the population. All runs began with 1990 data.

produce better regional estimates because of the higher resolution at which the modeling is carried out.

Of course, an additional advantage of the activity-based CA is that activities can be aggregated to any desired set of regions. Doing this for the electoral districts, which are the smallest units for which population data are readily available, allows us to produce a much more detailed map of prediction errors (figure 8.11). The smaller the regions, the greater the variation in errors that can be expected, and that effect is visible here. But the distribution of errors is good: on visual inspection, very little spatial autocorrelation is apparent. On the other hand, the errors are correlated with the type of location, with largely rural electoral districts having larger errors on average, electoral districts in periurban locations having somewhat smaller mean errors, and urban electoral districts having the smallest errors (table 8.6). It would be foolish to treat the activity predictions at the electoral district level as accurate, yet for areas just a little larger, on the order of half a dozen electoral districts, the predictions may well have a useful degree of accuracy. The UEP MOLAND application for assessing the adequacy of planned wastewater treatment facilities, discussed in chapter 7, is a clear instance where small-area predictions of activity levels would be helpful.

During the calibration process, in order to avoid overcalibration, the model was run to 2056 and the calibration was then adjusted to ensure a linear cluster size–frequency relationship. This final calibration, however, produced a surprising result for the 2056 land use pattern: urban development was largely in ribbons along roads (figure 8.12), a pattern that only began to emerge after about 2025 (see figure 8.6). Of course, there is no way to know for certain whether this is simply an artifact of the calibration or a likely future for the Dublin area. But it does show that simulation models can be useful in raising important questions for planners to consider. In this case, it would be reasonable to take the issue of ribbon development seriously since the predicted pattern for the Dublin area is very similar to the actual pattern in Flanders (figure 8.12 inset), and both regions share a history of lax enforcement of planning regulations.

Other Applications

Several applications to specific regions are underway in Belgium. As a preliminary exercise to those projects, the activity-based model, without network distances, was applied to the whole country. The settlement geography of Belgium is quite different from that of the Greater Dublin Region. Belgium contains an entire urban system and is thus polycentric, unlike the smaller region centered on Dublin. It is therefore a good test of whether the activity-based model is really generic. Only two comparable land use maps were available, for 2000 and 2006, both with a resolution of

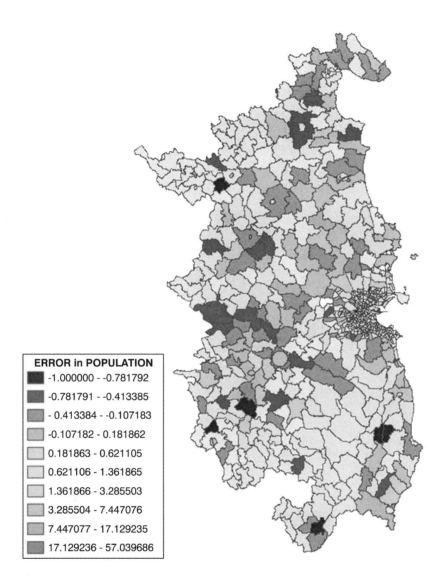

Figure 8.11
Error of predicted population by electoral district, Dublin, 2000.

Table 8.6
Root mean square errors of electoral district (ED) populations in rural, periurban, and urban locations

ED Predominantly:	RMSE
Urban residential	183.44
Urban other	542.59
Partly urban	562.31
Rural	1813.54

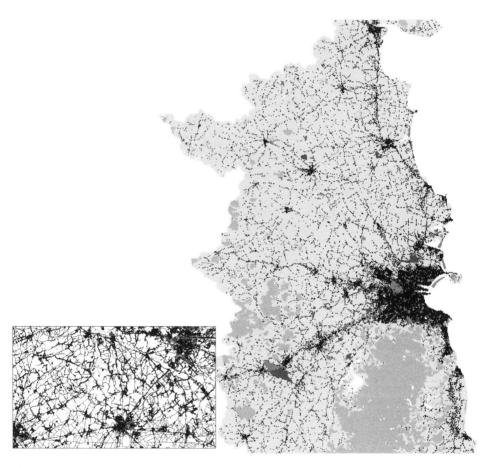

Figure 8.12
Simulated land use in Greater Dublin Region, 2056, showing ribbon development along roads. Inset: actual land use in part of Flanders, showing similar ribbon development.

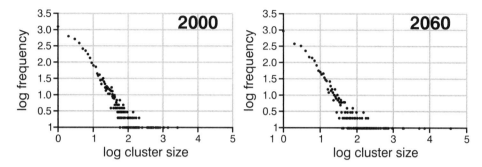

Figure 8.13
Cluster size–frequency relationship, Belgium: (*left*) actual, 2000; (*right*) simulated, 2060.

300 meters; the calibration period was thus relatively short—too short to give reliable estimates of the parameter values, especially since changes in land use and activity were minimal during this period. The calibration to land use was supplemented, however, with a calibration to the cluster size–frequency distribution, which, uniquely in Belgium, is *not* linear (see figure 8.13), probably as a result of the country's extensive strip development, which reduces the number of small clusters.

The land use maps used in the model included three urban categories: continuous urban fabric (essentially, dense urban cores), discontinuous urban fabric (largely residential), and a commercial/industrial class. A previous project had compiled population and economic data at the 300-meter resolution using a dasymetric mapping procedure, so that the project's activity data were good. Unfortunately, however, because a complete network map was not available, some link types could not be included in the model's local accessibility calculations, and thus some of the characteristic patterns of Belgian urbanization, especially strip development, could not be fully captured. Nevertheless, in general, the land use and activity density maps generated by the model seem reasonable, even over the long run to 2060, as shown in figure 8.14 (plate 11).

The national activity totals that were distributed by the model to produce these maps were taken from population and economic projections made for another study. The maps for 2060 suggest that the model is predicting substantial growth in all of the major urban regions in the northern two-thirds of the country. When, however, the density figures are summed by arrondissements (relatively small NUTS 3 units in the EU's system of standardized regional classification) and growth rates over the period 2000–2060 are calculated, the model predicts that the major urban centers of Wallonia will grow at a much slower rate than the Flemish centers, with Brussels growing at an intermediate rate. This suggests that the predicted growth of the Sambre–Meuse axis of Wallonia will involve more urban sprawl than the growth in

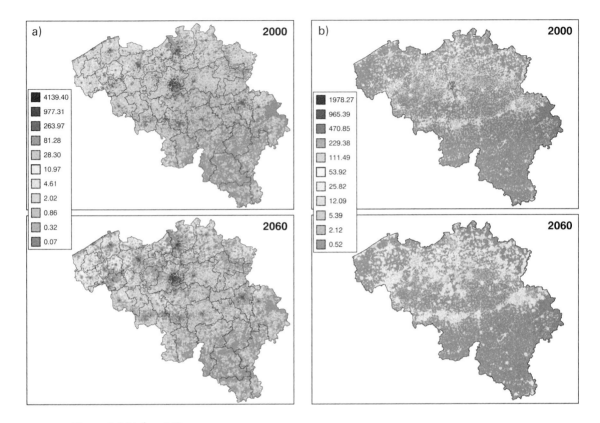

Figure 8.14 (plate 11)
Activity density 2000 (*top*); 2060 (*bottom*): (a) population; (b) commercial/industrial.

Flanders (White, Uljee, and Engelen, 2012). It is interesting to note that both faster growth in Flanders and relatively more urban sprawl in Wallonia, which the model produces purely on the basis of internal dynamics, are indeed current trends in Belgium. Although it would be unwise to treat this output as a prediction of the future of Belgium, it is suggestive of the insights that can be provided by models implementing various scenarios.

The Belgian whole-country application was preliminary to a larger project that has as one component the development of a model of Flanders (together with Brussels) at 100 meters resolution, using a newly developed database for both population and economic activities in which those data are available at that resolution. The activity-based model will be used to support spatial planning by the Flanders Region with the aim of better managing urban growth, environmental protection, and the quality of the lived environment, as described in chapter 11. Currently, improved

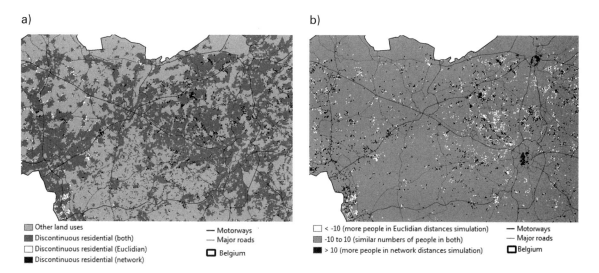

Figure 8.15
Effect of using network rather than Euclidian distances in the Antwerp-Brussels-Ghent triangle, 2060: (a) differences in land use; (b) differences in population density.

versions of the network distance module are being developed. Preliminary results show not only the effect of using network rather than Euclidian distances in the model (figure 8.15), but also the effect of both increasing congestion on the road network (figure 8.16) and the use of rail travel as an alternative transportation mode (figure 8.17). For legibility, only the Antwerp-Brussels-Ghent area is shown in these figures. When the model uses network rather than Euclidian distances, it predicts more residential land use in the Brussels-Antwerp corridor and less in the western part of the region (figure 8.16a). The differences are much less pronounced in the case of population densities, except that the use of network distances results in higher population densities in the central areas of both Antwerp and Brussels, but essentially no change at all in densities in the center of Ghent (figure 8.16b). If distances are treated as travel times solely during peak periods or solely during off-peak periods, rather than as some weighted average, then the results in terms of location patterns are fairly dramatic. The differences in land use are quite clear in figure 8.16a, with much more residential land use appearing in a ring around Ghent and much less in the Brussels periphery when peak period travel times are used (figure 8.16a). When we examine population densities, however, the picture is more nuanced, with a much larger area in the vicinity of the Brussels–Antwerp axis having lower densities, and a much larger area to the west having higher densities (figure 8.16b). Including the rail option in the time-distance calculations has only a very limited and localized effect on land use (figure 8.17a) and population density (figure 8.17b)

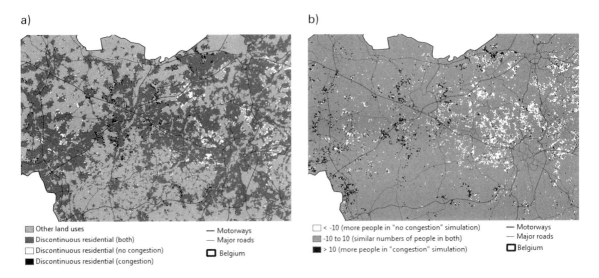

Figure 8.16
Effect of changes in effective network distances due to congestion in the Antwerp-Brussels-Ghent triangle, 2060: (a) differences in land use; (b) differences in population density.

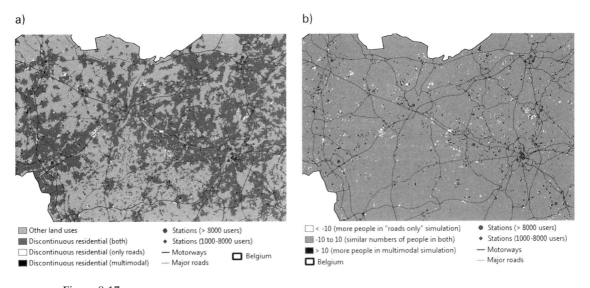

Figure 8.17
Effect of introducing the possibility of travel by rail in the Antwerp-Brussels-Ghent triangle, 2060: (a) differences in land use; (b) differences in population density.

patterns. All these comparisons are of results from simulations running a business-as-usual scenario for the year 2060, the strategic planning horizon for Flanders.

In general, the activity density maps corresponding to various planning-relevant scenarios are of more interest to planners than simple land use maps. Of even greater interest are various indicators and indicator maps produced from the land use and density maps. These will be discussed in greater detail in the context of an application of a MOLAND-class model to Flanders in chapter 11.

Our final example involves an adaptation of the activity-based model for use in a Belgian project on groundwater resources. The motivating concern is that climate change will increase the risk of groundwater drought, which could have serious consequences because the country depends on groundwater for industry, agriculture, and its municipal water supply. The project integrates the output of a regional climate model, a local meteorological simulation model, economic scenarios, land characteristics such as soils and slopes, an agricultural model, and a hydrological model involving runoff, infiltration, extraction, and groundwater flows. The agricultural model is central to this integration, providing the interface between climate and economics, on the one hand, and infiltration and runoff, which together determine groundwater recharge, on the other. Urban activities are also important because they may encroach on agricultural land or otherwise affect its use, and they also consume groundwater.

The agricultural model is a modified version of the activity-based CA. The mix of agricultural activities (crops and animals) on a cell is determined by expected yields (a function of soil type and weather), expected prices (exogenous), and the CA's neighborhood effect. The land use of an agricultural cell corresponds to the activity with the greatest expected value. Agricultural cells can have population as a secondary activity, which will affect yield, and an increase in population on them often precedes their conversion to an urban land use. Though not the case in the other applications, agricultural land uses are active in the Belgian groundwater application and have activities associated with them. Both urban and rural activities are modeled in the same CA, although the rules for the two are somewhat different—for example, the levels of agricultural activity, unlike those of urban activity, are unconstrained.

Densities of nonagricultural activities, whether on urban or rural land, are important not just because they affect productivity or yields. Since they are correlated with the proportion of a cell's land surface that is sealed or impervious (e.g., paved over), they can be used to predict the impervious fraction for future years, which is important in estimating the rates of infiltration and runoff. This use is indicative of the role played by the activity-based model in the larger project of which it is a part. Thus the model serves not only as an agricultural model, but also as a platform for integrating the other models and scenarios that, together, constitute a comprehensive model of the system. In general, many urgent environmental and planning problems can be effectively addressed only by integrated models embodying submodels drawn from a variety of fields. The technical problems of model integration are challenging but solvable. The institutional and social obstacles to effective collaboration are much more difficult to overcome.

The multiple activity variable grid CA-based model is essentially a parallel approach to addressing many of the same modeling problems that the linked models approach used in the MOLAND family of models is designed to deal with. But it does so more efficiently by collapsing the regional activity model into the CA-based land use model and thereby significantly reducing the number of parameters that must be calibrated. A fortunate consequence of this strategy is that the activities are modeled at the same high resolution as the land use. And although the predicted activity levels would not be meaningful at that resolution, when aggregated to somewhat larger units, they would be reliable enough to be useful for many purposes, and almost certainly as accurate as predictions made by any other technique currently available.

Of course, the quality of the predictions depends on the quality of both the model and its calibration. We can calibrate a model like the linked regional and CA-based models of the MOLAND class by calibrating each of the components separately, and then linking them and adjusting each calibration as necessary in an iterative procedure. If the models are not too tightly linked (and the regional and land use models are not), then their calibration process is effectively broken down into two relatively simple calibrations, and each model has been optimized to predict the phenomenon it deals with. In the case of a model like the activity-based CA, however, although there are fewer parameters to calibrate, and no need to mutually adjust two calibrations that were made separately, calibrating for good activity levels may make it impossible to achieve reasonable land use predictions, and vice versa. This may look like a calibration problem (and it certainly feels like one to the person doing the calibration). Such a trade-off is, however, a sign that the structure of the model is inappropriate. It should therefore be seen as an opportunity to improve the model. But here we anticipate the issues of calibration, validation, and verification that are discussed in chapter 9.

9
Issues of Calibration, Validation, and Methodology

There are trivial truths and the great truths. The opposite of a trivial truth is plainly false. The opposite of a great truth is also true.
—Niels Bohr

Bohr, in this well-known statement, was implying that the aim of science is to reduce great truths to trivialities. The question is, do our models represent science? Can we show that they are either true or false?

Calibration, validation, and verification of models of complex systems present large, open issues that are only beginning to be addressed by the modeling community. As long as models were, for the most part, "toy" models, designed to give only general insights into the behavior of a system, these issues were not pressing. But as models have become more specific to particular domains, with the goal of offering explanatory mechanisms or practical guidance to those involved in managing a particular system, the issues have become more urgent.

In the applications discussed in the previous chapters, the CA-based models were all calibrated and validated, but most end users gave these steps only perfunctory attention. The working assumption of most users is that the models are sound and will therefore produce reasonably reliable output; there is no reason to raise deep questions about validation. In the modeling community, however, we are not so sure. The basic concern, shared by many but often unspoken, is that it is not really possible to validate complex system models in a rigorous way. And although, to a degree, they are right, in a deeper sense, they are wrong. Complex system models belong to the realm of science; that their outcomes are typically ambiguous therefore poses a real problem if, as Bohr implied, the goal of science is to eliminate ambiguity and uncertainty. Paradoxically, the problem arises because the models are designed to capture the most basic aspects of reality—constant change and open futures—and open futures introduce ambiguity and uncertainty at the most fundamental level. Whatever other weaknesses they may have, our models are at least the right *kind* of model. In contrast, models like William Alonso's (1964) static equilibrium model of urban spatial structure, models that are unambiguously scientific in the conventional sense, give single predictions and are therefore easily testable. Of course, they are also deeply wrong.

Complex self-organizing systems are, by their very nature, both predictable and unpredictable. The fact that they are organized means that they have well-defined persisting structures with relatively stable properties. These structures have predictable behavior, at least locally and temporarily. On the other hand, these predictable structures come into existence and then disappear as the systems continue to organize themselves by passing through successive bifurcations. In general, the systems' choice of possible future structures is not predictable, at least not entirely. This is the problem of path dependence. Of course, the choices may often be influenced by appropriate interventions, and that is one of the major practical reasons to develop models of such systems.

Urban models, for example, give planners some ability to see the futures that are possible for the systems, and then, by means of "what if" experiments, to discover ways the systems might be nudged toward futures that are thought to be more desirable. But this very desirable quality of the models means that they are difficult to validate. By running a model many times, it is possible to map out the bifurcation points that the model encounters during the validation period, and thus reveal the various possible system states at the end of the validation period. But reality will show us only one outcome for that end date, and we have no way of knowing—other than intuition or the model—whether other possibilities existed then, and if so, what they were. Consequently, we are faced with a number of awkward possibilities of interpretation—awkward because we may have no way of deciding among them (see box 9.1). For example, if the model results are found to cluster around two distinct outcomes, this suggests that the model has discovered a bifurcation. If the data of the real systems fall within one of these clusters, then we need to decide whether the model is simply a bad model (or a good model badly calibrated) because it frequently predicts something quite different from what is observed, or whether, to the contrary, it is actually a good model that has been well calibrated and is revealing a real bifurcation in the system (figure 9.1). The only unambiguous outcome would be that the model fails to predict the empirical data at all, but, in that case, the model also fails the validation test.

Logically, the situation is no worse than it is in classical science, where it is also the case that it is possible in principle to disprove a hypothesis, but never to prove one true. On the other hand, classical science takes a positive result from a validation test in a well set up experiment to be relatively conclusive evidence that the hypothesis is true (but see Nuzzo, 2014) because only very unlikely and extraneous circumstances could lead to a false-positive result. In contrast, the very nature of self-organizing systems themselves ensures that both false positives and false negatives will be relatively frequent. With these systems, we are forced to recognize that,

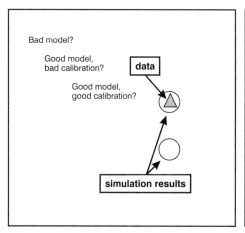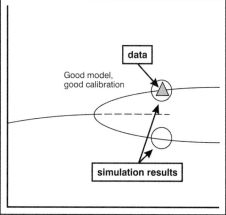

Figure 9.1
The ambiguity of simulation results. The model predicts two distinct possible outcomes, one of which coincides with the observed data (*left*). Is it correctly predicting both the data and the existence of a bifurcation (*right*), or is the unobserved cluster of outcomes the result of a bad calibration or a bad model because in reality there is no bifurcation?

Box 9.1
Overcalibration

> In addition to the possibilities mentioned in the main text, there is another that is even more problematic in terms of its practical consequences. If the model results are *always* close to the empirical data, then it is possible that there is no bifurcation and that the model is correct and well-calibrated. But it is more likely that the model is overcalibrated and would have predicted a bifurcation if it had been properly calibrated. This is especially likely to be the case when the predictions are of land use patterns, or of activity levels for small regions. In an excellent demonstration of this possibility, Daniel Brown and colleagues (2005) used an agent-based land use model to generate a series of land use maps for a region in Michigan. They treated these as a sample of all the possible landscapes that could occur if reality were rerun many times. The model revealed a bifurcation in that many of the maps showed a large cluster in the northwest, whereas others showed no cluster there, but rather one in the southeast. Next, they chose one of the maps with a cluster in the northwest to represent the "observed reality," that is, the single outcome that actually occurred. They then introduced a modeler who was clever enough to come up with a perfect model: it was identical to the one that generated the observed reality in the first place, as well as all the other possible realities. To calibrate the perfect model, the modeler used the only available data set, the "observed reality"—i.e., the map with the cluster in the northwest—to minimize the difference between the maps produced by the perfect model and the observed map. When the perfect model was run many times, it always generated a cluster in the northwest; thus the model looked very good. From our God-like perspective, however, we

Box 9.1 (continued)

know that it was wrong—that it was failing to reveal the other possibilities that could have occurred but did not—that is, the other branch of the bifurcation. Overcalibration transformed a perfect model into one that was erroneous and misleading.

It is difficult to avoid overcalibration because doing so means accepting a calibration that looks worse than it need be according to the objective measure used during calibration. One way to minimize the problem is to use a multicriterion, multiobjective procedure, which is more effective when at least one of the criteria has the property of stationarity. Overcalibration can be a serious issue in applications for planning or policy purposes. Since the future cannot be predicted precisely or in detail, one of the most basic and important uses of a model is to discover future possibilities inherent in the system, even if it cannot predict which one will actually occur. If some of the possibilities are more desirable than others, then policies can be implemented to make it more likely that one of the more desirable possibilities is the one that will actually happen. But, if the model does not predict those more desirable possibilities because it is overcalibrated, then the option of taking action to help make one of them happen is not available. If we end up on one branch of a bifurcation but would much prefer to be on the other, it is usually difficult, if not impossible, to make the jump. In physical terms, there is an energy barrier. Returning to the analogy of paddling our canoe upriver (figure 2.2), if we discover we have taken the wrong fork, we may have to portage over a mountain separating us from the river we want to be on. The difficulty of doing this is well illustrated in Werner Herzog's film *Fitzcarraldo*, in which a 320-ton steamship is hauled over a steep ridge to get it from one Amazon tributary to another (although in this case as well as in the actual nineteenth-century event that inspired the film, the herculean task was an intentional strategy to avoid impassable rapids rather than a desperate attempt to rectify a bad decision; see figure 9.1.1). For urban systems, the energy barrier may be measured by the economic costs of removing existing infrastructure to replace it with other facilities, as, for example, when cities like Seoul and Seattle decided to remove elevated highways and invest in other transport infrastructure. There were also, of course, major social and political costs involved.

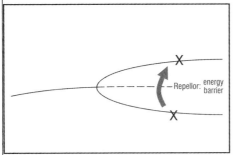 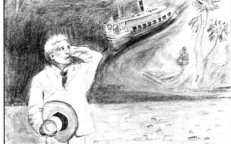

Figure 9.1.1
Crossing the great repellor (*left*); Brian "Fitzcarraldo" Fitzgerald and his steamship *Molly Aida* (*right*). Once past a bifurcation point it is difficult to reach the branch not chosen.

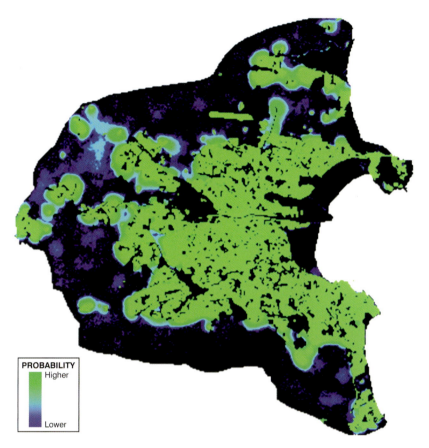

Plate 1 (figure 6.7)
Probability that a cell will be converted to an urban land use in Dublin simulation for 2008.

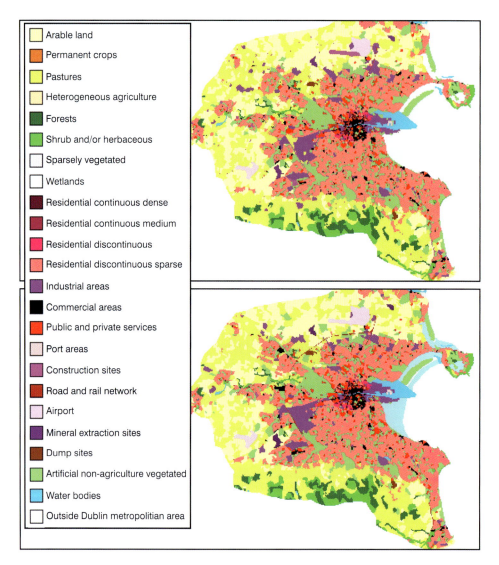

Plate 2 (figure 6.12)
Dublin application: (*top*) simulated land use, 1998; (*bottom*) actual land use, 1998.

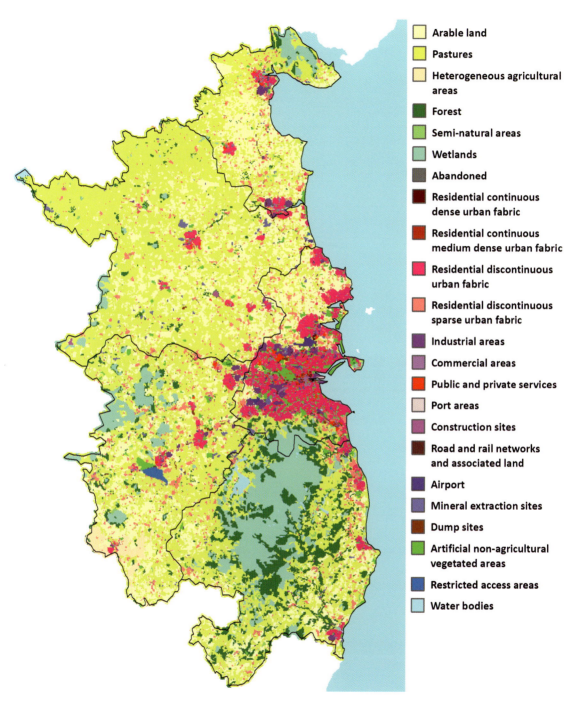

Plate 3 (figure 7.4)
Simulated land uses in GDR, 2026.

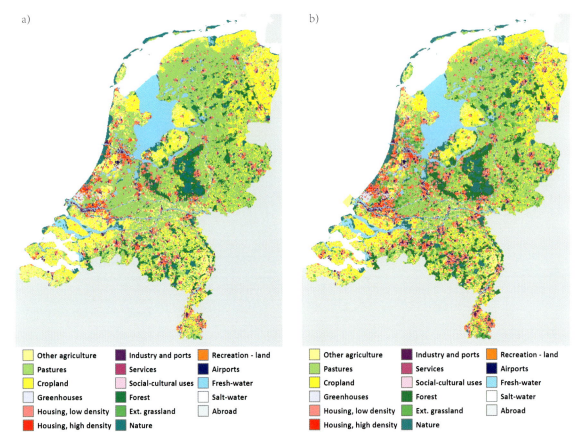

Plate 4 (figure 7.9)
Land use in Netherlands: (a) 2000 (actual); (b) 2030 (simulation). (Source: Netherlands National Institute for Health and the Environment [RIVM])

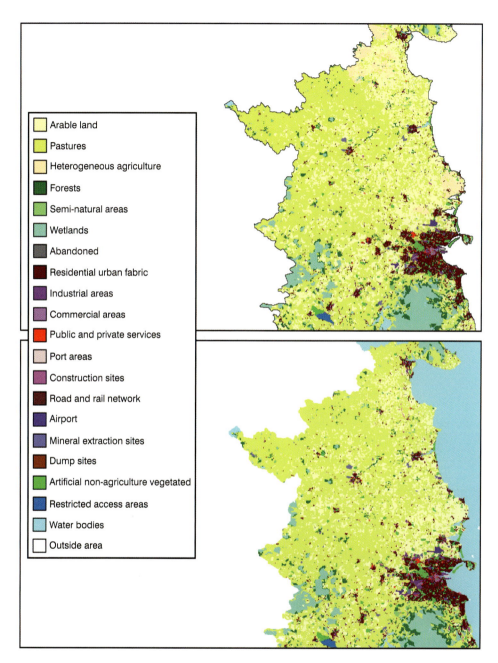

Plate 5 (figure 8.4)
Land use, Dublin, 2000: (*top*) simulated, using network distances; (*bottom*) actual.

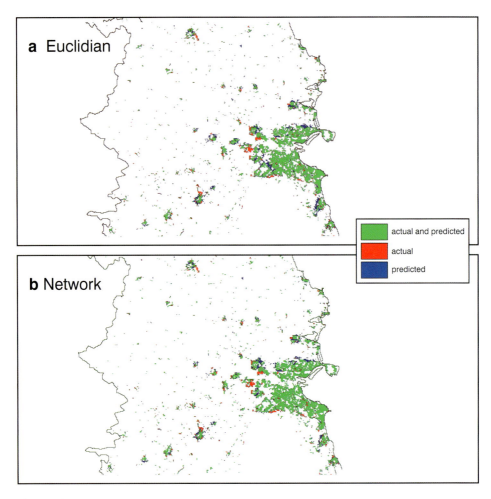

Plate 6 (figure 8.5)
Errors in simulated residential land use, Dublin, 2000: (*top*) simulation using Euclidian distances; (*bottom*) simulation using network distances.

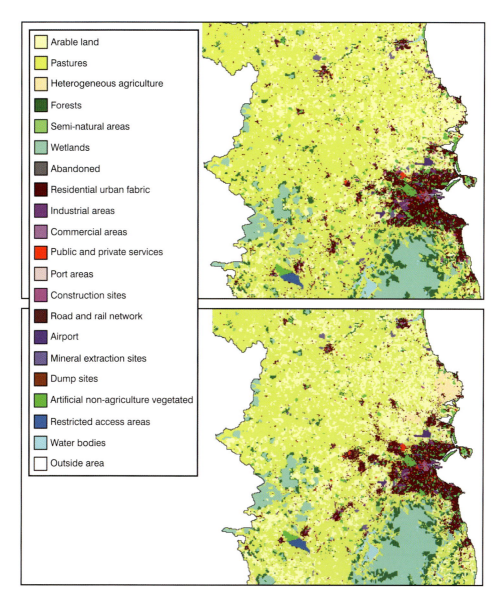

Plate 7 (figure 8.6)
Land use, Dublin, 2006: (*top*) actual; (*bottom*) simulated.

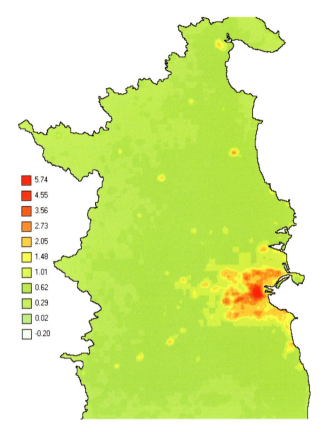

Plate 8 (figure 8.8)
Activity potential (population), Dublin, 2000, from simulation using network distances. Values are as calculated by equation 8.4.

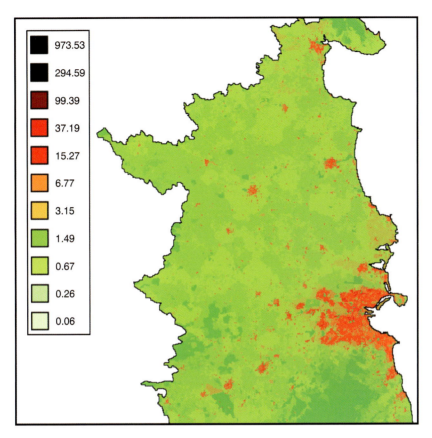

Plate 9 (figure 8.9)
Simulated population density, Dublin, 2000. Density is population per cell.

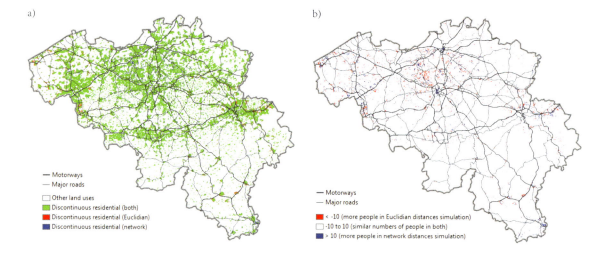

Plate 10 (figure 8.10)
Differences between Belgian simulations using network and Euclidian distances: (a) residential land use; (b) population density.

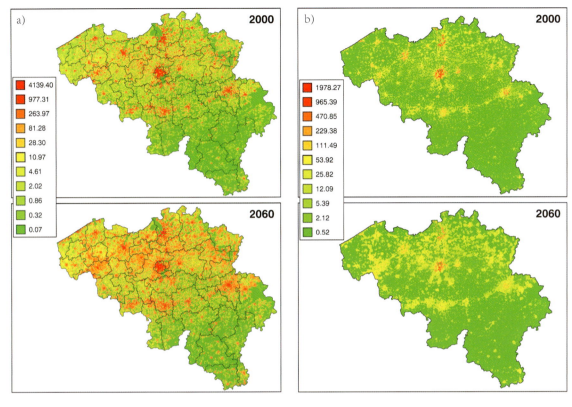

Plate 11 (figure 8.14)
Activity density 2000 (*top*); 2060 (*bottom*): (a) population; (b) commercial/industrial.

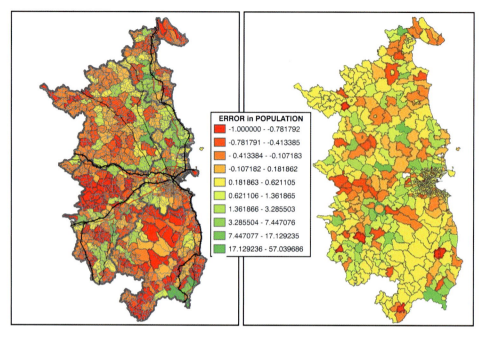

Plate 12 (figure 9.2)
Eliminating spatial autocorrelation in electoral district errors: (*left*) calibration optimizing population predictions at the county level that produced electoral district–level errors correlated with the transport network; (*right*) recalibration that eliminates the pattern in electoral district errors.

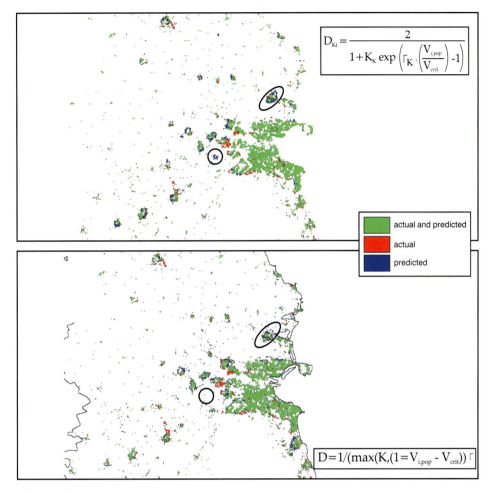

Plate 13 (figure 9.3)
Comparison of actual and predicted residential land use, Dublin, 2000, corresponding to two versions of the diseconomies equation as shown on figure panels. (*Bottom*) Version using the difference of potentials produces a better land use map (e.g., circled areas) and smaller errors in predicted county populations (RMSE = 3101) than does (*top*) the original version (RMSE = 5412).

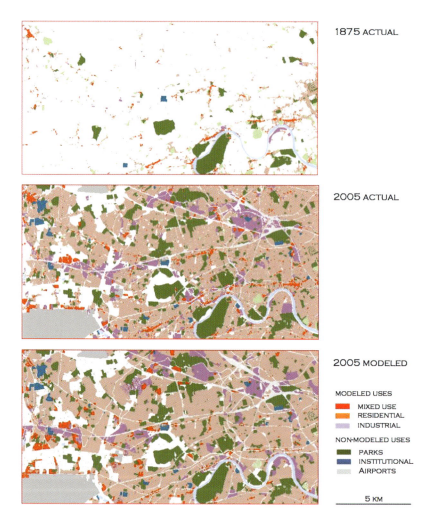

Plate 14 (figure 10.3)
Actual land use in west London, 1875 (*top*) and 2005 (*middle*); and simulated land use, 2005 (*bottom*), from the 1875–2005 simulation. (Simulation by Kiril Stanilov)

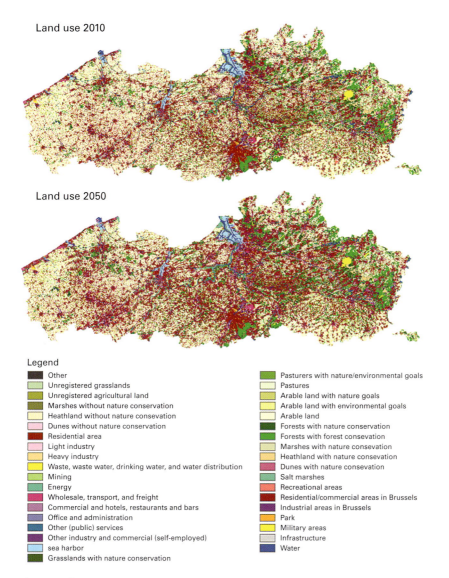

Plate 15 (figure 11.4)
Land use maps for Flanders and Brussels, 2010 (*top*); 2050 (*bottom*).

if we wish to do science, it will be a somewhat different kind of science because the phenomena we are dealing with are fundamentally different from those addressed by classical science. A different kind of science requires a different methodology, with different methodological standards. Instead of a few simple, elegant experiments, we will need many messy tests. And, instead of simple but strict standards, we will need multiple but loose ones.

A new methodology is emerging, but there are a number of problems that slow its progress. One of the most serious is a mindset that comes from classical science, and especially from technical fields like geographic information science (GIS) and remote sensing that are historically closely tied to modeling. In these fields, data and accuracy are both fundamentally important, as is testing to ensure accuracy. In modeling, these remain necessary, but they are of only secondary importance compared to how well the model captures the processes that drive the system being modeled. One way of determining whether the model represents the processes without relying on the same data that are used to calibrate and validate it is to take a reductionist approach and look at processes at a lower level than those being modeled. For example, to determine whether the influence functions are a reasonable representation of the aggregate behavior of individuals, we could look directly at the behavior of individuals who make locational decisions and see whether that behavior would collectively yield the influence functions. In human systems, if we go to the level of individual people, the relevant behavior is usually directly observable, and often relatively simple. This point will be developed further in chapter 10. Of course, to get some idea as to how well a model represents the processes being modeled, it is essential at some point to confront the model output with actual data. But placing too much importance on the data, or on the accuracy with which the model can reproduce the data, is likely to result in misjudging the quality of the model in the case of validation, or in overcalibrating it—a very serious problem (see box 9.1).

In order to avoid this trap, we must be guided by the basic reason for building the models in the first place: to understand the processes by which the system generates and transforms itself. This is the scientific goal. But the goal in applications is to use this understanding for predicting future possibilities in order to improve policy and planning. We do not plan for the past or present, the periods that are involved in calibration and validation; we plan for the future, for time horizons of ten or twenty years. Therefore, it is more important that the model predict the future correctly than that it perform well for past periods. This is the reason that split data sets are not useful in calibration and validation: both parts of a split data set, whether defined randomly or regionally, refer to a past time interval, whereas, for validation, we need data for a future period. The first methodological rule, then, is a paradoxical one: during empirical calibration and validation, modelers should give priority to the future—that is, to the period *after* the one represented by the data. Ton deNijs

(2009), who calibrated the application of the LOV (Environment Explorer) model to the Netherlands, is emphatic on this point: we model to understand the future, not the past, and calibration procedures should reflect this.

Calibration

The process of calibration itself raises several methodological issues that need to be addressed. Most notably, how do we design a calibration strategy that is appropriate for complex self-organizing systems, and how do we find appropriate standards and measures on which to base the calibration? The fact that complex systems are complex means that any adequate model of such a system, if it is not a toy model designed to investigate a specific property of the system, will itself necessarily be complex in certain respects, if only in its behavior. On the other hand, as the well-known expression has it, the best model is one that is as simple as possible, but no simpler. We believe that the models we have presented in the previous chapters satisfy this criterion. But because they are also designed as generic models to be applicable to a wide variety of urban and regional systems, they are more complex than they need to be for any particular application. Making a model's application as simple as possible but no simpler is the first task of the calibration process, which must eliminate as many parameters as possible by setting their values to zero, one or whatever value effectively removes them from the model. In many cases, eliminating parameters will have the effect of removing corresponding variables from equations or even eliminating functions or subroutines entirely.

Applying the rule of simplification, the top priority is to cull the sets of parameters that define the influence functions used to calculate the neighborhood effect. Each function is defined by up to eighteen parameters (including an inertia factor), and with N land uses in total, of which n are active, there can be up to $18nN$ parameters involved (these are the w_{khd} of equation 6.2). In the case of the UEP MOLAND application with twenty-three land use classes of which eight are active, that would be up to 3,312 parameters to specify the $nN = 184$ influence functions (influence functions are not defined for passive and fixed land uses). Working with that many influence functions would be difficult, to say the least, and the model would be unnecessarily complicated because, once calibrated, many of the functions would be found to have little effect. Therefore, the first step in calibrating the influence functions is to decide which ones are most likely to be significant and start the calibration using only those. The choice of which to include is a judgment that most modelers of urban and regional systems are well qualified to make on the basis of their domain knowledge combined with an examination of the relevant land use maps. After the calibration using the initial influence functions, errors in the simulated land use map might suggest that a few more influence functions should be added. In the end, an application with eight active land uses typically requires in the neighborhood of twenty influence functions, rather than 184. This still represents several hundred parameters, although, because they are essentially a clumsy way of defining fairly simple distance-decay functions, the effective number of parameters is much smaller.

In future versions of these CA-based models, it should be possible to further reduce the number of parameters in an influence function to four or five by replacing the weights with a mathematical function. A variable grid–based model would require two functions: one for the part of the curve corresponding to local influences and one for the long-distance interactions. We are currently investigating this possibility. In any case, whether by culling parameters during the calibration or by changing the model structurally to reduce the number of parameters, it is important to simplify the model as much as possible. Doing so not only makes it easier to work with; it also increases its Popperian "riskiness," and thereby increases our confidence that it is reliable, once it has been validated.

The influence functions are the heart of the CA-based models. Together with the accessibility parameters, they represent a generalization, to the cellular level, of the behavior of the underlying agents who are collectively structuring the urban system. The other parameters, such as suitabilities, essentially represent constraints on the dynamics generated by these parameters. An examination of the calibrated influence functions across a wide variety of applications around the world shows that they are almost always similar from one application to another suggesting that there is a degree of universality in the processes that structure cities and regions. This is a fascinating hypothesis that will be discussed further in chapter 10. But, at this stage, it is only a suggestion, not a result, because it has not been possible to make a rigorous comparison of the sets of influence functions. Several difficulties stand in the way, but the most fundamental one is that there is no assurance that the calibrations that we are comparing, made by different people using different methods and standards, are in fact comparable. Thus there is a real need for a standardized calibration procedure that would ensure not only better calibrations, but also comparable ones. An automatic calibration tool would serve this function well.

Automatic Calibration
Such a tool was developed for use with the integrated multiscale models like the UEP MOLAND model; it consists of two quite different calibration routines, one for the regional submodel and one for the CA submodel. Each submodel is calibrated independently by holding the parameters of the other constant; then each is recalibrated using the newly calibrated parameters of the other. The procedure is iterated several times; convergence is usually rapid because the links between the two submodels are relatively weak. The calibration routine for the regional submodel, though relatively conventional, is quite efficient, involving a golden mean search for optimal parameter

values and using the sum of squared errors of regional activity levels as the optimization criterion (van Loon, 2004; Engelen et al., 2005; de Nijs, 2009).

The automatic calibration of the CA submodel, on the other hand, is slower and more problematic. Although calibration of a two-state (urban, rural) CA-based land use model is relatively straightforward, once multiple active land uses are admitted, the calibration problem becomes much more difficult, and introducing a stochastic perturbation complicates matters further (Straatman, White, and Engelen, 2004; Engelen et al., 2005). The calibration procedure would normally focus on the cells with the largest discrepancy between the predicted deterministic transition potential and the actual land use and would then adjust the neighborhood influence functions to reduce the difference. The largest discrepancies, however, are usually due to the stochastic perturbation. The cells with these discrepancies must therefore be ignored or the calibration routine will, in effect, tune the parameters to predict a series of random numbers—hardly an efficient strategy.

The major problem with automatic calibration is that, even though the calibrated influence functions generally produce reasonably good land use maps when tested against the actual land use, they are occasionally wrong in terms of what is known about attraction and repulsion effects among land uses. For example, the automatic calibration might produce influence functions for residential land use that give good results, but the dominant function of the set might be one representing residential as being repelled by agricultural land use. This rule would force residential land use to the periphery of the urban area, the correct location, because its influence functions are too weak for it to be able to displace other urban land uses in order to get farther away from agriculture. Another, more plausible, influence function, however, representing residential land use as being most strongly attracted to other residential land, would also have the effect of locating residential land on the periphery of the city. Thus when two quite different influence functions have approximately the same effect, the automatic calibration routine may find the wrong one. This provides a good example of the limitation of automatic calibration tools. They may be able to tune the model to give good results over a test period, but for the wrong reasons. And if the model is wrong, regardless of how good the results of the calibration and validation seem, when it is run into the future—its proper use and purpose—the results will not be reliable.

At present, then, the automatic routine is not a stand-alone solution to the calibration problem. It can only be used with expert supervision, both to specify which of the possible influence functions should be used in the application and therefore calibrated, and to intervene if the routine begins to produce aberrant influence functions. Furthermore, at present, fine-tuning is always necessary because the optimization criterion is too simple—typically, a global measure of the similarity of the simulated and actual land use maps. But such measures, though convenient to use, are usually not very appropriate because most of them are not pattern based. This is a major problem (see box 9.2). Nevertheless, developing a reliable automatic calibration tool is a goal worth pursuing for several reasons. From the modeler's perspective, the most important one is humanitarian: a sound automatic procedure would put an end to days and weeks of tedious, Sisyphus-like labor. But an automatic procedure would also be useful scientifically. First, it would facilitate a less biased comparison of applications, and thus make it possible to determine whether the processes that generate the spatial structure of cities have universal characteristics. Second, it would probably lead to a much greater number of applications, especially by organizations that would not otherwise have the expertise to implement their own applications. Being able to click "calibrate" and have a model ready to use an hour later would certainly be simpler and much less expensive than hiring a consultant to do the job. And having a much larger sample of applications with standardized calibrations would increase the scientific value of the model as a theory-building tool.

Box 9.2
New Approaches to Map Comparison

> Kappa is a cell-based technique that compares the land use on two maps cell by cell to determine the level of agreement; it takes into account the fact that a certain number of cells will have the same land use simply by chance, especially in the case of the most common land use classes. It is popular because it summarizes the similarity of two maps in a single global measure; it is also easy to calculate from a contingency matrix. There were several technical problems with Kappa as it was originally proposed, but these have recently been corrected by R. Gil Pontius (2000, 2002) and Alex Hagen-Zanker (2008). Nevertheless, Kappa remains fundamentally inappropriate as the primary map comparison technique for simulation modeling because, as a cell-based technique, it is not spatial. Thus it assigns the same weight to small locational errors (e.g., a residential cell in the simulated map displaced one cell from the location of a residential cell in the actual map) that it does to large displacements, and the same significance to small classification errors (e.g., medium dense residential land use simulated on a cell that actually has dense residential land use) that it does to major ones (e.g., industry rather than residential).
>
> Hagen-Zanker and colleagues (Hagen-Zanker, 2008; Hagen-Zanker, Straatman, and Uljee, 2005; Hagen, 2003) have developed a variant version, fuzzy Kappa, that solves these particular problems by introducing a local window for evaluating disagreements between the maps. The window, in effect, adds a spatial dimension to Kappa, and as a result fuzzy Kappa is able to produce a cell space map of fuzzy similarity values, as well as a variety of similar maps showing various aspects of disagreement, such as disagreement due to omission (the land use is absent where it should be present) or to commission (the land use is present where it should not be) for various land use classes. Because the window is relatively small, however, structural similarities on all but the most local

Box 9.2 (continued)

scale are missed. Nevertheless, in introducing space and disaggregating the sources of similarity, the fuzzy Kappa approach represents a significant conceptual advance toward developing a useful tool for analyzing simulation results as they are expressed in a land use map. The fuzzy Kappa statistic itself, the measure of global similarity, can usefully be substituted for Kappa as a calibration objective. In most applications, however, it gives values that are similar to those of Kappa, which suggests that it is not capturing as much of the land use morphology as would be desirable.

Conrad Power, Alvin Simms, and Roger White (2001) introduced a polygon-based map comparison technique that compares two maps on the basis of their land use patterns rather than their cell-by-cell agreement. Like fuzzy Kappa, it is developed in a fuzzy logic framework. As implemented, it compares overlapping polygons on the basis of their degree of overlap, land use, and size, but it is possible to include other measures of polygon similarity, such as various shape measures. The technique produces a global similarity statistic, and, like fuzzy Kappa, it also gives a map showing degree of similarity.

The fuzzy Kappa and fuzzy polygon matching techniques were both developed in response to the need for better map comparison tools that arose with the advent of high-resolution CA-based land use models capable of producing realistic patterns. They are just a beginning, however. Alex Hagen-Zanker and Gilles Lajoie have continued to make progress in this area by developing a neighborhood-based approach, by implementing a method for creating appropriate neutral models of landscape change, and by creating a technique for integrating several map comparison criteria using wavelet analysis (Hagen-Zanker and Lajoie, 2008; Hagen-Zanker, 2008). Some map comparison techniques are appropriate for categorical data and others, for numerical data. The latter are useful for comparing maps of activity, or maps of the probability that a particular land use will occur. These techniques and others are collected in the Map Comparison Kit software, available for free download (http://mck.riks.nl/software).

Kappa and its variations, as well as the other techniques developed by Hagen-Zanker and Power, are metrics that specifically *compare* maps: they cannot be applied to a single map. Other metrics, however, designed to characterize a single map, can also be used to compare maps. The fractal dimensions discussed in chapter 5 are an example: used to calibrate the models in chapters 6–8, they have also been used to validate models by comparing the cluster size–frequency dimension or the radial dimension of the simulated map with the corresponding dimension of the reference map. Various patch-based metrics included in the FRAGSTATS package (McGarigalet al., 2002), widely used in landscape ecology, are another example. They characterize individual maps in terms of a global value for each metric, but these values can be compared with those of another map—even a map of a different area, which is not the case with true map comparison techniques. Patch-based metrics have occasionally been used to characterize the output of the CA-based land use models for planning purposes (Petrov et al., 2013; Agostinho, 2007), but they could also be incorporated directly into Power's fuzzy polygon-based technique mentioned above and thus become one criterion in a multicriterion map comparison technique.

Comparing Quantities and Comparing Maps

Calibration and validation depend on being able to compare the output of the model with measures of the real system. Although this sounds like an opportunity to bring in statistical techniques, the conventional statistical tests with their associated significance levels are, for the most part, either inapplicable or misleading; at best, they can be used descriptively. Most statistical hypothesis-testing techniques were developed for simple situations arising from known probability distributions. In more complex situations, where a multivariate analysis is required, causal variables must be independent of one another; otherwise, the derived parameter values and associated p-values are not well defined. But because the defining characteristic of the systems we are working with is feedback, the variables are always linked to one another through a complex causal network. In any case, researchers have increasingly come to realize that conventional inferential statistics are useful in an exploratory role but not in a confirmatory one (Nuzzo, 2014), that they are not as reliable as once thought, and that p-values do not in fact tell us much about the underlying reality.

In the case of regional activity levels, it is relatively easy to compare the output of a model with measures of a real system. An error measurement can be calculated for each region, and a global measure like the sum of squares of errors is a convenient summary statistic. Many calibrations, and essentially all automatic calibrations, use the global measure as the single objective to be optimized during the calibration and the only standard by which the validation is judged. Although it is always useful to have an overall measure of the state of the system, to rely exclusively on a global measure is not a good strategy because, by its very nature, such a measure hides problems with calibration and prevents qualifications to validation. For example, in an application where one region has much more activity than any other, or even, as in the case of the Greater Dublin Region (GDR), more than all other regions combined (County Dublin has twice the population of the other four counties combined), calibrating to minimize the sum of squares of errors (SSE) will lead to a result where regions have similar-sized absolute errors. But this means that the percentage errors will typically be much larger for the regions with less activity, whereas, in a region like the GDR, end users may prefer to have better predictions for the peripheral counties, where much of the future growth will occur, even if the error for County Dublin has to be slightly larger. In the case of the activity-based variable grid model, there is an additional complication. Since the simulation results can be aggregated to any set of regions, the error measurements used in calibration and validation can also be calculated for any set of regions. In practice, it is common to use only one set, but cutting this corner is not always a good idea. Thus, in early tests of the activity-based approach on data for the Greater Dublin Region, calibration and validation were carried out at the level of counties. But when the errors were

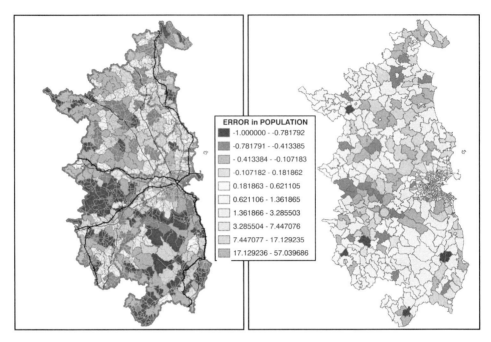

Figure 9.2 (plate 12)
Eliminating spatial autocorrelation in electoral district errors: (*left*) a calibration optimizing population predictions at the county level that produced errors correlated with the transport network at the electoral district level; (*right*) a recalibration that eliminates the pattern in electoral district errors.

examined at the much higher resolution of the 629 electoral district regions, it was found that they were correlated with major transportation corridors, indicating that the calibration was not optimal. A further calibration was carried out to eliminate this correlation, at the cost of a very slight degradation in model performance at the county level (figure 9.2; plate 12).

The application of the activity-based model to the GDR also gives us an example of how the need to optimize several measures at the same time may move the calibration procedure into the realm of model verification (we use the term *verification* here to refer to the question of whether the structure of the model, not just the set of parameter values, is sound). During the calibration of an earlier version of the model, one using a different equation for the diseconomies effect, there was always a trade-off between optimizing the population distribution (as measured by county populations) and optimizing the land use (as measured by the number of cells of residential land use in each county): it was possible to calibrate for a low error level in either one of these, but not in both. With a compromise calibration that left both population and land use with moderate error levels, a comparison of the simulated with the actual land use map for 2000 showed too much growth of residential land use around towns just beyond the urbanized area of Dublin, and too little growth on the periphery of Dublin itself (figure 9.3, bottom; plate 13). Changing the form of the equation representing the diseconomies effect to the difference of potentials version essentially eliminated the trade-off in the calibration, so that a single set of parameter values served to optimize both population distribution and land use, and at the same time reduced, but did not eliminate, the problem of wrongly located residential land in the Dublin area (figure 9.3, top; plate 13).

This improvement in the model structure was only possible because the same model predicts both land use and activities. In an approach using linked models, like the MOLAND model, where the links are relatively weak, the calibrations for both land use and activities can be optimized independently, and so it is less likely that structural problems will be revealed. We are benefiting here from Popper's principle of riskiness, which holds that the less probable it is, a priori, that a prediction will be true, the more confidence we can have in the model (or theory) making it if the prediction turns out to be true. The activity-based model is more risky because it predicts two quantities—population and land use—whereas the two submodels of MOLAND predict only one each. The earlier version of the riskier model failed (though not very seriously), and that failure provided the information necessary to improve the specification of the model.

The lesson from these examples is that calibration and validation of activities should almost always take a multicriterion, multiobjective approach, where trade-offs between objectives are explicit and can be adjusted to reflect the needs of the end user. A multiobjective approach also tends to bring balance to a calibration, and that in turn makes it less likely that the model, when run beyond the calibration period and into the future, will drift into extreme and unrealistic behavior. This is especially the case when one or more of the objectives have been shown to have a high degree of stationarity, like the cluster size–frequency distribution. Future progress toward minimizing the problem of overcalibration will depend in part on identifying more criteria that are relatively stable through time.

In the case of land use, a multicriterion, multiobjective approach is essential, although it is not entirely clear what the criteria and objectives should be. The problem is difficult because calibration and validation with respect to land use involve comparing a map produced by the simulation with an actual land use map for the same year, and there are potentially a great many criteria that could be used as a standard for comparison. Which ones should be used in any particular application will depend to a considerable extent on the purpose of the application: for example, in many ecological contexts, and some urban ones, it might be desirable to maximize patchiness or the availability of edges, whereas, for a model that is to be used in a number of applications with different purposes, a more generic criterion

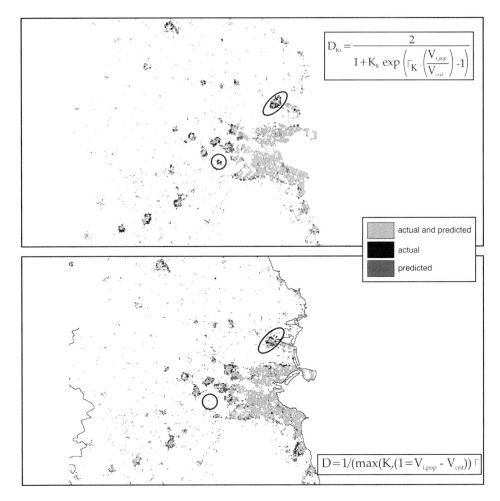

Figure 9.3 (plate 13)
Comparison of actual and predicted residential land use, Dublin, 2000, corresponding to two versions of the diseconomies equation as shown on figure panels. (*Bottom*) Version using the difference of potentials produces a better land use map (e.g., circled areas) and smaller errors in predicted county populations (RMSE = 3101) than does (*top*) the original version (RMSE = 5412).

would be appropriate. Decisions like these are only possible if a variety of different criteria have been both identified and incorporated into the map analysis tools. But it is only recently that new map comparison techniques based on appropriate criteria have even begun to be developed (see box 9.2).

The most commonly used method of map comparison, the Kappa statistic, borrowed from the remote sensing community, is not really appropriate for most applications involving land use modeling. Although, in recent years, the Kappa technique has been improved in various ways and has even acquired a local spatial element (Pontius 2000, 2002; Hagen-Zanker, 2008), its capabilities are still quite limited compared to those required to capture the range of qualities and patterns that can be seen in a land use map. Several approaches have been developed that give map comparisons based on patterns (Power, Simms, and White, 2001), pattern elements (McGarigal et al., 2002), and multiple criteria (Hagen-Zanker, 2008). And it is now accepted practice to characterize and then compare maps on the basis of the cluster size–frequency and radial dimensions. Nevertheless, because different processes reflect and respond to different landscape characteristics, it would be useful to have comparison metrics based on other criteria, and, as we model more processes, we will need to have new metrics that are appropriate to them.

The ultimate goal is to have an array of tools for making objective comparisons of maps, tools designed to capture the morphological features that we consider important when we look at a map. But, as Hagen-Zanker points out, it "is somehow ironic that with the purpose of making the validation of geosimulation models less dependent on subjective visual assessment and expert judgment, metrics are developed that are judged by essentially the same standard. Rather than eliminating subjectivity altogether, the border between objectivity and subjectivity has been redrawn" (Hagen-Zanker, 2008, p.162). Of course, there are good reasons for wanting objective metrics even if they do ultimately rest on subjective foundations. They are necessary for procedures like automatic calibration, and, by standardizing map characterizations and comparisons, they make it easier to identify universal characteristics in urban structure and the processes that generate them.

There is a way to move the border between subjectivity and objectivity even further back, and that is to use metrics that have been shown to correlate with urban qualities that are important in some respect, such as quality of life or economic growth. For example, it has been suggested by practitioners of the new urbanism that mixed-use neighborhoods promote walking, and health researchers have linked walking to lower obesity levels. Therefore, if we are using a land use model to assess various planning options, and one of the objectives is to encourage an urban form that will lead to lower obesity rates, then we should use the measure of local urban form that is most highly correlated with obesity rates. This is the sort of reasoning that underlies the selection of the FRAGSTATS metrics: they are all measures of landscape characteristics thought to be important for the functioning of ecosystems. The recent work by Xia Li and colleagues (2013) using landscape metrics as the evaluation criteria for calibrating a CA-based land use model by means of a genetic algorithm supports this conclusion. They find that use of landscape metrics gives superior results in validation tests. And recent research undertaken by Isabelle Thomas, Pierre Frankhauser, and others in the European network investigating the correlation of the fractal properties of cities with social, cultural, and economic characteristics is leading in the same direction (de Keersmaecker, Frankhauser, and Thomas, 2003; Thomas, Frankhauser, and Biernacki, 2008; Thomas, Tannier, and Frankhauser, 2008; Thomas et al., 2010). Our simulation models will be more relevant to end users once they are calibrated and evaluated using metrics that have been shown to be appropriate to the purpose of the application.

Methodology and Epistemology

The models discussed in this book are conceived of as scientific models, intended to capture in a generalized way the actual processes by which cities and regions structure and restructure themselves as they grow. As models of self-organizing systems, they are designed to show us how those processes generate a variety of urban forms under various circumstances. In other words, they are experimental tools for investigating the dynamical nature of cities and regions. In that sense they are a continuation by other means of classical location theory, which also sought to give a scientific explanation of spatial structure.

But they are also intended to function as applied models, models that can be used as tools by planners. In this role, they need to be highly detailed and able to provide output tailored to specific end-user requirements. There is a tension between these two reasons for modeling, but it can be an extremely fruitful tension. Scientific models typically start out as toy models. The first version of the CA-based land use model described in chapter 6 was essentially a toy model, with four land uses on a homogeneous cell space. Toy models can be very useful for exploring basic principles and understanding how they operate in the absence of complications; they serve as a virtual laboratory. But urban and regional systems are not only complex; they are also irreducibly complicated—they involve many factors in an essential way. Consequently, for a model to be an adequate representation of such a system, it must also be complicated to a certain degree. At a minimum, it must contain representations of the important subsystems, such as the economic, demographic, transportation, and natural systems. Furthermore, these must be reasonable, not pro forma, representations. Practical applications, where end-user needs must be satisfied, force the initial toy scientific model to evolve into a model that is as complicated as necessary to represent an urban system realistically. In other words, we are forced to build serious models rather than toys. It is these realistic models that have the greatest scientific utility, because they permit us to go beyond the level of understanding that is possible with toy models. Getting an application right amounts to an extended confrontation of the model with reality—an empirical grounding that is both multifaceted and detailed.

Not only does the scientific utility of the models increase dramatically when they become operational applied models; the end users also benefit from the fact that these models are, first of all, scientific ones. End users, unlike modelers in validation mode, are not interested in hindcasting; they are interested in prediction, in using the models for "what if" experiments. The reliability of a model's output is therefore of primary importance to them: the more reliable the predictions, the more useful the model, for if the output is *not* reliable, using the model can result in bad policy. But, as a scientific model, the model must be a good representation of the system it is modeling; and if it is, it is more likely to be reliable. The real danger comes when applied and scientific models are developed separately. The applied models are likely to be too simple, in order to make them easy to set up and use, and they may be less rigorously validated. They are also likely to be overcalibrated since overcalibration maximizes the measure of goodness of fit and makes the model look more reliable than it is, and this leads to overconfidence in the results.

The key to a successful methodology for understanding complex self-organizing systems seems to be multiplicity. A model that makes predictions about several phenomena using a single formal mechanism because it is riskier can be accepted with greater confidence once it has received empirical support. A model that has been calibrated and validated using multiple criteria and objectives is better supported and more likely to be an unbiased representation of the system it is modeling—again, in part, as a consequence of the riskiness principle. A model that has been successfully applied in multiple and varying situations is more likely to be a faithful representation of the type of system it is being applied to. And, finally, multiple overlapping models tell us more about a system than any single model, and the predictions and generalizations that are supported by more than one model are more robust, and therefore more likely to be true.

The multiplicity of successful applications is particularly important because not only does it constitute a relatively difficult test of a model, but it also tells us that all the cases to which the model was applied constitute instances of a single generic system. The successful applications of the linked regional CA-based model to Dublin, Flanders, the Netherlands, and Puerto Rico together indicate that the same underlying processes are generating the spatial structure in both cities and countries. We may treat this conclusion as a hypothesis in a theory of the spatial structure of cities and regions, to be further tested through more applications, but we may also increase our confidence in it by showing that other types of models lead to the same conclusion. In both cases, we are relying on the methodological principle of multiplicity.

Scientists traditionally value simplicity and precision. These are also important qualities in both urban and regional modeling and in the emerging science of urban systems. In general, however, these two qualities are less important than in the hard sciences, and in some cases, as we have seen, they can be counterproductive: too much precision during calibration, for example, can result in overcalibration. And simplification may well be the bigger threat: it results in toy models, and the majority of the hundreds of CA-based land use models that have been published over the last quarter century are of this sort. Although many of these models have introduced interesting variations on the CA approach, collectively, they have given us very few additional insights into the nature of urban and regional systems and the processes that drive them, and, individually, few of them are of any use in practical applications.

The proliferation of such models is no doubt partly due to the difficulties involved in creating large, complicated, but realistic models, but it is also likely to be due to the belief that scientific models must be simple and elegant. The urban modeling community could learn much from the example of atmospheric circulation models. In principle, the behavior of what is essentially a simple physical system with complex dynamics can be completely explained by the relevant laws of physics. Indeed, Edward Lorenz (1963) rediscovered the mathematical phenomenon of deterministic chaotic dynamics while experimenting with a simple, three-equation model of the atmosphere, one that embodied essentially all the physics necessary to understand its dynamics. Yet, as long as atmospheric scientists limited themselves to simple models, they were unable either to show exactly how various atmospheric phenomena emerged or to accurately predict the weather. It was not until they made their models much more complicated by disaggregating them spatially to ever higher resolutions, integrating other phenomena such as clouds and aerosols, and coupling them to other models, in particular, oceanic circulation models, that they achieved real success. The large complicated models gave them a much deeper scientific understanding of what is going on in the atmosphere and, as a consequence, they also yielded the practical benefit of more accurate weather forecasts.

Of course, urban systems are more complex than the atmosphere. Up to a point, their dynamics are analogous to those of the atmosphere (Warntz, 1965, 1967; Coffey, 1981), which is why analogous dynamical models can be used to understand both systems. But, unlike the atmosphere, urban systems are created, maintained, and changed by human agents who have characteristics not shared by molecules of nitrogen and oxygen. In particular, people change the rules of the game, whereas the molecules in the atmosphere cannot change the laws of physics. To account fully for the creative role of people in an urban system would require not just an agent-based model, but also an evolutionary model in which new types of agents emerged endogenously. This is necessary because people create new kinds of agents, like governments and corporations, that act in the system, and because they also change both their own behavioral rules and those of the agents they create. In other words, they change the very structure of the systems we are trying to model. It is quite possible to design evolutionary models (e.g., Straatman, White, and Banzhaf, 2008), but, to this point, none have been designed for urban systems. The fact that these rule-changing and evolutionary phenomena are not included in our models limits both the prediction horizon of the models and our ability to estimate their future degree of predictability because evolutionary phenomena undermine stationarity. But stationarity is never completely lost, so there is always some predictability. Multiple applications of a variety of models over longer time spans should increase our knowledge of stationarity in urban systems and improve our ability to find it.

In the context of complex dynamics complicated by structural changes to the system, no single test or result of a model is ever really conclusive, and many are not much more than suggestive. But, cumulatively, they result in a winnowing of both models and the generalizations suggested by the models; thus we are left with a set of models in which we have a substantial degree of confidence and a set of general results that we can treat as the basis of a theory of urban and regional systems. This messy process of conjectures and refutations—of building, testing, using, modifying, and occasionally discarding models—amounts, in fact, to a methodology based on evolutionary principles. Given that we are dealing with systems that are evolving by moving through a tree of bifurcating possibilities, an evolutionary methodology is probably the only possible one. It would replace a methodology based on the logic of definitive tests.

The development of an evolutionary methodology is a pragmatic response to urgent problems. At present, it is happening on an ad hoc and somewhat covert basis. Modelers drop old approaches that seem irrelevant or impractical and find new ones, but they usually do not call attention to the process. They fear that when they adopt practices that deviate from the conventional ones they leave their work open to the criticism that it does not meet generally accepted scientific standards. This fear is justified: for example, we know of a case where a simulation model has been rejected in favor of a regression-based approach, which comes with tests of significance and therefore can apparently be trusted. The value of having an explicit, overarching methodology appropriate to complex self-organizing systems is that it would both legitimate current practice and accelerate the development of new methods. Having a general methodological framework in place would act as an invitation to researchers to develop it further. A coherent methodology is, however, more than a collection of practices; it must have an appropriate philosophical framework. Complex self-organizing systems have received considerable attention of a philosophical nature, and this is useful support for the emerging evolutionary methodology. But both the conventional philosophy of science and the epistemology that underlies it remain not just inappropriate, but antagonistic.

Mainstream scientific epistemology is essentially an epistemology of physics, and it attempts to show how knowledge can be justified as certain. The position that the role of epistemology is to show how knowledge can be known to be certain, which goes back to the roots of Western philosophy, is pervasive and nearly universal—there are virtually no alternatives in the literature. Consequently, it exerts a powerful influence. It underpins the orthodox methodology of science that developed in concert with the physical sciences. This methodology calls for theories to be mapped onto mathematics or logic to show that they are free of contradiction, and then for quantified empirical tests of the theories so that confidence levels can be established. Such a strategy has not, however, worked so well in the social sciences. Only in economics are theories typically formalized mathematically, but these theories are rarely tested empirically. In the softer social sciences, such as sociology or human geography, to the limited extent that they still consider themselves to be sciences, an empirical approach based on inferential statistics is considered the gold standard; theories, if they exist at all, are rarely, if ever, formalized.

In any case, the contradiction-free status of mathematics and logic is possible only because they are ideal, formal systems without time; thus the only systems that can be mapped into them are those in which time can be eliminated. This is not a problem for most of physics: the laws are time reversible, which means, in effect, that they are independent of time (Prigogine,1997; Prigogine and Stengers, 1979, 1984; Smolin, 2013). The exception is in thermodynamics, where time is not reversible and cannot be eliminated, and, as we saw in chapter 2, it is thermodynamic systems that we are concerned with. They are also the systems that led to the development of an alternative to the prevailing philosophical paradigm: evolutionary epistemology.

A relatively recent development in the philosophy of science, evolutionary epistemology grew out of the later work of Karl Popper (1982) and was further developed by Donald Campbell (1987) and W. W. Bartley (1987), among others. It proposes an epistemology that is appropriate not only for the physical sciences, but also—and especially—for the biological and social sciences. Its basic position is that the creation of knowledge is an evolutionary process, a process embedded in time, and therefore one whose description cannot be mapped into a timeless formal system like mathematics or logic (although the description may contain mathematical and logical expressions). Consequently, and contrary to the standard epistemology, philosophers cannot have a God-like, global view of knowledge creation from outside time. Furthermore, the new epistemology takes the position that knowledge creation is not just analogous to biological evolution; biological evolution is itself knowledge creation. This position may seem radical. Bartley (1987) points out that knowledge about the environment has been accumulating since life first appeared. It is encoded endosomatically in the organisms themselves. The appearance of new species represents the accumulation of new knowledge about the system, as well as a change in the system itself. As the system evolves, some knowledge becomes false and is eliminated through extinction.

On the other hand, the embodiment of knowledge can also be more explicit. As Robert Rosen (1991) has pointed out, a universal characteristic of life seems to be that any living entity embodies a model of itself and its relationship with its environment. At the most basic level, an organism's DNA may be understood to encode such a model: the DNA consists of instructions for generating the organism, and the organism so created always has the means for detecting relevant features of its environment and responding to them in appropriate ways. But more evolved species have additional means for modeling themselves and their environment, including, in our own case, computer-based simulation models. In other words, every organism knows something about itself and its environment, and some know more than others. As we move from simple life-forms like bacteria to more complex ones like ourselves, the nature of the knowing becomes less implicit and more explicit, and the means for knowing become more elaborate and varied. In consequence, the number and variety of things that can be known also tend to increase.

This is the basic premise of evolutionary epistemology: that both what can be known and the way it can be known depend on the evolutionary history of the organism and its environment. It has immediate implications for our knowledge of complex systems. Normally, it is assumed that, in principle, *all* possible branches of a bifurcation tree can be mapped. But evolutionary epistemology implies that this is not the case. As we move farther out on the branches stemming from branch A of a bifurcation tree, it becomes more difficult to know anything about the structure of the branches stemming from branch B. More powerful theory may tell us more about the structure of subtree B, but we can in principle know less about it than we can about the structure of subtree A because we will lack some necessary means of knowing that we would have acquired had we taken branch B in the first place. From another point of view, it is those unknown means of knowing which would have been one of the causes of existence of the further branches of B. In a sense, this is an example of Stuart Kauffman's (1994) finding that the shape of the fitness landscape itself depends on the behavior of the species adapting on it.

With our species, knowledge is encoded not only endosomatically but also externally, in devices such as books and computers. This is Popper's "World 3," and, as he points out, this knowledge is no less a part of the natural world than the prehuman knowledge encoded in all living organisms, and it impacts the world just as the appearance of new species does (Popper, 1982). Furthermore, this explicit knowledge appears by the same kind of evolutionary process. This implies that evolution itself, in a generalized sense, is the proper foundation for epistemology. From this perspective, epistemology can never provide a methodology for guaranteeing knowledge. At most, it can provide guidelines for making the evolutionary process of knowledge creation more effective—but that is perhaps an even more valuable contribution. By providing an appropriate framework for an evolutionary methodology, this new epistemology would increase confidence in—and lend legitimacy to—our methods of modeling complex self-organizing systems.

10
Emerging Theory

We have presented several models covering various aspects of urban and regional morphology. Although they are scientific models in the sense that they are based on what we know about the processes that shape cities, given their emphasis on realism and the numerous applications directed at planning and policy issues, they might be considered to be more practical than theoretical. To what extent, then, do they represent an advance in the theory of cities and regions?

Writing about ecology and population biology in heterogeneous environments, a close analogue to the field represented by the models in this book, Richard Levins (1968) defined a theory as a cluster of models and their robust consequences. In Levins's view, a single model cannot cover every aspect of a complex system. In particular, no model can simultaneously optimize generality, realism, and precision. It is therefore useful, if not essential, to have several overlapping models that individually emphasize one or two of these qualities, so that, together, they cover all three. The CA-based models we have presented seem to aim for all three. They aim for generality—to be applicable to any city or region—and judging by the variety of applications, this claim seems to be justified. They are relatively realistic, dealing with a variety of processes, activities, and underlying factors known to characterize cities, while their output, in the form of maps and predicted values of various variables, is convincingly like what we see in real cities. And from the high resolution of the input data to the detail in the output, precision seems to be one of their most striking characteristics—think of the difference between the CA output of the Dublin area at a resolution of 100meters and the concentric zones of land use produced by William Alonso's (1964) model of urban spatial structure. But, as we have pointed out before, the precision is spurious: the output appears to be detailed and specific, but that is simply a consequence of using numerical modeling techniques; and the realism lies in the quality of the patterns produced, not in their specific details.

There are several reasons for the spurious precision. The most immediate one is stochastic perturbation. Beyond that is the imprecision of our knowledge of the proper values for the calibrated parameters: if we overcalibrate, they are wrong; if we de-tune the calibration, there are few constraints to ensure that we move toward better values. Finally, there are the bifurcations inherent in the dynamics of the model: the small local ones appear simply as more random variations in the output. Because it is either unrecognized or ignored, spurious precision may be one of the biggest problems in applications for planning and policy, especially since the apparent precision and realism of the models are perhaps the characteristics that most attract potential end users.

Our deeper understanding of the nature and causes of spurious precision comes from the theory of complex self-organizing systems, and the fact that our models are instantiations of that theory; our models are also instantiations of a more limited theory, the theory of cities and regions as self-organizing systems, a theory that, at present, is largely implicit. But we can use the models to begin to construct an explicit version of that theory. As Levins says, the model is the basic unit of theoretical investigation.

The three CA-based models and the model of central places are all representations of processes by which cities and regions evolve their spatial structure. In that sense, collectively, they represent the formal core of a theory. They perform quite well in generating the great diversity of forms that can be seen in actual urban and regional systems. Although in part this is due to the constraints built into the particular applications when the models are initialized with the particular maps and data sets corresponding to the application, it is also inherent in the operation of the models themselves. This was demonstrated when the basic CA-based land use model was run on an isotropic plain: in repeated runs, it produced a wide variety of urban forms, each one distinct. This is important because any model of a complex self-organizing system must, first of all, be able to generate complexity and diversity. In contrast, the models of classical location theory, developed when it was thought that formal theory should express universal laws, fail this test.

Robust Consequences

Ilya Prigogine, Hermann Haken, and others have shown us that the universal laws of physics generate, under conditions far from thermodynamic equilibrium, systems that are ordered over various temporal and spatial scales, but because the scales are always finite, we cannot look for universal laws governing these systems. We can, however, look for a theory and therefore some predictability. The structures that are relatively long lasting are the ones we characterize as having the property of stationarity. And if they appear in almost all instances, for example, in virtually all cities, then these structures in some sense play the role of universal laws. These are the robust consequences of the models that, together with the models themselves, constitute the theory.

We have the models. Do we have any robust consequences? In previous chapters, we have identified several:

- The clustering-dispersal bifurcation dependent on the distance-decay parameter
- The bifractal radial dimension
- The linearity of the cluster size–frequency relationship
- The decomposition into two distinct scales—local and long distance—of the distance-decay effect
- The (possibly) universal similarity of the influence functions

These regularities arise for different kinds of reasons, and some of them are better supported than others. Each is robust in the sense that it appears in most or all of the applications of the model that generates it, and some are robust in the stronger sense that they are also generated by more than one model. Furthermore, in principle, they can all be supported by economic and behavioral theories. We will examine each of them in greater detail.

The Clustering-Dispersal Bifurcation

As we saw in chapter 4, the clustering-dispersal bifurcation arises directly from joining the economic theory of the firm with the spatial interaction theory of consumer behavior within a system dynamics framework. Businesses competing with one another for spatially dispersed consumers will, as the dynamics unfold, end up clustering together or dispersing widely through the region depending on the spatial behavior of the consumers as described by a distance-decay parameter. In the simplest case, with no economies or diseconomies of scale and a uniform distribution of consumers, when the distance exponent, n, in the spatial interaction equation has a low value ($n < 1.2$, approximately, in a gravity equation) central place activities will move into a few large clusters; when the value is large ($n > 1.7$ approximately), they will disperse. In more complex, realistic cases, the spatial patterns become more varied and complex, but these all represent expressions of the basic bifurcation under varying conditions and constraints. In the dynamic central place model, the bifurcation arises in the dynamics of the system, but the underlying economic and behavioral causes are explicit. The bifurcation is well supported empirically, and the grounding in economic and spatial interaction theory gives us further confidence that the phenomenon is real, especially since empirically derived values of the key parameter, n, correspond to the values necessary to produce the bifurcation.

The bifurcation phenomenon is marginally robust across models in that it can also be partially reproduced by the multiple activity variable grid CA-based model. This model, like the dynamic central place model, has dynamics that are shaped by distance-decay functions—in this case, represented by the influence functions in the neighborhood effect. Otherwise, it is quite different. There is no explicit representation of the economics of the situation—no calculation of revenue, cost, profit, or loss—and therefore the dynamics are not based on these. Furthermore, there is no explicit representation of competition among the centers. The (implicit) revenue received by commercial activity depends only on its location, not on the location of other commercial cells (box 10.1). Despite these differences, the model generates reasonable distributions of commercial activity in its applications, as does the dynamic central place model. But to get a better idea as to whether the CA-based model is actually able to reproduce the bifurcation phenomenon, it was set up to mimic the conditions of the basic experiments of the central place model: uniform population density over the cell space, commercial activity initially located in a scattering of small clusters, and the weights of the influence function for the effect of population on commercial activity set to describe a gravity equation with a distance exponent of either 1 or 2. In the low-exponent case ($n = 1$), commercial activity always ended up in a single cluster toward the center of the map. In the high-exponent case ($n = 2$), activity also moved to a single cluster, but the cluster was rarely in the central part of the map, as it always was in the low-n case. Thus the CA-based model reproduces one aspect of the bifurcation—the clustering at the center of the map when n is low versus no such tendency when n is high. But it fails to reproduce the other aspect, the multiplicity of clusters when n is high.

The more important lesson from this comparison is that it would be useful to introduce more economics explicitly into the various CA-based models. The multiple activity CA-based model already takes several steps in this direction, with activities represented by their quantities, not just by their land uses, and with a component representing diseconomies of agglomeration. But this component is better understood as a surrogate measure, just as transition potentials can be considered a surrogate measure of land prices. If land prices were modeled explicitly, then they could be used directly as an expression of diseconomies, perhaps in conjunction with congestion levels as calculated by a linked transportation model. And if clusters were identified dynamically during run time, the dynamic central place model could be

Box 10.1
Comparing the Treatment of Commerce in the Multiple Activity CA-Based and Dynamic Central Place Models

> In both models, commercial activity is attracted to population, represented in the variable grid model by a neighborhood influence function in which the weights are set to describe a gravity equation with a distance exponent of either 1 or 2 (hence the gravity expression in the equation for V_K below). Commercial activity is induced to cluster in the variable grid model by an influence function for the effect of commercial on commercial activity that has positive weights (w_{di}) at short distances. In the comparison

Box 10.1 (continued)

simulations, both models were given fixed and uniform population densities over the cell space, and commercial activity was initially located in small clusters scattered over the map. A comparison of the most relevant parts of the models can be represented somewhat schematically as follows:

CA-Based Model

$$V_k = \sum_{i \in C} \left(\frac{w_{di} S_i}{S} \right) + \frac{\left(\sum_i \frac{P_i}{d^n_{ki}} \right)}{(P)}$$

(no cost equation)

$$S_{(t+1)k} = \frac{S V_k}{\sum_k V_k}$$

Dynamic Central Place Model

$$R_k = r P_k \sum_i \left\{ \frac{\left(\frac{S_i}{d^n_{ki}} \right)}{\left(\sum_j \frac{S_j}{d^n_{ij}} \right)} \right\}$$

$$C_k = c S_k$$

$$S_{(t+1)k} = S_k + g(R_k - C_k)$$

where

Σ_i is over all cells
$\Sigma_{i \in C}$ is over only cells in the given commerce cluster,
Σ_k is the sum over all cells with land use = commerce
V_k = activity potential
S = total commercial activity, and
P = total population
w_{di} = influence weight applied to commerce at distance d
R = revenue
C = cost
g = growth parameter.

Note: in this CA experiment, V_k reduces to the neighborhood effect since suitability, accessibility, zoning, and diseconomies are all set = 1.

inserted to represent the dynamics of the commercial sector. These changes would make the model more realistic, probably improve its performance, and almost certainly make it more useful for a variety of applications.

The Bifractal Radial Dimension

The bifractal nature of the urbanized area, shown by the kinked area-radius plot, is, in a sense, not so surprising since the inner zone is the area within which urbanization is essentially complete, with a dimension value of 1.90–1.95 (2.0 being the maximum), and the second zone, with a much lower value, simply represents the area into which the city is growing, where urbanization is underway but not complete. As the city grows, so does the inner zone, and the second zone shifts outward. Although one table published by Pierre Frankhauser and Roland Sadler (1991) shows that the radial dimension of Berlin grew from 1.36 in 1875 to 1.81 in 1945, maps and an analysis published elsewhere by Frankhauser (1990) suggest that these values confound the first and second zones as well as a third, rural zone, and that the dimension of the inner zone remained stable for the entire period. Although it is obvious that growing cities must have a zone in which growth is underway, it was surprising that this zone should show up so clearly in the Berlin radial analysis. It was even more surprising that many, though not all, individual land uses should also show this bifractal structure. The fact that the inner zone slopes for the various specific land uses are quite different from one another shows that statistically, though not very visibly, cities are characterized by concentric zones of different land uses, as the classical land use theories predict.

The stationarity of the bifractal nature of the urban area makes it useful as a supplementary check on the quality of model calibration, as some calibrations do not maintain the bilinear form of the area-radius plot if run long into the future, or, if they do maintain it, the slope of the second zone may drift away from values that have ever been observed for real cities. The plots for individual land uses are not so helpful since they are not always stable over time, as shown by the analysis for 1956–1998 for Dublin (table 5.3). On the other hand, in their sharply differing slopes, they do show that each of the several land uses is relatively concentrated in a particular concentric zone, an arrangement that is predicted also by the Alonso-Muth model (Alonso, 1964; Muth, 1969) and observed in actual cities, as shown in table 5.3. In any case, since they can easily replicate the radial structure observed in actual cities, CA-based models are, in a sense, providing a formal explanation of it.

The Linearity of the Cluster Size–Frequency Relationship

That the cluster size–frequency relationship for any urban land use is loglinear for almost all cities and regions is evidence of self-organization. Inverse power laws, of which this is an example, have long been taken as a signature of self-organizing processes. Thus Stuart Kauffman (1994) finds power law avalanches of evolutionary change in his Boolean network models, and Per Bak (1994, 1996; see also Bak, Chen, and Wisenfeld, 1988) finds a power law distribution of avalanches in his sandpile models, as we saw in chapter 2 and in chapter 5. The stationarity of the cluster size–frequency relationship is useful for testing and constraining calibrations, but those practical uses depend on the relationship having a deeper significance.

As a city or region grows, most of the clusters of particular land uses—or, at a higher level of aggregation, of urbanized land—will also grow. But if that is all that is happening, the small clusters will become larger, leaving progressively fewer small clusters; in other words, the relationship between cluster size and frequency will evolve from a linear one to one that is convex from above. The only way that a linear relationship can be maintained is for sufficient numbers of new clusters to appear, so that there is always a supply of small clusters available to grow. This seems to happen naturally in urban systems, as small new residential developments appear in rural areas, for example, or new commercial zones are established in residential areas. But it is not entirely clear why. In the case of new commercial clusters in residential areas, for example, there is a functional explanation: people need places to shop, and commercial establishments need customers. In the case of new residential areas in the countryside, it is not as clear what the functional explanation might be—perhaps that land is sufficiently cheap there to make it attractive to develop. In any case, we can attribute some of the decisions that establish new clusters simply to the heterogeneity of the agents involved, in terms of tastes, desires, and needs. So even though we cannot explain every case, it is not at all surprising that new clusters appear. What is surprising is that they appear in just the right numbers to keep the cluster size–frequency distribution linear over the long run. Of course, there are exceptions. As we saw in chapter 5, the distribution for Belgium is convex rather than linear. But, in this case, the convexity seems to arise from the linear development pattern (figure 10.1) that characterizes the country combined with the high density of urbanized land use in the northern half of the country (essentially Flanders together with Brussels): there are relatively few locations on the road network where a new urban cell would not be adjacent to an existing one, and existing clusters are so close to one another that new clusters quickly merge with them as they grow. In the extreme limit, when the entire country is urbanized, there can be only one cluster; it seems Belgium has taken a first small step toward this outcome.

But why, in less extreme circumstances, would the dynamics keep the distribution linear? Complexity theory suggests that systems evolve to a critical state, where they just maintain their structure, which can then be described by a power law. This seems to be happening in cities, but unlike avalanches on the sandpile, it is not at all obvious in what sense a city is in the critical state needed to maintain the power law distribution of clusters, or what would keep it there. A city is essentially a bottom-up system,

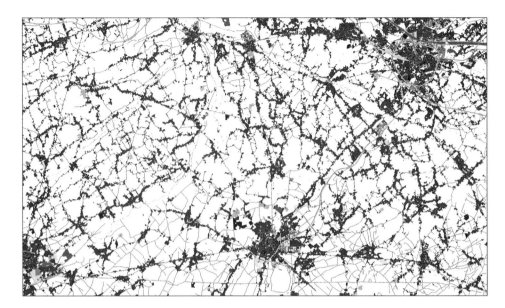

Figure 10.1
Part of Flanders, showing the high-density ribbon development typical of Belgium. (Source: Flemish Institute for Technological Research [VITO])

with spontaneous decisions by a variety of actors generating its structure. To understand the maintenance of urban criticality, we will need to understand how it emerges from the individual decisions of the myriad of actors. If we take cells to be agents, with their behavior described by the CA transition rules, then, in a sense, the CA-based models show how that happens, in the same way that Prigogine's simulation at the level of molecules colliding with one another shows how convection cells emerge from Brownian motion (Prigogine and Stengers, 1984): the models show that large-scale structures do emerge from individual local interactions, even if we find it difficult to generalize or explain the process beyond what is already implicit in the models. But, in fact, the CA-based models do not show us that much because the crucial parameter for generating a critical state is the one controlling the degree of stochasticity in the system, which we have interpreted as representing heterogeneity among the agents or their behavior, and we have tuned that parameter to yield the state of criticality represented by the linear cluster size relationship. In other words, we have buried the explanation in the calibration process. We must still understand how agents, by interacting among themselves, are led to adjust their characteristics and their behavior in such a way that, collectively, their actions lead the system to a state of criticality.

Agent-based modeling of the sort undertaken by Juval Portugali and Itzhak Benenson (1995, 1997; Portugali, Benenson, and Omer, 1994; Portugali, 2000) can handle the first part of the problem by showing how agents change their nature and their actions in response to their interactions with one another, but it is not clear that it can address the second part, the issue of how these changes in the agents are tuned. Part of the answer may lie in the emergence of cultural norms, and especially in the regulation of behavior by government and other organizations. If agents are individually too heterogeneous in their actions, so that the system is unable to structure itself, then regulation can tune their behavior back to the level necessary for criticality. But this can only be a small part of the answer because it assumes that agents are, on average, overly diverse or extreme in their actions, and there is no reason to believe that this is the case.

The Decomposition of the Distance-Decay Effect into Two Distinct Scales
Calibration of the multiple activity variable grid model of chapter 8 led to the discovery that the influence functions for the neighborhood effect have a distinctive form: in the nearby part of the neighborhood, out to approximately one kilometer, the weights are very large, but diminish rapidly with distance. Beyond, out to the edge of the modeled region, they are very small, but decline only slowly with distance (table 8.1 and figure 8.2). In part, this pattern reflects the fact that there are only a few cells in the inner part of the neighborhood (eighty-one in the example of figure 8.2), as opposed to nearly 200,000 in the rest of the region, and the weights are multiplied by the amount of activity in the cells; thus, if the inner neighborhood is to have any impact at all, it must be weighted heavily.

Nevertheless, the kink is real. The transition is sudden, and although the inner weights can show a variety of patterns after calibration, very similar to the patterns of weights seen in the MOLAND-type cellular automaton with a 196-cell neighborhood, the weights of the outer zone can be approximated by a standard distance-decay function like a gravity equation. This suggests that people and organizations making locational decisions assess in quite different ways the immediate neighborhood of a potential site and its location within the larger region. This is intuitively plausible because, in their immediate surroundings, what they might consider important would be factors such as whether the area is attractive or ugly, or has compatible land uses, or reasonable levels of commercial activity. At larger scales, these factors would be less important, and what might matter would be general accessibility to what the region offers—employment opportunities, shopping areas, parks, and other people. We may treat this as a general hypothesis about the perception and evaluation of the urban environment by the agents who make locational decisions, and, as a hypothesis, it deserves further investigation.

In this case, we are using a model that has been calibrated to give good predictions to reveal indirectly something about the underlying agents who are generating the patterns, in other words, to characterize the patterns not by what they are, but by what it takes to generate them. In this sense, the model becomes an investigative tool, somewhat like a data-mining technique. The model has suggested a hypothesis, and it is a characteristic of a good model—and especially of the theory that it instantiates—that it both resolves existing questions and raises new ones. The same is true of the next robust consequence of the model.

The (Possibly) Universal Similarity of the Influence Functions
The influence functions are the core of the CA-based models. They represent in a summary way the behavior of the underlying agents that are collectively structuring the urban system. Collectively, across a variety of applications, they may therefore offer the possibility of gaining some insight into the degree of universality of the processes that generate the urban structure. The two most important characteristics of the influence functions are the shape of their curves and their height above the distance axis. The shape, especially as characterized by slope and curvature, essentially determines the kinds of locations and patterns that emerge—for example, it determines how tightly clustered a particular activity will be. The height determines the relative competitive power of the various active land uses: the stronger ones are able to displace others, and of course this is also an important factor influencing the emerging land use patterns.

Interestingly, the shapes for the curves of particular land use classes tend to be quite similar across many applications. Comparing them, however, is difficult for several reasons. First, land use class definitions tend to vary from one application to another. For example, one application may use four residential categories, whereas another may use only one; or one may use a single industrial-commercial class, whereas another may separate them into distinct classes. Nevertheless, the apparently incompatible classes can usually be brought into an approximate correspondence, and then the similarities become clear. In figure 10.2, some of the functions have been rescaled by the factor shown in order to make it easier to compare the shapes. Dublin and the Pordenone region have relatively similar curves; the functions for Lagos are a bit flatter.

Perhaps a bigger difficulty than incompatibilities in land use classes is the lack of control over the calibrations that generated the curves shown. The various applications were calibrated by different people using informal procedures and standards that are not fully documented, so that similarities or differences could be due to differences among the calibration procedures used and thus tell us little about underlying urban processes. For example, a common way to begin a calibration is to copy influence functions from another application and then modify them. If the

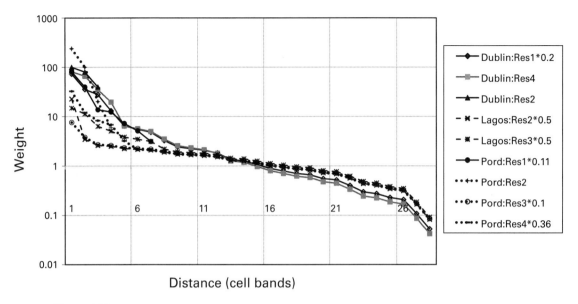

Figure 10.2
Similarity of influence functions: Dublin, Lagos, and the Pordenone region of Italy.

calibration is a lazy one, then the result will be a bias toward similarity of the functions across applications. A necessary first step toward a more rigorous evaluation of the similarity of influence functions is a method for standardized calibrations; an automatic calibration tool would serve this function well.

Nevertheless, the problems of comparison notwithstanding, the similarity of the influence functions across a variety of applications is striking and merits further investigation: if there is a substantial degree of universality, at the most practical level, it would facilitate calibration procedures, including the development of practical, reliable automatic techniques; it would also increase our confidence in the output of the models by suggesting that calibrations should remain more stable than we might have thought. And, from a theoretical perspective, it would suggest that people as well as businesses and other organizations behave in essentially the same way everywhere when making locational decisions, implying that cultural differences have relatively little influence on the structuring of cities and regions, at least at the level of generality represented in the models. This position is supported by Kiril Stanilov and Michael Batty (2011), who hypothesized that, if there were in fact a substantial degree of universality in the factors that determine urban morphology, then it should be possible to simulate the development of land use patterns over a long time span without updating the influence functions. In an application of the model described in chapter 6 to an area of west London over the period 1875–2005, they found that this was indeed possible (figure 10.3; plate 14). By examining land use patterns at approximately twenty-year intervals as established from Ordnance Survey maps and other sources, they found that a single set of influence functions produced a very reasonable prediction of land use patterns over the entire course of the 130-year period, as this part of London developed from an area that was largely rural to one that is densely urban.

But Where Is the Theory?

The best way to gain a deeper understanding of the possible universality of the influence functions would be to investigate their origin using an individual-based modeling approach. At the level of the individual-based model, the heterogeneity of agents and their behavior can be represented explicitly and realistically, not just as a perturbation on a single deterministic function that represents their average behavior. Such a model would allow us to investigate how and, more importantly, under what conditions, influence functions that are relatively stable across both time and space can emerge from individual behavior.

The problem of the origin of higher-level rules and regularities is a general one. It is one of the central concerns of the theory of self-organizing systems, and in particular it is the focus of the work of Haken and his Synergetics group at the University of Stuttgart (Haken, 1973, 1983). It is the problem of how higher-level structures, organizations, and regularities emerge from the collective behavior of lower-level entities, with the higher-level entities then constraining or "enslaving" the behavior of the lower-level ones so that they act coherently. The CA-based models of cities and regions are themselves examples of the application of the general theory, but they really involve only two levels—the level of cell dynamics and that of the emergent spatial structures. There has been almost no research into the individual-based origins of the cell-level dynamics. Only the work of Juval Portugali and Itzhak Benenson based on models that integrate individual- and CA-based techniques, work that is focused on understanding the spatial structure of land use, ethnicity, and socioeconomic status in Tel Aviv, makes some link between the individual and raster levels (Portugali and Benenson, 1995, 1997; Portugali, 2000), but even that work is not aimed directly at showing how rules at one level are derived from the collective application of rules at a lower level. Such a derivation would amount to a kind of verification of the upper-level model. Given that statistical validation will always be problematic and inconclusive when used for complex systems models, it is particularly important that the models be supported in other ways. Verification by derivation from lower-level models is one such way, and potentially an important one.

Another way of strengthening the models is to introduce more location theory into them directly. The dynamic central place model is essentially an embedding of

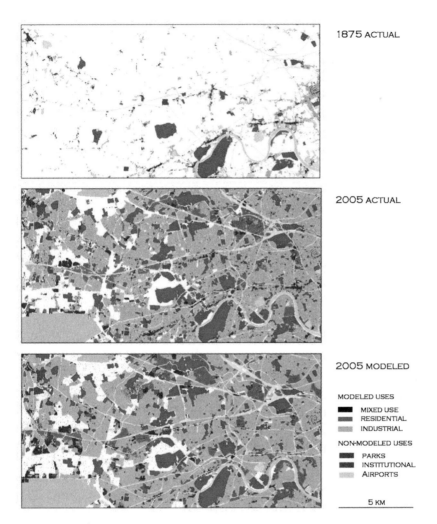

Figure 10.3 (plate 14)
Actual land use in west London, 1875 (*top*) and 2005 (*middle*); and simulated land use, 2005 (*bottom*), from the 1875–2005 simulation. (Simulation by Kiril Stanilov)

some of the economics used in retail location theory into a dynamical framework. MOLAND-type models link a classical spatial interaction–based model of activity migration to a CA-based land use model, whereas the variable grid cellular automaton embeds it directly into the CA transition rules, with the result that more quantities can be predicted, and, arguably, predicted more accurately. Much of location theory is potentially valuable by virtue of being a rich repository of economic principles in a spatial context. In its present form, however, it has been abandoned by everyone except location theorists because it produces predictions that are too unrealistic to be useful. Specifically, its static equilibrium framework is highly inappropriate to a dynamic, evolving world. Furthermore, it is formulated mathematically rather than algorithmically; therefore, its models have to be kept simple enough, for example, by postulating an isotropic plain and radial symmetry, that the equations can be solved. Without a solution to the equations, the theory can make no predictions and hence has no content. Both of these severe limitations are removed, however, if the equations are embedded in a dynamic model like a CA-based land use model, where they are in an algorithmic context in a very nonisotropic space, and where the solution is not a final state, but a year-by-year trajectory of the system into the future. Geoffrey Caruso and colleagues (Caruso, Rounsevell, and Cojocaru, 2005; Caruso et al., 2007) have integrated the Alonso-Muth land use model with a CA-based model, thus bringing economics explicitly into the CA approach to land use dynamics. There is scope for much more of this sort of integration. Bringing economics into the cellular automaton would provide explanatory and functional depth to the CA transition rules, specifically to the influence functions that are a part of those rules, just as an individual-based model would.

Returning to the question of the theoretical content of our CA-based and dynamic central place models, we have three robust predictions about urban systems that are consequences of the models in the sense intended by Levins: the clustering-dispersal bifurcation, the bifractal radial structure, and the linear cluster size–frequency relationship. In addition, the models implicitly establish several general characteristics the underlying agents must have in order for urban systems to be as we observe them. First, the existence of two distinct scales for the distance-decay effect implies that the agents must evaluate their immediate neighborhood on the basis of different criteria than those they use to evaluate the larger region around them. Second, the apparently universal similarity of the influence functions suggests that agents everywhere are broadly similar in the way they evaluate the space around them and act on that evaluation. Finally, agents must be relatively heterogeneous. In a model, this heterogeneity must have some explicit representation. If implicit agents are represented only by average behavior, as in economics and classical location theory, models are not able to give a reasonable representation of the self-organization of a city or region.

These five, or six, robust predictions may seem a relatively meager harvest of theory from the urban models. But remember Levins's definition of a theory as consisting of both the robust predictions and the cluster of models that generates them. In our case, it is the models themselves that embody the essentials of the theory. And, as Levins claims elsewhere, when dealing with complex self-organizing systems, the most important characteristic of a theory is not that it should result in the discovery of universals because, in a strict sense, there are none to discover, but that it should account for differences (Levins, 1968, p. 6). The only true universal to be found in these systems is that they are highly complex and diverse and tend to become progressively more so. This is the fundamentally important characteristic that conventional urban theory completely fails to capture. The urban models that form the core of our theory capture this characteristic by giving a formal, executable description of the processes that generate urban and regional structures. That representation is sufficient to predict not only several observed quasi or candidate universals, but also the great complexity within cities and the diversity among them.

As an instantiation of the general theory of complex self-organizing systems, our theory of urban and regional systems predicts both their regularities and their complexity; it also shows us the structure of their unpredictability. By predicting the bifurcations that a system is likely to encounter, it shows the future not as a single prediction but as a collection of possible futures. These possibilities exist, and they are the reason that the theory as embodied in the models is useful in practical applications. In addition to showing planners possible futures, it gives them a platform for performing "what if" experiments to determine which interventions are more likely to nudge the system toward a future that is considered more desirable. It is certain that social, cultural, or technological develoments will change the system as modeled into another, somewhat different system in the future. Although our theory cannot predict these changes, it can, through "what if" experiments, facilitate an exploration of their consequences.

11

Modeling in Support of Spatial Planning and Policy Making: The Example of Flanders

(with Lien Poelmans)

Thus far, we have given only brief examples of applications of the models presented. In this chapter, we provide a more extensive treatment of applications of the integrated regional CA-based model described in chapter 7. The setting is Flanders, one of the three constituent regions of the federal state of Belgium. In recent years, several departments of the Flemish government have begun to use the integrated model—in a version called the "RuimteModel"—to support spatial planning and policy development. Because the applications all have distinctive characteristics, together, they give a good idea of both the problems and the advantages of using the model in various types of planning situations. Most of the planning problems touch in one way or another on the need to preserve open space and the natural environment in a very densely settled region.

The Goal: Sustainable Spatial Development

Space is essential for the provision of goods, services, and amenities such as agriculture, industry, education, housing, parks, and leisure facilities, as well as for regulatory functions such as carbon dioxide sequestration, drinking water storage, and flood control. Space is also essential for the conservation of ecosystems, biodiversity, landscapes, and cultural heritage. But available space in Flanders is extremely limited. Flanders is among the most urbanized regions of Europe. With over six million people living, working, and engaging in leisure activities on some 13,500 square kilometers (~5,200 square miles), the population pressure on space is very high. Both cartographic and statistical sources show that the proportion of land in Flanders occupied by urban functions and infrastructure was nearly 27% in 2006. This was greater than that for Belgium as a whole, just under 20%, and far above the average for the European Union, 4.4%, and for individual member states like Spain, 2% (Prokop, Jobstmann, and Schönbauer, 2011). Moreover, on the basis of updated, more detailed maps, this proportion was estimated to have risen to 32% in 2013. Projections show that the population of Flanders will likely reach some 7 million by

2050. Unless policies change, the urbanized area will expand, too, at a rate of 6 hectares (~15 acres) per day. Thus proactive management of the use of space as a valuable and limited resource is of paramount importance if further loss of agricultural and natural land is to be avoided. This is where spatial planning has a role to play.

Spatial planners are no longer the sole guardians of space. Increasingly, they are joined by colleagues active in environmental management, nature protection, the provision of housing, the regional economy, and transportation. The problem for planners, however, is that nobody knows how society, and hence land use, will evolve over the next forty or fifty years. How strong will the effect of climate change be? How fast will sea levels rise and how serious will the problem of flooding become? Will fossil fuels be depleted, and if so, will there be adequate alternatives? What will the world economy look like? Will international bodies like the European Union, the United Nations, and the World Trade Organization become more important? Or will more decisions be made at the local and regional levels? How will these changes affect mobility, internal and external migration, housing demand, and patterns of urbanization? In short, what will all this mean for the land that we have available in Flanders?

Uncertainties such as these underline the importance of sustainable spatial development, which requires a fair distribution of burdens and benefits both within the present generation and between present and future generations. In other words, appropriate spatial development policies must be based not only on the relevant science but also on appropriate social choices between real, not illusory, alternatives. Therefore, planners need to explore potential development paths so that these choices can be made in light of the best possible indications of their long-term consequences. In this context, spatial models have an important role to play, allowing users to perform "what if" experiments under various scenarios of the global future and of specific policy and planning options to suggest the variety of possible consequences in each case. Through the bifurcation tree of possible futures associated with each scenario, these models can show planners how environmental quality, the carrying capacity of ecosystems, the economy, and the quality of life may evolve in the future under various circumstances. Given the challenges involved in spatial planning for a not-so-predictable future, it is sensible to formulate policies with two planning horizons. To achieve the sustainable spatial development of Flanders, planners have therefore proposed a 2020 horizon for short-term goals and corresponding implementation measures, a horizon less than two legislative terms away, and a 2050 horizon for strategic goals, ones that provide the context for the short-term policies. These two planning horizons were adopted by the Flemish Ministry of Spatial Planning in 2009.

Spatially explicit scenarios play a prominent role in policy preparation in the domains of environmental management, protection of natural areas, and spatial planning in Flanders. The most important of these are the integrated scenarios developed in the Environment Outlook 2030 MIRA-S-2009 and the Nature Outlook 2030 NARA-S-2009 studies. A version of the three-level integrated land use model discussed in chapter 7, the RuimteModel, was used to analyze and visualize the spatial outcomes of both scenario studies (Maes et al., 2009; Gobin et al., 2009). Spatial scenarios have also been adopted as an analytical instrument in spatial planning practice as part of the new Flanders Spatial Policy Plan (Beleidsplan Ruimte Vlaanderen or BRV), initiated in 2010. Over the next few years, the BRV will become the primary instrument for spatial planning in Flanders. Currently, its development is in the second of three phases, which should result in a more-detailed expression of the general principles and objectives presented in the *Green Paper Spatial Policy Plan* (RWO, 2012), which was produced in phase one. The BRV is intended to be the foundation of a spatial planning policy that will result in the sustainable spatial development of the Flanders Region. With the Flanders Spatial Policy Plan, planners and policy makers are hoping to break with the past, to overcome the inertia that has characterized the planning history of Flanders.

A Brief History of Spatial Planning in Flanders

For many centuries one of the most intensively developed agricultural areas of Europe, Flanders was also one of the first regions to develop a major nonagricultural sector, one based on textiles. This led to the development of a dense network of relatively small but compact urban nuclei (Pirenne, 1937). The intensive nature of Flemish agriculture was made possible by the fertility of the soil and facilitated by the fact that the land is flat, which means, however, that it is also suitable for the construction of housing and other urban land uses. As the industrial revolution swept across Flanders, the landscape changed dramatically, with a rapid expansion of housing and industry beyond the urban nuclei; in other words, urban sprawl appeared. The early development of a system of public transport by train and streetcar made it possible for businesses to bring in workers from greater distances. Employers and other members of the establishment preferred that workers remain scattered in the rural areas "under the church tower," as was said at the time, rather than concentrate in the urban areas where, away from the influence of the church, they might be less docile (De Decker, 2011). This avoided the creation of large slums and associated health problems, while also tending to constrain social unrest and opposition to the harsh conditions in the factories. Commuting became a part of the culture; the roads connecting the small urban centers became the preferred location for residential development. These roads fulfilled two principal functions that made them cost effective: they facilitated the flow of traffic to the urban centers, and they became the axes along which electricity, telephone, water, and other services could be provided efficiently. Notably, however, the residential strips along them (see figure 10.1) allowed people to live on plots sufficiently large to permit small-scale food production. Thus suburbanization and ribbon development, now so typical of Belgium, became facts (Wouters, 2013). The rise in the use of the private car between the two world wars intensified this phenomenon dramatically: ever greater distances to the urban centers could be covered easily, and thus cheaper land was within reach.

Unlike most other European countries in the 1930s, Belgium had no laws or regulations to restrain this urban sprawl. On the contrary, initiatives in this respect were nipped in the bud by landowners who could profit by selling land to those in need of housing. During World War II, the German occupation government organized the reconstruction of destroyed areas under a centrally controlled, planned initiative. After the war, therefore, most Belgians associated central planning and urbanism with the occupation and fascism and thus rejected them (Uyttenhove, 1989). Whereas other countries, such as the Netherlands, had spatial planning policies in place and opted for reconstruction based on systematic, large-scale projects, reconstruction was left to individuals in Belgium. Thus the De Taeye law of 1948 provided funds to enable individuals to acquire land for their houses, which they were allowed to build anywhere and in any way. Planning regulations were prepared by bureaucrats in the national government, but their implementation was the responsibility of municipal representatives, who were careful not to offend the voters who elected them by denying building permits. The regulations thus remained a dead letter. As a result, haphazard, scattered development spread across the countryside, especially in densely populated Flanders. At the same time, urban core areas began to decay because it was cheaper to construct outside the towns than to renew their downtowns.

Although the first Belgian legislation on spatial planning, the 1962 Law on Urban Planning, was a sound piece of legal work, it was not practically implemented until fifteen years later, in 1977, when "Sector Plans" were drawn up covering all land in Belgium. The plans defined, on topographic maps and in associated textual documents, the *destination* or eventual permitted use, of all parcels of land, hence the legal development potential in each specified area, whether residential, residential expansion, industrial, agricultural, natural, or any other type. Implementation of these plans marks Belgium's transition to more systematic and orderly spatial development. Primarily intended to protect the scarce remaining green spaces from speculators, the Sector Plans provided a partial answer to the rampant postwar suburbanization and were consistent with a growing interest in the environment and nature and with a growing concern about the quality of Belgian agriculture. Where not superseded by newer plans, they still determine the ultimate permitted use of land at the parcel level.

On the downside, however, the Sector Plans institutionalized the spatial separation of functions—for example, residential areas from workplaces—thus increasing the demand for transportation and encouraging suburbanization. The Sector Plans were also static and could not adapt to changes in society. They were to be updated after ten years, but that never happened. And because the Sector Plans stipulated what went where, but rarely how and when, space allotted to specific destinations was usually taken in as soon as possible. In particular, the Sector Plans designated extensive areas of land occupied by agriculture as available for residential and industrial expansion. Agricultural land was thus systematically and rapidly converted into urbanized land, especially on the periphery of towns—exactly the opposite of what was intended when the Sector Plans were drafted. What the Sector Plans lacked, most of all, was a guiding spatial planning policy, an overarching perspective. That perspective came with the Flanders Spatial Structure Plan (Ruimtelijke Structuurplan Vlaanderen or RSV).

In the meantime, Belgium continued its evolution to a federal structure. In 1980, the three constituent regions—Flanders, Wallonia, and Brussels—became responsible for formulating and implementing their own policies on land use planning. As a consequence of approval of the Flanders Spatial Structure Plan (RSV) in 1997 and the Decree on the Organization of Spatial Planning in 1999, two new planning tools were introduced: the Spatial Structure Plan, which defines the overall vision of spatial structure, and the Spatial Implementation Plan, which describes how that vision will be realized in practice. By law, the Flanders Region, its five provinces, and its 308 municipalities were all to develop their own structure plans as well as implementation plans to fit within the policy options stipulated in the structure plans. The subsidiarity principle, which is common in EU policy making, applies. This means that the plan at each lower administrative level is embedded within the plan at the next higher administrative level. Thus the spatial structure defined at the level of the Flemish Region can be refined and rendered more specific—but not contradicted—at the provincial and municipal levels as a function of local conditions. Also, each level of government exercises powers specific to its level.

In addition to the formulation of structure and implementation plans, strategic projects were launched to achieve the vision laid out in the Flanders Spatial Structure Plan (Geldolf et al., 2013). Defined as an area-oriented project with an integrated spatial approach that enhances the quality of the spatial structure across both sectoral and administrative lines, a *strategic project* had to be carried out in the short to medium term, at least in principle. It was hoped that the implementation of strategic projects would increase the support for planning in general and spatial planning in particular, but funding for the projects was both insufficient and slow in coming, which made it difficult to get the projects off the ground.

With the approval of the Flanders Spatial Structure Plan in 1997, a major step was taken toward an effective strategic spatial policy. The RSV formulated a vision for the sustainable spatial development of Flanders, which involves both respect for the carrying capacity of the land and a commitment to achieving spatial quality, especially in the lived environment. The RSV aims to intensify the urban areas of Flanders while protecting and enhancing its rural areas. It has four basic objectives:

1. To selectively expand urban areas both through creation of multipurpose nodes, with economic functions and amenities bundled together, and through optimal use and management of the existing urban structure;
2. To maintain and, where possible, strengthen rural areas by concentrating housing and nonfarm workplaces in small urban nodes in the countryside;
3. To counter the scattering of economic activities by promoting the development of industrial parks and ports as an engine for economic growth;
4. To create spatial conditions for improving public transport by concentrating activities that require transportation at locations accessible by public transport, thus optimizing use of the existing transportation infrastructure.

Initially, there was broad support for the Flanders Spatial Structure Plan, which was generally recognized as necessary, but, during its implementation, this support faded, and a consensus emerged that a new instrument, more focused on strategic planning, was needed. In 2010, an evaluation of the RSV (Voets et al., 2010) concluded that, though it had made an important contribution to improving the spatial structure of Flanders, the RSV had not adequately achieved its ambitious goals; in particular, it had not shifted development trends to the extent hoped for. Although residential density had increased, the urbanization of rural areas continued at an unacceptable pace, and the pressure on open space had not been reversed. RSV programs to concentrate economic activity in industrial nodes had met with only partial success, and those for improving the transportation infrastructure, strengthening public transport, and solving the traffic problems had not really begun.

The spatial policy instruments of the Flanders Spatial Structure Plan were insufficient to achieve the desired spatial policy objectives. The development of structure plans and implementation plans at the three administrative levels was cumbersome and time consuming. Certainly, the task stretched the technical and financial capabilities of the smaller municipalities to the limit. Because provinces and municipalities often failed to make full use of their freedom to produce plans in line with their own conditions and ambitions, the result was structure plans with a lack of vision, the opposite of what the RSV intended. Consequently, planning with the RSV all too often remained limited to producing the plans themselves. Too little progress was made in involving citizens and other stakeholders in formulating and implementing the plans. Moreover, the RSV had only very limited success in its intended role of coordinating the development and implementation of other governmental programs and policies with a bearing on spatial structure. In various policy areas with a pronounced spatial character such as housing, mobility, agriculture, nature, and the environment, the responsible organizations continued to implement their own programs and develop their own policies without regard to the spatial consequences. A new approach, one more focused on strategic planning, was thus called for. The result was the new Flanders Spatial Policy Plan (BRV), initiated in 2010 but not yet finalized or implemented.

The Flanders Spatial Policy Plan builds on the Flanders Spatial Structure Plan, yet it also aims to deal with the current challenges of spatial planning in Flanders. Sustainable spatial development is still the main objective, but the emphasis is not on making plans alone but on actual results in the field. The BRV promotes the principle of *thin planning*: plans are to be developed only when required and for areas, objectives, and projects that are actually in play. The BRV's project-oriented approach is characterized by a more pronounced involvement of civil society actors sharing responsibilities. The objective is to put more thought and effort into a spatial policy based on a strategic spatial vision for Flanders. The various tiers of government are to draw up concrete action plans in which government, market players, and citizens collaborate, set priorities, earmark budgets, and proceed to the final physical realization of the planned actions. The BRV thus shares certain similarities with the outcomes-based planning system in New Zealand. Finally, continuing in the tradition of the Flanders Spatial Structure Plan, the Flanders Spatial Policy Plan has a strong academic foundation. A large group of scientists, consultants, and others are collaborating with administrators to develop the conceptual framework. The public at large has been consulted by means of modern social media to solicit its vision for Flanders in 2050. The response has been massive. This does not mean, of course, that there is a single clear vision supported by all, or that it is straightforward to turn the suggested ideas of a vision into a definite plan. On the contrary, difficulties have currently slowed the process. In the meantime, the spatial planners have been strengthening the scientific basis for their work. In particular, they have sponsored the creation of a high-resolution land use database for Flanders, the development and implementation of RuimteModel Flanders (a version of the model described in chapter 7), and formulation of a vision for 2050 using scenarios developed with that model.

Setting Up and Calibrating the RuimteModel for Flanders

Data Requirements and Acquisition
The RuimteModel land use model discussed in this chapter is an advanced application of the model described in chapter 7. It represents spatial dynamics in Flanders

at three geographical levels: the *global* level of the combined Flanders and Brussels Regions, the *regional* level of the twenty-two arrondissements of Flanders plus Brussels, and the *local*, cellular level of the some 1,375,000 cells of the regular grid covering the territory of the two regions. The RuimteModel makes extensive use of statistical and geographic information system (GIS) data available from administrative bodies within the Flemish and Belgian governments. At both the global and regional levels, the model deals with the population, employment in twelve aggregated economic sectors, and land claimed by six classes of agriculture and eleven of nature. At the cellular level, land use is modeled for thirty-seven land use classes, five of which are static in the model.

The development of the RuimteModel started in 2006 with the aim of supporting scenario exercises and other prognostic applications in Flanders. Since 2009, it has been used in several policy exercises carried out for departments of the Flemish government dealing with the environment, nature, transportation, and flood risk management. Impacts of current, intended, or optional policies were assessed to improve the quality of policy making, planning, and management. Developed in 2011, the version of the RuimteModel discussed here was set up to run simulations for the period 2010–2050 in order to meet the requirements for scenario evaluation. The first step was to identify the most important factors that were likely to drive the development of Flanders during the forty-year simulation period; values for the variables and technical parameters describing these factors were established on the basis of current data combined with scenarios of future trends. Since the RuimteModel is to be used as a tool for policy support, it is essential that it run on the same, official data that are used by other official domain models and by the government agencies that might employ the model. Thus the data used in the model are all from official Flemish or Belgian federal sources, or derived from them.

A baseline or business-as-usual (BAU) scenario was developed by assuming the continuation of currently observed trends and existing policies, and the model was calibrated using that scenario. Also used in this exercise were forecasts of socioeconomic trends that became available as the result of modeling exercises both in the Environment Outlook MIRA-S-2009 (Van Steertegem et al., 2009) and the Nature Outlook NARA-S-2009 (Dumortier et al., 2009) programs and with the PLANET (Desmet et al., 2008) and the SELES (Gavilan et al., 2007) models. Developed by the Belgian Federal Planning Bureau (FPB) to model the interrelationship between the economy and transport in Belgium, PLANET is used to compute the long-term (2030) needs for transportation of both people and freight, to simulate the effects of transportation policy measures, and to carry out cost-benefit analyses of the measures. Developed by the Flemish Environment Agency (VMM) in collaboration with the Flemish Administration for Agriculture and Fisheries (ALV) to provide insights about the yield, income, and environmental pressure of agricultural activities, the Seles model includes some fifteen agricultural and horticultural activities and nine animal husbandry activities, which together cover the complete agricultural sector in Flanders. The main assumption underlying the model is that individual farmers are striving to maximize their profits subject to constraints set by environmental legislation, subsidy systems, and other factors.

The business-as-usual (BAU) scenario provides a means for examining the consequences of anticipated changes in the population and economy for the land use patterns in Flanders over the period 2010–2050. The drivers for this scenario include projections of population size, employment in the twelve aggregated economic sectors, and areas in use for agriculture and nature. These were obtained by combining data from various administrative and statistical sources in Flanders, starting with the projections for the total population size at the arrondissement (NUTS 3) level, which were available from the Federal Planning Bureau by five-year age cohorts and by gender for each arrondissement in Belgium. According to these estimates, the population of Flanders is expected to grow by some 720,000, from 6,251,983 in 2010 to nearly 6,972,000 in 2050; the population in the Brussels Region, by some 220,000, from 1,089,538 to just over 1,310,000. These projections are characterized by relatively high population growth rates due to labor migration, particularly for the Brussels Region, and by aging in Flanders (Maene, 2011). The RuimteModel works with the total population size to derive the demand for residential land use. The population projections are also used to generate employment figures, although refinement of the projections in terms of gender and five-year age cohorts is still needed to estimate the size of the active population of persons between the ages of 15 and 64 and to properly apply long-term projections for the economic participation rate in the model. Projections for the economic participation rate were obtained from the Flemish Statistics Institute at the regional (NUTS 1) level for the period to 2030 (Pelfrene, 2005). They are expressed as the fraction of employed persons relative to the total size of the potential labor population by gender and five-year age cohort. The gradually stabilizing increase of the participation rate, particularly for women over the age of 50, was assumed to remain constant after 2030 in the RuimteModel. Combining the population size projections with those for the participation rate gave estimates of the size of the active population at the regional level—that is, for the Flemish and Brussels Regions—according to region of residence. A recent estimate of interregional commuting in Belgium (ADSEI, 2011) was used to translate these results to region of employment, assuming constant interregional commuting rates for the period 2010–2050. This correction required using employment projections for the Wallonia Region as well. The resulting estimate was that a very modest growth of employment in Flanders could be expected: from 3,226,000 in 2010 to 3,500,000 in 2050.

With respect to the regional employment projections, the output of the PLANET model (Desmet et al., 2008) had to be modified for use in the RuimteModel. First, the composition of the aggregated economic sectors in the PLANET model did not entirely match those of the RuimteModel. Based on a detailed analysis of the disaggregated economic sectors in both models, the PLANET figures were reclassified so that they matched the RuimteModel sectors. Second, because PLANET computes outputs until 2030, whereas the RuimteModel does so until 2050, the forecasts of the PLANET model were extended to 2050 on the basis of the expected evolution of the population structure and labor participation rates. Employment in the *harbors* economic sector required special attention. Data from the National Bank of Belgium (Van Claude, 2009) were used to separate harbor activities from the other economic activities and to avoid the double-counting of harbor employment. Thus the calculation of the estimated jobs in the various economic sectors for 2010–2050 at the level of the individual arrondissements involved a complex algorithm requiring data from various sources. Figure 11.1 shows the evolution of the sectoral structure of the economy over the 2010–2050 period. Except for a gradual increase in the *other services* sector and a corresponding decrease in *light* and *heavy industry*, that structure remains remarkably stable.

Calibration of the Spatial Interaction–Based Regional Submodel

The total population and employment per sector at the level of the arrondissements in 2010 is used to initialize the spatial interaction–based regional submodel. The parameters of the regional submodel are then calibrated so that the RuimteModel

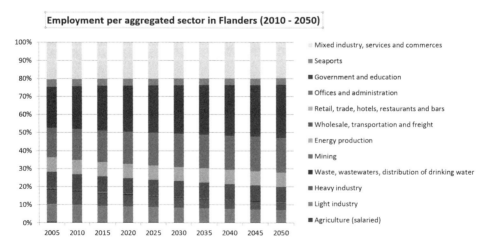

Figure 11.1
Employment in Flanders by sector as percentage of total, 2010–2050, in business-as-usual scenario.

will generate as precisely as possible the same output as the PLANET model. The results of this calibration are good: the RuimteModel can predict the population and the activity levels in each sector and arrondissement with an accuracy greater than 96%. It thus outperforms a "constant share" model, which has an accuracy of 92%, although these calibration results indicate only that the RuimteModel can generate an outcome close to that of PLANET. To the extent that the forecasts of the PLANET model are in error, then this calibration procedure forces the RuimteModel to replicate PLANET's errors. Nevertheless, as previously mentioned, this calibration strategy is preferred by policy makers because it enhances the compatibility of the results of the various models.

The forecasts of the land requirements for the nature classes were based on work done by the Institute for Nature and Forest Research (INBO) under the Nature Outlook NARA-S 2009 scenarios (Dumortier et al., 2009). On the advice of experts at INBO, it was decided to assume that policy goals set with respect to land for nature would be met in 2050 rather than in 2030, as was originally assumed in the NARA-S-2009 reference scenario. This was done for two reasons: first, earlier projections turned out to be overly optimistic with respect to the pace at which areas for protected nature develop; and, second, there is no Flemish or EU requirement to increase the amount of land for protected nature beyond the objectives incorporated in the NARA-S-2009 reference scenario. Hence no changes in policies are to be expected. The regional totals of land requirements for new nature areas are allocated to the individual arrondissements on the basis of suitability in areas zoned for nature expansion, as determined from the suitability and zoning maps in the model.

The SELES model generates forecasts of agricultural land uses under the Environment Outlook MIRA-S-2009 scenarios for the eight agricultural zones of Flanders. These totals are first disaggregated to the level of municipalities and, next, aggregated to the level of arrondissements, as required by the RuimteModel. In the process, the areas are also aggregated to the five agricultural activity classes used by the RuimteModel (Gobin et al., 2009). Agricultural land use in the SELES model involves only land officially registered by farmers. Agriculture has traditionally been the net supplier of land for all other functions in Flanders. Thus, in order to know the total area available for agricultural activities, the RuimteModel was run once to determine the area remaining after subtraction of the land assigned to residential, economic, and protected nature classes. Contrary to the assumptions made in the MIRA-S-2009 and NARA-S-2009 scenarios, the demand for unregistered agricultural land, owned mostly by individuals engaged in hobby gardening or in raising horses and sheep, was kept constant between 2010 and 2050. Current trends show that such land is not as easily given up as land used by productive farming, for which the income generated by farming has to outweigh the value of the land on the market if it is to remain in agricultural use. This is confirmed by data showing that the area occupied by unregistered agricultural land has remained constant over time. Registered agricultural land, in effect, a residual category—land left over after all other land use demands have been met—was thus considered to be the net provider of land for urban expansion. Within the agricultural land use classes, it was assumed that productive grasslands occupied a fixed proportion of total agricultural land as a result of the EU subsidy policy.

The RuimteModel includes the cell-density submodel described in chapter 7 (Box 7.1), which adjusts the amount of land occupied per inhabitant and per person employed in each of the twelve economic sectors during the course of a simulation. Density is adjusted on the basis of several factors, including an autonomous trend in density, demand for land compared to the availability of land, and the availability, suitability, and accessibility of zoned land. The importance of each factor is controlled by at least one parameter, which is calibrated on the basis of observed trends. As part of the business-as-usual scenario, the assumptions built into the MIRA-S-2009 reference scenario apply. This results in a continuing decline in the activity density of both residential land use and most economic sectors. Toward 2050, the decline in these densities comes more or less to a halt.

The transportation infrastructure is represented in the RuimteModel by the networks of roads, railroads, and navigable waterways, as well as railroad stations and bus stops, buses. This infrastructure determines the accessibility at the regional and local levels. A fairly simple transportation submodel computes the distances between the centroids of the arrondissements based on a generalized cost function that takes into account travel times and costs. Of course, the transportation system is not fixed; planned changes such as completion of the "missing links" in the road network are taken from sources such as the Flanders Spatial Structure Plan or from the investment program of De Lijn, the Flemish bus and streetcar company. During a simulation, these changes are incorporated in the submodel's network representation at the expected time of completion, thus changing the effective distances between arrondissements. Currently, this submodel considers only private transport over the road system. In the future, it may be replaced by a more sophisticated four-stage multimodal transportation model currently being developed by the Flemish Transportation Center, thus making the RuimteModel into a full land use–transportation interaction (LUTI) model operating at high spatial resolution.

Calibration of the CA-Based Land Use Model

Based on the forecast population, the number of jobs in each economic sector, and the amount of land needed per person or job, the cell-density submodel calculates the amount of land required for each land use in each arrondissement. These requirements are passed to the CA-based land use model, which then allocates them over the cell space of the arrondissement. The local level of the RuimteModel relies heavily on a variety of high-quality data sets to calculate accessibility, suitability, and zoning maps for the various land uses. But perhaps the most critical GIS layer in the model is the land use map of Flanders, which must be of the highest possible quality. Compiled explicitly for use in the RuimteModel because no existing land use map of sufficiently high quality was available, the map is now also being used in a variety of other contexts. Although the RuimteModel represents land use at a resolution of 1 hectare (~2.5 acres), the land use map was first compiled at a resolution of 10 meters (~33 feet) in order to facilitate aggregation for use for a wide variety of purposes. A GIS procedure compiles the land use map from some fifteen high-resolution GIS layers, among which are the CADVEC for cadastral information, the Biological Valuation Map (BWK), and the Agricultural Parcel Registry (EPR; Van Esch et al., 2010). In addition, information with respect to the location of individual businesses in Flanders is incorporated, enabling a representation of parcels occupied by economic activities as aggregated into twenty-one categories defined on the basis of the NACE industrial classification codes. This information is obtained from the Flemish Registry of Companies (VKBO) and made available by the government agencies responsible for updating it: Enterprise Flanders (Agentschap Ondernemen) and CORVE (Flemish E-government Coordinating Unit).

Other GIS-based data used in the model describe the physical state of Flanders, its institutional status, and finally its transportation infrastructure. This geographical information is used to compute the suitability of each 1-hectare cell for each of the land uses modeled. The physical suitability is based on information with respect to relief, soils, and susceptibility to problems such as erosion, inundation, and noise pollution. The zoning or policy status is determined in part by the Spatial Accounts (Ruimteboekhouding) of the Flemish Spatial Planning Administration, which synthesizes the currently approved spatial implementation plans of the RSV and the Sector Plans that still apply. It also incorporates the Natura 2000 nature protection areas as well as the areas that are part of the Flemish Ecological Network (VEN).

Calibration of a cellular automaton normally requires a minimum of two high-quality land use maps, produced using identical methodologies, at the beginning and end of a period sufficiently long that a significant amount of land use change has occurred—in Belgium, such a period would be at least ten years. But because such data are not available for Flanders, another calibration procedure was adopted. To begin with, the CA influence functions were copied from the version of the RuimteModel applied in the MIRA-NARA scenario studies (Maes et al., 2009; Gobin et al., 2009) and adapted to account for the different resolution (100 meters as opposed to 150 meters in the earlier application) as well as for differences in the definitions of the land uses modeled. Next, all inertia weights were set to zero. Finally, these inertia-free influence functions were calibrated on the basis of a zero-growth scenario, a purely technical scenario, covering some ten years, in which it is assumed that the population, employment, activity densities, transportation system, policies, and all other factors remain constant. Therefore, any changes in the land use pattern generated by the model over the ten-year period must result from the influence function rules alone. The purpose of the exercise is to find a set of influence functions that can preserve the initial spatial pattern over the entire duration of the run. This may seem simple, but in the self-organizing context of the model, where any small change may be amplified in a cascade of further changes, the goal is difficult to achieve. The resulting rule set can be considered the genome of the spatial structure in that it has all the information required to replicate the land use pattern. The rule set resulting from the zero-growth scenario is then tested for its capacity to generate changes in the spatial structure that are very likely to happen when growth is introduced to the model, changes that include the expansion of residential, industrial, commercial, or service land use in areas designated in a Spatial Implementation Plan for these uses within a given period of time. Limited to selected areas, the tests are used to fine-tune the calibration in what amounts to an artificial historical calibration. The larger calibration process also involves a series of analyses and manual corrections of the rule set. For example, a cross tabulation is performed to test the location of land uses with respect to the accessibility, suitability, and zoning maps for each land use to ensure that the land uses are consistent with those maps.

The calibrated model is run forward in time to validate its capacity to generate realistic land use patterns in 2050. As an indication of the quality of the 2050 simulation, the rank-size distribution of the urban clusters in both the initial state (2010) and the final state (2050) are compared. All urban land use classes are combined into a single urban class, and the size of each urban cluster is determined. For many distributions, George Zipf and others (Zipf, 1949; Gabaix and Ioannides, 2004) postulate that the number of clusters of size equal to or larger than S ($P(Size \geq S)$ is proportional to $1/S$. This seems indeed to be the case for the Flemish urban system in 2010, where the relationship is close to linear over the full range of cluster sizes, although, as we saw in chapter 8, the cluster size–frequency distribution is convex. The distribution for 2050 remains very close to that of 2010, suggesting that, by this measure at least, the calibration of the CA-based model is producing reasonable results (figure 11.2).

Application of the Model to Flanders: The Business-as-Usual Scenario

Although the primary output of the RuimteModel relevant for spatial policy is its sequence of land use maps, the model also produces a number of user-defined indicators based on land use that emphasize specific characteristics of the forecast development of particular interest to the model's users. Like land use, the indicators are computed on a yearly time step; they are made available as maps that are easy to

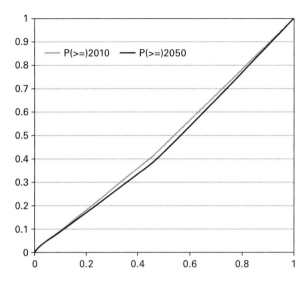

Figure 11.2
Zipf plot for urban clusters on initial (2010) and simulated (2050) land use maps of Flanders. P(>=) indicates proportion (y-axis) of clusters with a size S greater than or equal to 1/S (x-axis). Zipf's (empirical) law states that this relationship is linear and constant over time.

read and interpret, but they are also aggregated by arrondissement and for the whole of Flanders as graphs showing the evolution of the indicated characteristics over time. In this section, in addition to land use, we discuss four indicators: degree of urbanization, cluster size of urbanized areas, cluster size of open spaces, and urban pressure on agricultural land.

Land Use
The business-as-usual (BAU) scenario, when run to 2050, predicts a significant expansion of urban land use. This can be seen in the graph in figure 11.3 but is more dramatic in the land use maps, where the dark colors representing the urban residential, industrial, commercial, services, and infrastructure land use classes dominate the land use map of figure 11.4 (plate 15) (*bottom*). For this and subsequent map figures in this chapter, figure 11.3 is a reference map showing the location of the cities mentioned in the text, as well as the transportation network. The expansion of urban land is remarkable: urban land use grows by 108,201 hectares (~420 square miles) from 364,528 hectares in 2010 to 472,729 hectares (~1,825 square miles) in 2050. Averaged over the whole forty-year period between 2010 and 2050, this is some 2,705 hectares (~10 square miles) per year. The "land take" (Prokop, Jobstmann, and Schönbauer, 2011) of the residential areas in Flanders and Brussels is slightly over 6 hectares (~15 acres) per day, whereas the combined land take of the

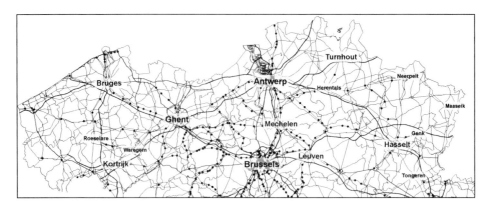

Figure 11.3
Reference map of Belgium showing cities mentioned in text and transportation network.

industrial, commercial services, and infrastructure sectors amounts to around 1.4 hectares (~3.5 acres) per day. This expansion of the urban land consists not only of suburbanization on the periphery of cities like Antwerp, Ghent, and Kortrijk, but also of new urban development in the more or less "rurban" regions in Flanders between the main urban centers. Clearly, the main transportation axes, in particular motorways (superhighways) and waterways, facilitate this urban development and seem to generate urban corridors between the larger cities. Also, the central part of Flanders is under pressure from residential development in the BAU scenario, particularly in the area to the east of Mechelen and north of Leuven, although the phenomenon can be observed generally in the "Flemish diamond," the area marked out by Antwerp to the north, Ghent to the west, Brussels to the south, and Leuven to the east. This urban expansion generally happens at the expense of registered agricultural land, whereas the area occupied by the eleven natural land uses shows a small increase toward 2050, which takes place mainly in the eastern arrondissements such as Maaseik, Hasselt, and Turnhout.

Degree of Urbanization

The indicator *degree of urbanization* is calculated as the percentage of cells with a land use in one of the urban classes (specifically, residential, the twelve nonagricultural economic land uses, and infrastructure) in a circular area with a radius of 1.5 kilometers (~1 mile) centered on the cell. The higher the value of the indicator, the more a cell is surrounded by urban land uses. The overall degree of urbanization in Flanders as measured by land use increases from 27% in 2010 to 35% in 2050. Figure 11.5 shows that the degree of urbanization was already high in 2010 in the agglomerations of Antwerp, Ghent (see figure 11.5 inset top left), and Brussels. By

Modeling in Support of Spatial Planning and Policy Making   267

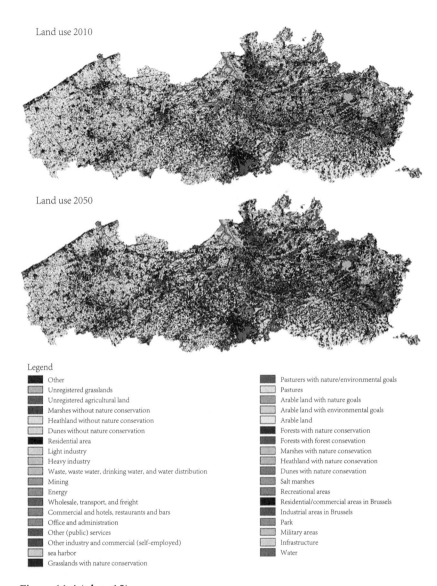

Figure 11.4 (plate 15)
Land use maps for Flanders and Brussels, 2010 (*top*); 2050 (*bottom*).

268   Chapter 11

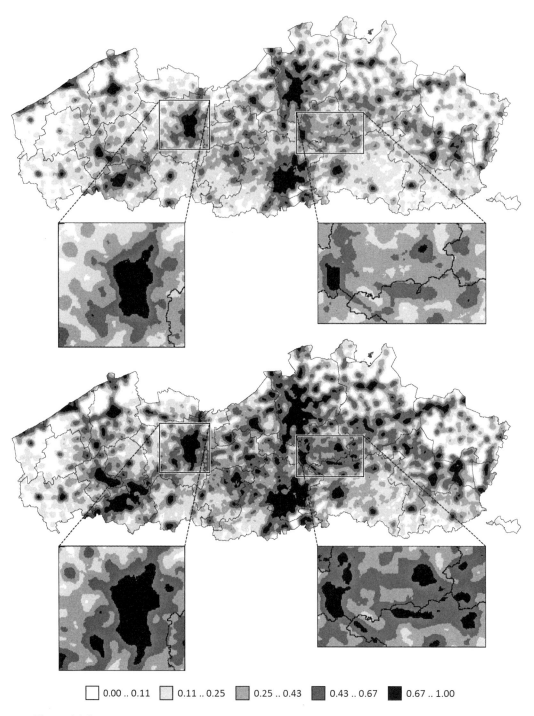

Figure 11.5
Degree of urbanization for Flanders and Brussels, 2010 (*top*); 2050 (*bottom*), ranging from 0.00 (not urbanized at all) to 1.00 (completely urbanized).

2050, these agglomerations have expanded considerably and are growing into one another. This is clearly the case on the north–south axis running from Antwerp to Brussels, where the city of Mechelen merges with Antwerp. A similar phenomenon of merging cities can be observed in the northeast–southwest axis running from Neerpelt in the north of Limburg Province to Mechelen and in the east–west axis running from Genk to Antwerp. These axes intersect at Herentals, where substantial new urbanization is observed. In the southwest, the cities of Kortrijk, Waregem, and Roeselare have grown into one conurbation linked by the local motorways and canals. Toward the year 2050, the degree of urbanization is also progressing in more rural areas captured by the outward expansion of the cities, such as the region mentioned earlier to the east of Mechelen and north of Leuven (see figure 11.7 inset bottom right) and in the Flemish diamond.

Cluster Size of Urbanized Areas
An urban cluster consists of all urban cells that are contiguous in the rook directions, and its size is measured as the number of cells it contains. Each cell in the cluster is then assigned the size of the cluster as its indicator value. The indicator *cluster size of urbanized areas* confirms the conclusions drawn from the indicator maps for degree of urbanization. The existing urban clusters generally expand (figure 11.6). Typically, smaller clusters (smaller than 1,000 hectares or ~4 square miles) grow and thus move up in the hierarchy to become part of the next higher class. On the map, this clearly results in more clusters of the largest class (larger than 1,000 hectares) growing toward and into one another. As a result, the main urban axes become strongly accentuated; this is shown even more clearly by this indicator than by the degree of urbanization indicator. The north–south Antwerp–Mechelen–Brussels axis is intensified over the simulation period, but so are the other urbanization axes. Large urban clusters are also seen to grow in the Flemish diamond to the west and east (see figure 11.6 insets bottom left, bottom right) of the Antwerp–Mechelen–Brussels axis.

Cluster Size of Open Spaces
The indicator *cluster size of open spaces* assigns to every cell occupied by a land use in the aggregated *open space* class the size of the cluster it belongs to; the open-space class combines eleven natural and six agricultural classes, as well as the military, recreational, water, and parks land uses. Contiguity is broken by all transportation infrastructure other than local roads. This is nicely demonstrated in the indicator maps by the generally smaller clusters along the motorways, waterways, and railroad lines between the main agglomerations (figure 11.7).

Despite the decrease in the area of open space, clusters of open space grow larger until 2020 (figure 11.8), and, as a consequence, the number of open-space clusters

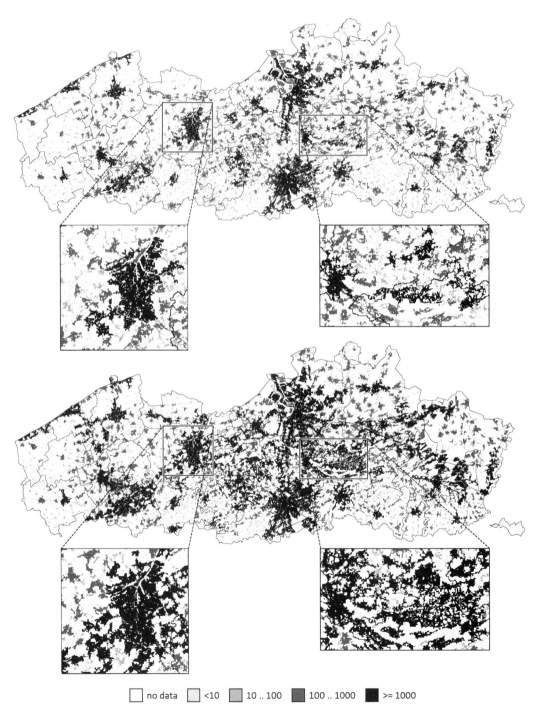

Figure 11.6
Cluster size of urban land for Flanders and Brussels, 2010 (*top*); 2050 (*bottom*).

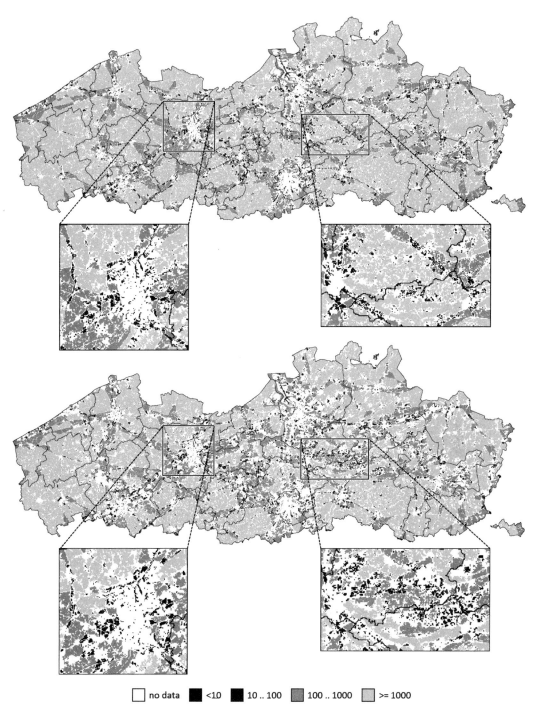

Figure 11.7
Cluster size of open space for Flanders and Brussels, 2010 (*top*); 2050 (*bottom*).

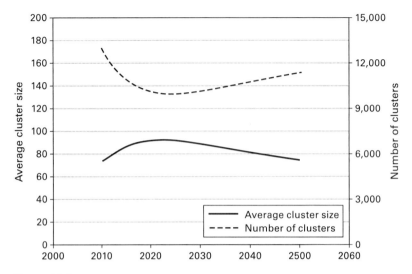

Figure 11.8
Average cluster size and number of clusters of open space in Flanders, 2010–2050.

decreases. This effect is caused by suburbanization in the neighborhood of already urbanized cells, causing small clusters of open space in between the urban cells (mainly agricultural land) to disappear. The larger clusters of open space in the neighborhood of urban cells are less affected by the urban expansion. On the other hand, in the period 2020–2050, the number of clusters of open space increases and the clusters become smaller, hence the open space is increasingly fragmented. This is solely due to the expansion of urban land use. This development can clearly be observed in the center of Flanders (figure 11.7). Nearly all clusters of the largest size (larger than 1,000 hectares) disappear from the Flemish diamond. This is very conspicuous in the area to the east of Mechelen (see figure 11.7 inset bottom right). The arrondissements in the far western and northern parts of Limburg and Antwerp Provinces, where large clusters of protected natural reserves persist, are less affected. The western part of Flanders is also less affected by urban expansion.

Urban Pressure on Agricultural Land
Computed as the percentage of urbanized cells in a circular area with a radius of 1.5 kilometers centered on each cell occupied by an agricultural land use, the indicator *urban pressure on agricultural land* makes no distinction between the various urban land uses: they are all weighted equally. The higher the value of the indicator, the more the agricultural land is enclosed or fragmented by urban land uses. The agricultural activity therefore can be assumed to be under pressure from urbanization.

Figure 11.9 shows the highly fragmented nature of agricultural land in Flanders. The areas of contiguous agricultural land in 2010 are largely confined to the western part of the region and to parts of the southern fringe. Even less contiguous agricultural land remains in 2050. Within the 1.5-kilometer neighborhood around the agricultural cells, the mean percentage of the cells that are urban is 44% in 2010. By 2050, the proportion reaches 67%. This is another measure of the ongoing pressure of urbanization on agricultural land. In 2010, agricultural land is most under pressure of urbanization in the Flemish diamond; this is even more the case in 2050. Only in the far western part of Flanders does a large agricultural area relatively free of urban pressure persist. Most other agricultural areas are under major urban pressure.

Conclusions

The business-as-usual scenario shows the many changes that land use in Flanders may undergo if the expected population growth becomes a reality and spatial policies remain unchanged. Extensive urbanization and suburbanization of the rural areas would become a fact. A growing need for land for both residential and economic uses is propelling these processes. Much agricultural land has been lost to urban expansion since 2010, and even more will be lost or under urban pressure in 2050. Other consequences evident in the simulation results but not discussed in this chapter are the high costs for infrastructure such as the distribution networks for gas, electricity, and drinking water; increased costs for solid waste collection and the maintenance of road infrastructure; and significantly increased demands on the transportation system, with a concomitant degradation of service standards. Thus the business-as-usual scenario leads to a future with higher costs, degraded performance of the transportation system, and a significant loss of agricultural land combined with widespread urban sprawl. These outcomes are most likely the consequence of the declining activity densities that are assumed in all sectors except services. Clearly, such development is not sustainable in Flanders given the already high pressure on the available land. In the next section, we examine the results of a simulation run with a scenario designed to evaluate the consequences of a policy measure aimed at reducing the land take.

Toward a Land Take–Neutral Flanders in 2050

As part of the Flanders Spatial Policy Plan, the RuimteModel analyzed an alternative to business-as-usual development, namely, *land take–neutral* development, an option inspired by the *Green Paper Spatial Policy Plan* published in 2012, which states: "Continuing to consume a finite resource like open space is no longer feasible. We wish to evolve towards a spatial development in which the total built-up area no

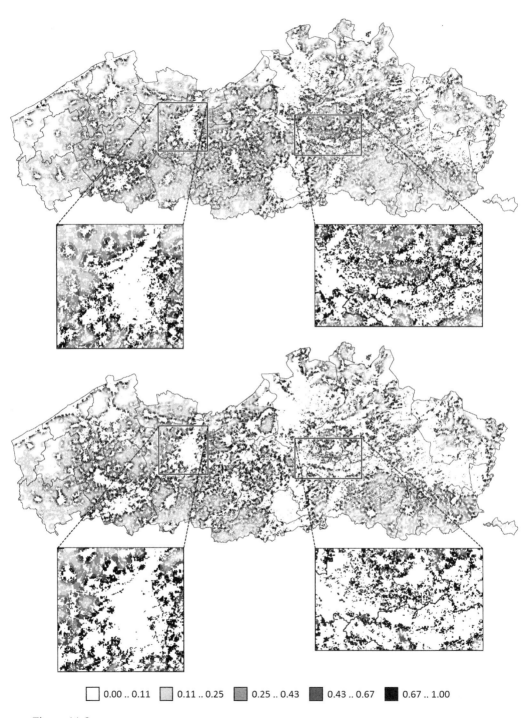

Figure 11.9
Urban pressure on agricultural land in Flanders, 2010 (*top*); 2050 (*bottom*), ranging from 0.00 (no pressure at all) to 1.00 (maximum pressure).

longer increases" (RWO, 2012, p. 23), and "To make this transformation possible, we want to use the existing built environment more efficiently and intelligently for housing, work, shopping and recreation.... That brings Flanders into line with the Roadmap to a Resource Efficient Europe" (p. 21). Indeed, the EU's Soil Thematic Strategy (COM (2006) 231), adopted September 22, 2006, aims for a zero land take, that is, for zero loss of agricultural and natural land areas because of urban expansion.

In order to analyze the feasibility and consequences of such an option in Flanders, a land take–neutral scenario (LTN) was developed and compared with the business-as-usual (BAU) scenario described in the previous section. In the LTN scenario, it is assumed that the current level of land take of some 7.4 hectares (~18 acres) per day is reduced to a level of 3 hectares (~7 acres) per day in 2020 and further reduced to 0 hectares per day by 2050. An analysis of land take in Flanders since 1990 reveals that LTN development may well be possible. Yearly data obtained from the cadastral registry show a clear decline in land take over the 1990–2012 period (figure 11.10, left). Although a simple exponential regression line suggests that a reduction to 1 hectare (~2.5 acres) per day in 2050 may be the long-term result of this decline, such a trend line does not take into consideration three significant factors. First, the population of Flanders is expected to grow by another 750,000 people by 2050. Second, since 1990, the population density of Flanders has decreased by some 12 inhabitants per hectare (~3,100 per square mile; figure 11.10, right), a trend that is expected to continue, but less strongly, under business-as-usual conditions. And, third, expansion of residential areas is responsible for some two-thirds of the total land take in Flanders. The result of these three factors combined is BAU development in which land

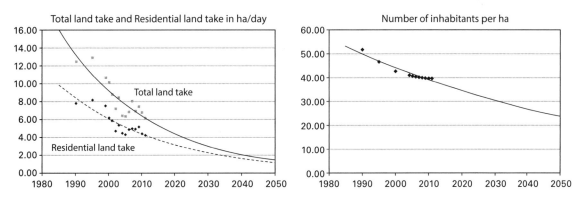

Figure 11.10
Trends in residential activity in Flanders, 1990–2012: (*left*) total land take and residential land take in hectares per day; (*right*) residential density (inhabitants per hectare).

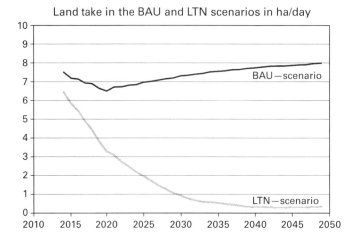

Figure 11.11
Land take in Flanders in hectares per day according to business-as-usual (BAU) and land take–neutral (LTN) scenarios.

take falls somewhat until 2020, mostly because of the aging population, but then starts to rise again (figure 11.11).

For the analysis discussed here, no effort is made to define the possible policy and planning measures that would be capable of generating the increased population and employment densities that the land take–neutral scenario requires in both the currently urbanized area and in newly urbanized areas. Rather, it is simply assumed that appropriate measures can be found. The increases in density specified in the scenario are greatest at the outset, but fall at a constant rate over the 2010–2021 period and then at a declining rate until 2050. Whereas in the business-as-usual scenario, densification is entirely controlled by the appropriate submodel of the RuimteModel itself, in the land take–neutral scenario, the submodel is forced to follow the trends imposed, although the densities are slightly modulated by the dynamics of the model (figure 11.11).

To assess the effects of a land take–neutral policy, the RuimteModel is run with both the BAU and LTN scenarios for the period 2010–2050. To facilitate the comparison, the same indicators are computed for both scenarios. As table 11.1 shows, the BAU scenario results in a strong increase in urban land uses, from 26.70% of total land uses in 2010 to 34.63% in 2050 (see also figure 11.4; plate 15). In comparison, the LTN scenario results in a very modest increase, from 26.70% in 2010 to 28.81% in 2050. The differences between the scenarios are most pronounced in the land areas between the larger agglomerations of Flanders, that is, those most subject to suburbanization and urban sprawl. This is clearly demonstrated by the indicator degree of urbanization (figure 11.12).

Table 11.1
Evolution of urban land use in Flanders in business-as-usual and land take–neutral scenarios, 2010–2050

Scenario	Hectares	Urban (%)
2010 (actual)	364,528	26.70
BAU scenario 2050	472,729	34.63
LTN scenario 2050	393,386	28.81

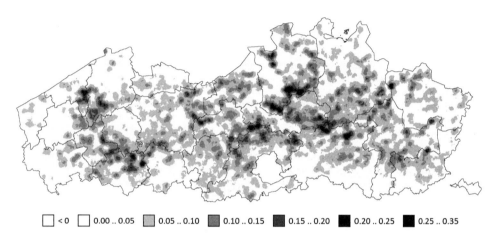

Figure 11.12
Differences in indicator *degree of urbanization* between BAU and LTN scenarios for Flanders and Brussels.

The degree of urbanization in the Flemish diamond and in the Antwerp-Brussels-Hasselt triangle is nearly 25% less under the LTN than under the BAU scenario. The same phenomenon can be observed in areas to the north of Kortrijk and to the southwest of Bruges; which are shown to be under high pressure of urbanization in the BAU scenario. This reduction in urban sprawl is reflected in the increased integrity of the open spaces. Figure 11.13 shows the differences in size of the open-space cluster to which each open-space cell belongs between the two scenarios for 2050. In the LTN scenario, larger clusters of open space persist throughout Flanders, but the effect is most pronounced for the area between Antwerp, Brussels, and Hasselt, with clusters that are as much as 2,400 hectares (~9.5 square miles) larger in size. Preserving open spaces in highly urbanized areas like Flanders is vital for recreation, nature protection, and agricultural activity.

The consequences of an LTN policy for agriculture are clearly shown by the indicator *agriculturally sensitive area*. As defined by the Flemish Ministry of Agriculture.,

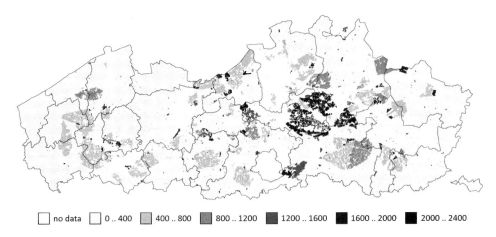

Figure 11.13
Differences between LTN and the BAU scenarios in terms of cluster size of open spaces for Flanders and Brussels.

it expresses on a scale of 0 to 10 the value attributed to each agricultural parcel, based on the physical, economic, and social characteristics of the parcel itself and the value to the farmer to whom the parcel belongs. Under the land take–neutral scenario, the loss of agriculturally sensitive area is clearly less than under the business-as-usual scenario (figure 11.14). This difference is most pronounced in the western part of Flanders and in the areas to the southeast of Antwerp and the northwest of Brussels. The loss of agricultural land has consequences for ecosystem services provided by the agricultural sector, and especially for the output of the agricultural sector. An indicator of the value of output of each agricultural parcel is calculated as a function of its soil quality and its use as either arable land or permanent grassland; its potential food production is expressed in monetary terms. Potential production values are based on data provided by the agricultural sector (Broekx et al., 2013). They range from 790 to 1,579 euros per hectare (~320 to 640 euros per acre) for grassland and from 1,233 to 2,188 euros per hectare (~500 to 885 euros per acre) for crops. Clearly, cells that are converted to urban land use lose their capacity to produce food. The difference between the two scenarios with respect to this indicator is shown in figure 11.15. The total yearly average loss for Flanders amounts to about 126 million euros in the BAU and about 39 million euros in the LTN scenario.

The four indicators discussed show the clear benefits of land take–neutral development with respect to the preservation of open spaces and agriculturally sensitive areas, the reduction of suburbanization and urban sprawl, and the production of food. On the other hand, LTN development assumes densification, and it remains to

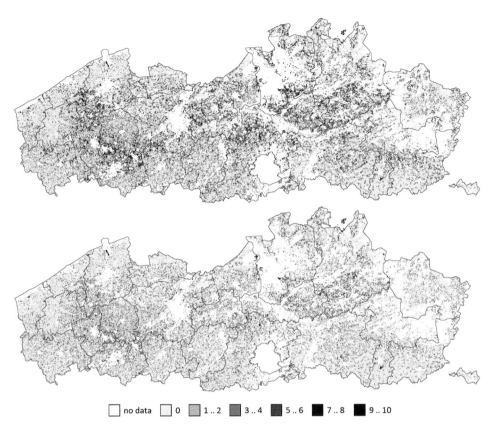

Figure 11.14
Value per cell of agriculturally sensitive area lost in Flanders: (*top*) BAU scenario: (*bottom*) LTN scenario; index of values ranges from 0 (no value) to 10 (maximum value).

be seen whether the required densification is feasible in Flanders. To address this issue, an additional indicator was developed, one showing the population density associated with each residential cell. The initial (2010) residential density is calculated by means of dasymetric mapping (Mennis, 2003), which allocates the population of the 9,182 statistical sectors of Flanders to the cells in the *residential* and the *mixed residential, industry, and commerce* land use classes (see figure 11.4; plate 15). For each consecutive year in the simulation interval, the population densities are updated in line with the output of the regional model. For newly developed residential and mixed residential, industry, and commerce cells, population densities are computed as the median of all inhabited cells in their immediate surroundings, a circular neighborhood with a radius of 300 meters (~0.2 mile). Cells that are no longer occupied by residential or mixed residential, industry, and commerce land use

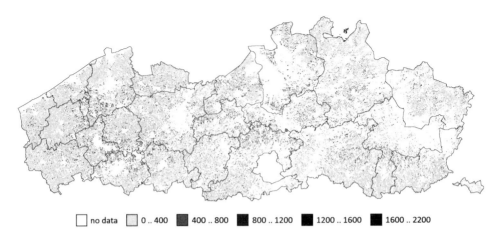

Figure 11.15
Differences in potential food production (in euros per hectare) in Flanders between LTN and BAU scenarios. Cell values are LTN minus BAU.

lose their population. Finally, conservation of mass is enforced, with the population densities per cell rescaled so that the sum of the population in all the cells of an arrondissement is equal to the total population of the arrondissement as calculated in the regional model.

For the whole of Flanders, population density in 2010 was 24.7 inhabitants per hectare (~6,400 per square mile). In the business-as-usual scenario, the population density drops to a value of 21.1 (~5,500 per square mile) in 2050. In contrast, it increases to 25.5 (~6,700 per square mile) in the land take–neutral scenario. This means that LTN development requires an increase of the population density of only 0.8 persons per hectare (~200 per square mile), or slightly more than 3% on average over the forty-year period from 2010 to 2050. Although, at first glance, this seems possible, as the map in figure 11.16 shows, the increase in density is not evenly distributed over the territory. The LTN scenario results in significantly higher densities in nearly all urban centers. The increase is most pronounced in the centers of the larger agglomerations such as Antwerp, Brussels, and Ghent, but also in midsized cities located in areas under particular urbanization pressure such as Leuven, Ostend, Mechelen, Tongeren, and Hasselt. Increases in density of up to 50 inhabitants per hectare (~13,000 per square mile) may be required in these urban centers. In contrast, nearly all of the locations experiencing a reduction in density (not shown on the map of figure 11.16) are those which do not urbanize in the LTN scenario even though they do so in the BAU scenario.

From this comparison of scenarios, we might conclude that a land take–neutral development seems feasible, requiring an increase in population density that is

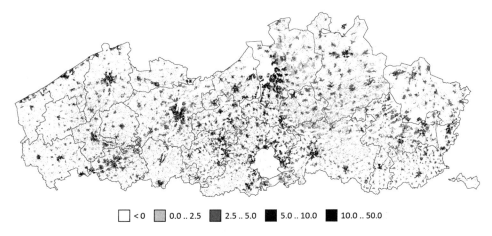

Figure 11.16
Differences in population density for Flanders and Brussels between LTN and the BAU scenarios. Cell values are LTN minus BAU populations.

possible, even in the urban cores. Indeed, over the course of forty years, it should be feasible to renew the housing stock while increasing the population density by as much as 50 inhabitants per hectare (~13,000 per square mile) in some sections of the urban cores, but generally less than 25 inhabitants per hectare (~6,500 per square mile). The resulting densities would still be low compared to those in neighboring countries and certainly compared to those in densely populated cities elsewhere in the world. The benefits would be experienced most strongly in the remaining open spaces of Flanders. Whereas business-as-usual development would seriously fragment and consume open spaces, land take–neutral development would leave more open space and have less of an impact on farming, recreation, and nature protection. It is expected that other effects of LTN development not yet addressed will be in the near future. These include the impact on investment needed to build new or maintain existing infrastructure for the distribution of electricity, water, and gas and for the collection of waste water and solid waste, as well as on mobility, the use of energy, carbon dioxide production, and human health.

Although scenario comparisons play an important role in supporting both analytical and visioning exercises in spatial planning, when it comes to making firm decisions on which areas should be designated or developed for a particular land use, spatial optimization is a more appropriate technique. A spatial optimization tool was developed incorporating the RuimteModel as one of the core modules. The modeling exercise discussed in the next section was carried out for the province of Limburg in the eastern part of Flanders.

Seeking Locations for New Business Parks in Limburg Province: The RUBELIM Application

As discussed in the introductory section, spatial planning in Flanders is currently directed by the Flanders Spatial Structure Plan (RSV), according to which the Flemish Spatial Planning Administration is tasked with assessing the need for land for new business parks, among other types of functions, and with determining where in Flanders such land is to be found or freed up. The administration can also require individual provinces to locate the needed land, however, and in the exercise discussed here, it required Limburg Province to find some 447 hectares (~1.75 square miles) of land for the development of business parks of "regional importance" in sixteen of the province's municipalities. *Regional importance* refers to business parks of a size larger than 5 hectares (~12.5 acres), in principle occupied by larger companies of a national or regional scale, distributing their products over larger areas, and located in municipalities with distinct urban characteristics, namely, "small towns" and "small-scale economic centers." In contrast, local business parks have a local importance, serve local markets, are generally smaller, attract smaller-scale activities, and fall under the full authority of the municipalities, the third and lowest hierarchical level in the RSV. Limburg Province decided to address the question with a scientifically rooted, quantitative approach. In support of this exercise, a spatial optimization model based on the RuimteModel, the OptimizationTool, was developed to find the locations, and stakeholders were invited to join in the exercise and define the various socioeconomic criteria used for selecting the areas for business parks, to supplement the spatial criteria defined in the Limburg Spatial Structure Plan or derived from other legally binding documents, such as Natura 2000, which defines protected natural areas. The OptimizationTool consists of three coupled modules, as depicted in figure 11.17.

The allocation module provides the general conditions for alternative solutions to the location of the business parks. It specifies the alternative solutions by means of a suitability map for business parks and sets of weights for the local accessibility parameters. This module is thus, in a sense, simply a tool for generating part of the input necessary to initialize the RuimteModel. It is important, however, because its suitability maps and accessibility parameter sets represent alternative hypotheses about what constitutes a good location. Although these could be generated by competing analyses of the requirements of business parks, in the present case, they were generated by various stakeholders, such as developers and environmental groups. The allocation module thus performs the vital function of providing a medium for stakeholder participation.

The RuimteModel is the core module. It finds the actual locations for the business parks that correspond to the alternative solutions generated by the allocation

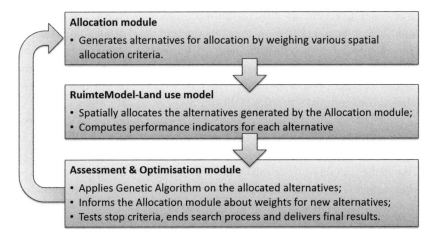

Figure 11.17
Three linked modules of the OptimizationTool.

module. In addition, for each solution, it computes spatial performance indicators for the resulting land use map.

The assessment and optimization module applies a genetic algorithm to all the alternative solutions generated and evaluated by the RuimteModel. The genetic algorithm generates new weights to create superior alternative solutions in the allocation module. By cycling through the three modules, more alternative solutions are found for the location of new business parks that better fit the specified criteria.

For the purpose of the exercise, the RuimteModel was adapted in several ways. First, an additional land use, *new business parks*, was introduced. The influence functions for this land use were based on those for light industry, commerce, and services, with a blended set of influence weights to reflect the fact that the new business parks must function as good locations for all three types of activity. In a more significant modification, the time loop of the CA-based land use model serves not to advance time in a dynamic land use model, but rather to implement an iterative solution to the optimum location problem. Accordingly, all land uses are kept stable in their initial state except for the new business parks, which are introduced one by one as a demand for the appropriate amount of land, for example, 20 hectares (~50 acres). The gradual introduction prevents instabilities in the calculation of the transition potentials. At this stage, the model converts the cells with the highest transition potentials to the new business park land use, but these cells are not necessarily contiguous. A realistic solution, however, requires that they be contiguous. The contiguity problem is solved at a later stage of the solution process, which will be discussed shortly.

Each alternative solution generated by the allocation module consists of one suitability map and a set of weights for the accessibility submodel. For all solutions, the same zoning map is applied, thus reflecting the hard zoning constraints that must be adhered to (see table 11.2). The zoning map is binary and distinguishes areas where business parks can be developed from those where their development is forbidden. The total excluded area amounts to 70,621 hectares (~275 square miles), which is some 30% of the territory of Limburg Province (figure 11.18, left). The suitability map represents the fitness of the territory for business parks (figure 11.18, right). It is a weighted sum of physical, ecological, socioeconomic, and spatial planning criteria, each represented by a GIS layer covering the entire territory of the province (see table 11.3).The parameters of the accessibility submodel represent the importance given to the proximity not only of transportation infrastructure, specifically roads, railroads, high-speed streetcars, bus stops, waterways, multimodal logistic terminals,

Table 11.2
GIS layers to zoning map for *new business parks* land use in Flanders

Areas from which *business parks* land use is excluded	
Flanders Ecological Network	Natura 2000 Special Areas of Conservation
Recreation areas	Open-space corridors
Silence areas	Cultural heritage areas
"HogeKempen" national park	Protected landscapes
Flood-prone areas	(Ground)water storage and extraction areas
Destinations according to zoning plans	

Table 11.3
Criteria used as input to calculate suitability map for *new business parks* land use in Flanders

Suitability criteria	
Available business park area in municipality	Proximity to town centers
Distance to urban areas	Nearby population density
Nearby number of unemployed	Nearby Ford workers
Protected green areas	Slope of terrain
Confirmed agricultural zones	Agriculturally sensitive land
Distance to commercial centers	Distance to existing business parks
Ecological corridors	Water storage and exploitation areas
Cultural heritage areas	Natura 2000 Special Areas of Conservation
Open-space corridors	Flood-prone areas
Silence areas	

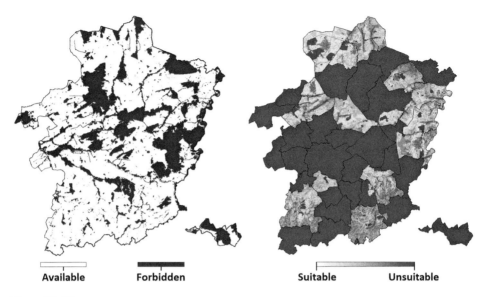

Figure 11.18
Zoning and suitability for the land use *new business parks* in Limburg Province: (*left*) zoning map (development in dark areas is forbidden); (*right*) suitability map (lighter areas are suitable; darker areas are unsuitable). Municipalities that are not to receive a business park are assigned uniformly low suitabilities.

and bicycle paths, but also of energy distribution infrastructure, such as high-voltage power stations and gas pipelines.

By giving different weights to the map layers or the accessibility parameters, the RuimteModel generates fairly different suitability and accessibility maps, and thus alternative solutions for the location of new business parks. The first trial solution is generated with equal weights, and the model then computes the associated spatial configuration and a set of performance indicators for the configuration. Performance indicators involve overlay operations (e.g., to establish the amount and location of sensitive agricultural area lost), buffer operations (e.g., to compute the number and location of unemployed people within 5 kilometers or ~3 miles), or distance-decay computations (to determine proximity to the urban centers, high-voltage transformer stations, and other relevant nodes). They assess the appropriateness of the locations of the nearby business parks against criteria derived from the Limburg Spatial Structure Plan, such as protection of open-space corridors, safeguarding of silence areas, or avoiding flood-prone areas, and criteria formulated by the stakeholders, such as protection of agricultural land, proximity to waterways, and proximity to former Ford workers. The last criterion was important because the Ford Motor Company was scheduled to close its car assembly plant in Genk in December 2014, and did in fact do so, with the result that some 10,000 people working for Ford or local companies supplying components lost their jobs.

Rather than applying all criteria simultaneously, which would lead to a single set of optimal locations, the decision was made to determine optimal locations with respect to four different scenarios: environment, employment, logistics, and knowledge centers (table 11.4). The term *scenario* is used here to represent a particular focus in the optimization exercise. The environment scenario is focused on preventing the loss of valuable agricultural and natural land. Thus it favors locations in or near already urbanized areas. The employment scenario is directed at maximizing conveniently located employment opportunities, so locations near population

Table 11.4
Criteria applied in five allocation scenarios

Environment	Employment
Agriculturally sensitive land	Population within 5 kilometers (~3 miles)
Open-space corridors	Unemployed within 5 kilometers
Silence areas	
Confirmed agricultural zones	Proximity to cycling network
Natura 2000 Special Areas of Conservation	Proximity to bus stops/railroad stations/Spartacus stops
Cultural heritage areas	
Flood-prone areas	
Water storage and conservation areas	

Logistics	Knowledge centers
Proximity to existing business parks	Proximity to commercial and service centers
Proximity to railroads	Proximity to existing business parks
Proximity to cargo routes	Proximity to railroad stations/Spartacus stops
Proximity to high-voltage transformer stations/pipelines	Proximity to logistics terminals
	Proximity to waterways
	Plus:
	Available business park area in municipality
	Criteria considered in all scenarios
	Proximity to motorway entrance/exit points
	Proximity to primary/secondary roads
	Slope of terrain
	Protected green areas
	Spatial policy map
	Attraction to urban areas, repulsion from town centers

concentrations, especially concentrations of unemployed people, as well as locations that are easily accessible by public transport are highly ranked. The logistics scenario favors the location of business parks near the main transportation and other infrastructure. The logistics-plus scenario is a variant that avoids creating additional business parks in municipalities that have not yet used up the area available in existing business parks. Finally, the knowledge centers scenario seeks locations for knowledge-intensive activities such as business incubators or university spin-off companies; locations in the vicinity of existing business parks, commercial and service centers, universities and other tertiary-level institutions, as well as those near public transport are most likely to be chosen in this scenario. For each scenario, the Ruimte-Model computes all performance indicators for each alternative solution and passes these on to the assessment and optimization module, which applies a genetic algorithm to assess the performance of the weight sets used in the alternative solutions for the scenario and generates improved weight sets. The new weight sets are returned to the allocation module to begin a new iteration. A typical exercise involves several thousand iterations and thus also the generation and assessment of several thousand alternative solutions for each scenario.

In the next step, the OptimizationTool applies a Pareto optimality procedure to find the best solution for each scenario. Optimal solutions are those located on the Pareto frontier, which consists of those solutions not dominated by any other solution. A solution S_1 dominates S_2 if S_1 equals or outscores S_2 on all criteria. In the OptimizationTool, the Pareto frontier is reduced in size by applying minimum threshold values for each criterion. Solutions are considered only if they score better than the threshold value for all criteria.

For each scenario, the OptimizationTool produces a map with Pareto frequencies representing the number of times a cell is occupied by the new business park land use in solutions that belong to the Pareto frontier. Figure 11.19 shows the Pareto frequency maps for the municipality of Tongeren, in the south of the province, for the four scenarios. In general, the same cells show up with high-frequency values in the areas immediately adjacent to existing business parks in all four scenarios. This is not surprising because proximity to existing business parks was a criterion in all scenarios, either directly, or indirectly through the employment-related criteria in combination with the influence functions in the RuimteModel. Furthermore, existing business parks are generally well located with respect to the criteria used in the exercise. On the other hand, each scenario also highlights some locations as particularly attractive that do not stand out in the other scenarios, typically the result of criteria that are specific to the particular scenario. For example, the strong clusters in the more northerly part of the map in the knowledge centers scenario are due to the criteria favoring access to high-speed streetcar stops and proximity to commercial and service centers, whereas, in the logistics scenario, the strong clusters in the

288 Chapter 11

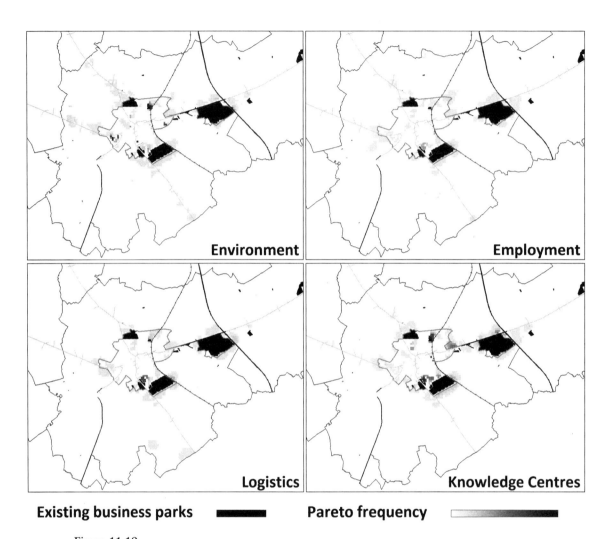

Figure 11.19
Pareto frequencies for Tongeren municipality for environment, employment, logistics, and knowledge centers scenarios.

remote locations to the south are due to the proximity of high-voltage transformer stations.

Although the Pareto optimality maps are interesting, they are not directly useful in solving the new business park location problem because the cells in a cluster representing a new business park are often somewhat scattered, whereas a business park would consist of a compact cluster of fifteen or twenty contiguous 1-hectare cells. A cluster algorithm was therefore developed that defined clusters of the required size with the highest total Pareto optimality scores while respecting the contiguity requirement. To provide options for spatial planners and municipal authorities, both the best and second-best clusters were identified in each of the four scenarios. Figure 11.20 shows the results for 20-hectare business parks in Tongeren municipality according to the logistics scenario.

For the spatial planners of Limburg Province, the end results of the RuimteModel analysis looked quite realistic. Some locations were identical to those they had identified prior to the exercise; others were new and relatively unexpected. The planners were reassured by the fact that the model supported their original candidate sites, but they were also pleased to be provided with reasonable alternatives that had not previously been identified. Both the results and the methodology were presented to the political, administrative, and technical organizations active within the province of Limburg, as well as to the mayors of the municipalities concerned. The results

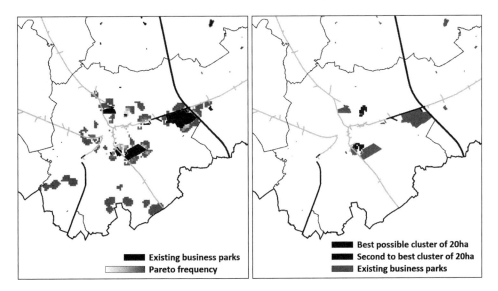

Figure 11.20
Best and second-best locations for business parks of 20 hectares (~50 acres) in Tongeren municipality under logistics scenario.

were accepted and moved to the implementation phase. The spatial planning department of Limburg Province now actively supports the municipalities ready to invest in the development of one of the two alternative locations identified in the exercise. Municipalities can request financial assistance for the development of the approved new business parks.

The next phase of the RUBELIM project will consist of a similar exercise, but will involve all municipalities in the province and focus on municipal business parks about 5 hectares in size. Although the OptimizationTool will be applied as it is, the criteria will be modified to focus more on the particular locational characteristics of these small local business parks. Collaboration with the municipalities will be intensified, with each municipality invited to introduce spatial optimization criteria taken from planning documents such as the municipal Spatial Structure Plan.

Supporting Participatory Planning Processes

In the examples just described, the RuimteModel was used in a relatively traditional way to provide information to support decision making by planners and other governmental officials. Spatial planning is rapidly becoming less of a top-down procedure, however; planners are increasingly expected to act as facilitators and guardians of good planning principles in a process involving a variety of experts and stakeholders, many of whom have strongly conflicting agendas. In these situations, it may be extremely difficult to reach a consensus and thus arrive at an acceptable solution. A modeling tool introduced into a planning process with strong stakeholder participation can be highly effective in helping the various parties move toward a common position, because the model provides a framework that excludes proposals involving hidden contradictions, while revealing possible solutions that the participants may not be able to find on their own. More generally, a model can provide a common framework for discussions among stakeholders.

A good example is provided by the successful use of the OptimizationTool in the implementation of Flemish biodiversity policy. Flanders, as part of an EU member state, must adhere to the Natura 2000 biodiversity policy, meaning that it must ensure the protection of forty-six habitat types of European importance in thirty-eight Special Areas of Conservation (SACs), covering 104,888 hectares (~400 square miles) or close to 8% of the total area of Flanders. The SACs are highly fragmented into some 400 subareas, which are under severe pressure from agriculture, infrastructure, and urbanization. The areas and subareas must be delineated and managed in such a way as to satisfy a large number of criteria determined at the European Union level to ensure that the protected habitats remain healthy. Although many of these criteria are physical, biological, ecological, or environmental in nature, some are socioeconomic, and, in any case, socioeconomic activities may have a major impact on whether the other criteria can be met. Given the large number of conservation areas involved and the multiplicity of criteria to be satisfied, as well as the variety of stakeholders and the diversity of their interests, finding an optimal set of habitat conservation areas is a problem that requires more than a good discussion or the expertise of a planner to resolve. Moreover, at the technical level, it is a difficult spatial allocation problem that must be handled at a resolution of 1 hectare (~2.5 acres) in order to capture its essential spatial characteristics. But it is also an allocation problem that must take into account the interests and concerns of the stakeholders in order to be acceptable.

In Flanders, the Agency for Forest and Nature (ANB) is responsible for the implementation of biodiversity policy. The implementation exercise was carried out in close collaboration with other government departments, especially those responsible for agriculture, spatial planning, the environment, and transportation infrastructure, but also in consultation with stakeholder organizations representing farmers, landowners, the forestry sector, industry, and water supply, and with nongovernmntal organizations involved in nature protection. The stakeholders all had very particular requirements. For example, having to extract groundwater for municipal and industrial use, the water companies did not want any areas of humid habitat in the vicinity of their pumping cones to be designated for protection because that would restrict the amount of water they would be allowed to extract. Many of the stakeholder requirements conflicted with one another; as a consequence, the implementation exercise, which had been ongoing for a number of years, had made little progress toward identifying the actual areas to be set aside as protected habitats. When it was suggested that a model be used to provide technical support, all parties agreed that, rather than carrying on with negotiations that seemed to be leading nowhere, the OptimizationTool would be used to compute a global optimum, one reflecting both their concerns and the biophysical constraints. Most important, the parties agreed to accept the global optimum as a definitive solution. Under the deadlines fixed by the European Union, they had only nine months left to find a solution, enact it into law, and submit it to the EU.

To start the OptimizationTool exercise, the stakeholders were invited to develop optimization criteria that would reflect their interests and concerns, and they were assisted in this process to ensure that the criteria were sufficiently well defined to be implemented in the modeling tool. Each stakeholder was limited to two spatial criteria. Together with the biophysical criteria, implemented with the assistance of the Research Institute for Nature and Forest and the Flemish Agency for Forest and Nature, the spatial criteria were then introduced into the OptimizationTool. Intermediate results were computed, presented, and discussed in biweekly meetings with all parties involved. Meanwhile, additional information was gathered and better algorithms were developed to capture the complex biophysical requirements. At first, the stakeholders found it difficult to understand the complexity of the modeling and optimization methodology and were skeptical of both the methodology and the results. They criticized the ANB for inadequate baseline data and for the poor quality of the intermediate results. During discussions, positions tended to be polarized, with the stakeholders, on one side, opposing the ANB, on the other. Nevertheless, the OptimizationTool approach retained sufficient support that all parties were willing to continue with it. Gradually, as the data improved and the criteria provided by the stakeholders evolved toward a complete and definite set representing the precise characteristics that concerned them, the results were taken much more seriously. The stakeholders started to understand the effects of the solutions for their respective sectors and began to negotiate among themselves on the basis of each new round of optimization results. Interestingly, the parties rapidly came to understand that a global optimum really meant compromise by all stakeholders—that negotiating for better conditions in one location for one stakeholder would automatically mean worse conditions for that same stakeholder, or another one, in another location. With that understanding, the stakeholders rather quickly accepted the results of the optimization exercise as the best they could achieve.

Shortly after agreement was achieved, the results were enacted into law by the Flemish Parliament. The process described, from the introduction of the OptimizationTool to the vote in parliament, took less than a year. Given the complexity of the issue, the stakes involved, and the time devoted to it, this can be considered a real success. Currently, the Natura 2000 exercise has moved on to the next phase, actual implementation on the ground. The OptimizationTool is again being used in this exercise. It has been modified so that it can delineate the optimal parcels of land to be purchased for the conservation of the various habitats at the level of the 400 SAC conservation subareas. This process involves the same agencies and stakeholders, and even the same people. In fact, they were the ones who together decided to continue using the OptimizationTool.

Conclusions and Further Research

Work with the RuimteModel started in early 2007 as a proof of concept for the feasibility of using CA-based land use modeling in Flanders to support planning and policy development. By 2009, both the Environment Outlook 2030 and Nature Outlook 2030 relied on the RuimteModel for inquiries related to expected land use changes and their effects on biodiversity and environmental quality indices. In addition, the business-as-usual scenario described in this chapter has been used in the development of the flood risk policy plans being prepared by the Flemish Environment Agency (VMM). The identification of sites for new business parks and the facilitation of stakeholder negotiations to arrive quickly at an agreement on the location of habitat conservation areas as required by Natura 2000 demonstrate that a land use modeling tool can indeed be usefully integrated into formal planning processes.

Although evidence is accumulating that complex scientific instruments like the RuimteModel can be applied to solve practical planning problems, introducing the modeling approach into the everyday planning process still presents a number of challenges, most notably, bridging the gap between the practical concerns of spatial planners and other decision makers, on the one hand, and the theoretical and technical world of modelers, on the other; both sides must learn to speak each other's language and to understand each other's problems. Modelers soon discover that the ability to forecast land use change is not, in itself, sufficient to support decision making. Rather, the functionalities, variables, parameters, and output of the models must be immediately relevant to the decision makers so that scenarios can be defined and run that are straightforward to interpret. The ability to compute custom-defined indicators is certainly a step toward making the models into flexible decision support tools; making them more transparent and intuitive, especially with respect to matters like embedded assumptions and uncertainty propagation, will convince more potential users to trust the models and apply them as part of the decision-making process.

12
Paths to the Future

The family of models described in this book represents an evolution from relatively simple models of a single phenomenon to complex integrated models handling a variety of phenomena. The basic constrained CA-based model captures the local endogenous spatial dynamics of land use as they are driven by exogenous growth and modified by the spatially inhomogeneous landscape. The integrated models, in which domain-specific models from other fields such as economics, transportation, and hydrology are linked dynamically to the land use CA, come closer to a comprehensive representation of urban and regional dynamics. Finally, the multiple activity variable grid CA-based model integrates material from location theory, regional science, demography, and economics, as well as from physical and human geography within the CA itself. This may seem to be a "Franken-CA," and in a sense it is, but even though it may not appeal to purists, it has real advantages. It provides a relatively comprehensive high-resolution representation of the spatial dynamics of a city or region, and being a CA, it remains computationally efficient. As a unitary model of several phenomena rather than a collection of coupled models, each dedicated to a subset of the phenomena, it has fewer parameters, and being more risky in the Popperian sense, it is more likely to be reliable once validated. Furthermore, its structure reflects the unitary nature of the city. In that sense, it begins to reunite the fragmented knowledge we have from a variety of special-purpose models rooted in different disciplines.

The models and applications we have presented, together with the work of urban modelers such as Juval Portugali and Itzhak Benenson, Keith Clarke, and Xia Li, among others, demonstrate the feasibility and utility of modeling cities and regions as complex systems that are integrated wholes. The models give good insights into the way cities and regions organize themselves over time, and increasingly, they are able to provide practical guidance to planners and policy makers. But there are several impediments to further progress. The community of urban and regional modelers is quite small, dwarfed, for example, by the number of modelers addressing the dynamics of the atmospheric system. Furthermore, the obvious client community consisting of urban, regional, and transportation planners is largely unaware of the possibility of using these models, and our experience to date suggests that it will be a lengthy process to capture their interest. The danger is that, in the absence of a sizeable client community, modelers will retreat to building toy models of only academic interest. At present, however, the process is at least moving in the right direction, with increasing numbers of planners willing to give the models a try.

Moreover, some inherent characteristics of the models themselves raise issues that impede the widespread acceptance of modeling by potential end users, most fundamentally, the issues of predictability and validation. As we saw in chapter 9, the models are only quasi-predictive, reflecting the quasi predictability of the phenomena being modeled, which, in turn, makes them difficult to validate. These issues tend to make potential end users hesitate when considering whether to use the models. Of course, these issues go far beyond urban and regional modeling; they arise in any field in which complex self-organizing systems are modeled. We consider that fortunate because it means that the problems that these issues present will not have to be solved by urban and regional modelers alone. Ecologists, to take one example, are already dealing with them, as are some philosophers who look at the methodological and epistemological problems posed by biology.

Because the problems of predictability, validation, and acceptance by a client community are closely related, we believe that solutions will emerge gradually from modeling practice and be codified into a methodological protocol, with philosophical support from evolutionary epistemology. Once it is recognized that quasi predictability implies quasi validation, a methodological argument can be made that confidence in a model increases with the number of successful applications. Thus validation and application are mutually reinforcing. Of course, the question of confidence is crucial. If potential users have no confidence in a model because of doubts about validation, they are unlikely to use it, and efforts to achieve cumulative validation will be stillborn. On the other hand, as philosophers and others begin to grapple with problems arising in the science of systems with open futures, that is, systems that are, by their very nature, only quasi-predictable and subject to emergence, they will systematize and legitimize the best practices of the modelers working on these systems. Because these issues affect the future of urban and regional modeling, we examine them here in greater detail.

Quasi Predictability and the Evolution of Models

The integrated, comprehensive models we have presented are, in a sense, an attempt to regain a holistic understanding of cities and regions, but one based on a formal, computational approach. There seems to be a widespread belief, however, that large, complex models are unreliable because their behavior cannot be completely understood, their calibration is arbitrary, and they cannot be validated. As we saw in chapter 9, this attitude can be traced, in part, to a belief in the standards of classical scientific methodology, a methodology that is not really appropriate for research on complex self-organizing systems. The models that seem to be the most "scientific" when judged by these standards probably embody the least science. For example, a simple CA-based model of urbanization—one with two states, transition rules extracted from remotely sensed data by a neural network, and validation using a split data set—would seem to be a safe bet because all steps, including the validation test, are quantified, and the model structure is simple enough to be transparent. But, in fact, it is little more than a description of land use change in a particular situation. It incorporates almost nothing, explicitly, about the processes generating urbanization. It is unlikely to be reliable when used beyond the calibration period. Furthermore, it adds little to our understanding of urbanization and its spatial manifestations, which are driven by the complex interplay of the various social, economic, political, and technological phenomena that characterize a city, and which are, at a deeper level, the result of all the varied, complex interactions of the individual people, companies, and organizations that make up the city. That is why we need comprehensive, integrated models, ones that represent all the essential aspects of a city or region.

But the complexity of such models comes at a price, one that at present we cannot quite afford. The heart of the problem is prediction. Models that integrate the treatment of a variety of phenomena within a complex self-organizing systems framework do not fit the classical scientific paradigm of validation anchored by a significance test, a paradigm that requires them to make predictions that can be compared quantitatively with empirical observations. As we have seen, complex self-organizing systems are only quasi-predictable, and one of their essential characteristics is the presence of bifurcations, which complicates the notion of predictability and makes simple, rigorous empirical tests impossible. There is widespread ignorance of this phenomenon, even among specialists on validation. For example, Robert Marks (2007), in a formal treatment of validation, classifies as "complete but inaccurate" a model that produces all behavior observed in the real system but also some other behavior as well. But, as we have seen, a model of a system subject to bifurcations *must* produce unobserved behavior or it is both incomplete and inaccurate.

In a sense, the real problem is that the current formal protocols for model and theory validation, developed to deal with phenomena that could be isolated experimentally or statistically and that are governed (or could reasonably be assumed to be governed) by universal laws, are inappropriate for models of complex systems. Although a few complex systems, notably, the atmospheric-oceanic system, are also governed by universal laws, those laws operate in a regime that produces complex or chaotic dynamics. Biological and social systems, on the other hand, even though they may ultimately be dependent on universal physical laws, are characterized by behavior that is largely independent of those laws, which is to say, the laws are responsible for the existence of processes of self-organization, but the nature and outcomes of the self-organization processes are largely unconstrained by those laws. And even though these systems often exhibit quasi-law-like behavior, such behavior is a manifestation of the process of self-organization: the systems must have a sufficient degree of organization and predictability to continue to exist, but they cannot have complete predictability because to continue to exist they must constantly adapt and evolve. And because these systems are, in a sense, creative, models of them must reflect the strategic indeterminacy of this creativity, and methodological protocols must support it.

Until a more appropriate protocol is developed, complex systems models will seem suspect to some. On the other hand, as we saw in chapter 9, the outlines of a protocol for verifying and validating complex systems models are beginning to emerge. Multiple tests of a model on a variety of analogous cases (e.g., a variety of cities) constitute one useful approach, one which also provides an indication of the degree of universality of a model (Pérez, Dragićević, and White, 2013; Refsgaard and Henriksen, 2004; Rykiel, 1996). The degree of correspondence between model output and empirical data is also an issue. Traditional criteria for significance tests assume that the closer the correspondence, the higher the degree of validation; but, as we have seen, if the predictions of a complex systems model are too similar to the data, the model is probably overcalibrated. It seems unlikely that a standard can be developed for the optimal degree of divergence between predictions and test data, but using multiple criteria in validation tests is one practical way around this problem. In any case, a model that performs well on a variety of tests is more worthy of our confidence than one that is validated on only a single test criterion, even if that single result is better than the result of any of the individual tests in the multicriterion approach. And the model's calibration process can itself be part of the model's verification. As we saw in chapter 9, if there is a trade-off during the calibration so that an improvement in model performance on one criterion results in a degradation of performance on another, then the model structure contains a misspecification; therefore, a model that can be calibrated *without* performance trade-offs has already passed a structural test. All of these procedures are ways of accommodating quasi-predictability. As applications of complex systems models become more common, we may expect that a formal methodological protocol will begin to emerge.

Whatever the shape of an eventual formal methodology for the validation and verification of complex systems models, it seems certain that repetition will play a central role. A single definitive test is not a realistic possibility when dealing with complex systems. Understanding the degree to which a model captures the essentials of a real system requires multiple applications in a variety of settings. The most important output of a complex systems model is a mapping of the bifurcation tree of possible system futures, and since any particular city or region has only a single history, that is, a single path through the implicit bifurcation tree, an application to a single city or region can only confirm that the model can generate that path. If the model can be successfully applied to a number of cases, then, its ability to generate an approximately correct bifurcation tree for any particular city is supported. If generic types of bifurcations, such as the agglomeration-dispersal bifurcation, can be identified, then validation can be made more explicit. In any case, the essential point is that robust validation depends on multiple applications.

Of course, models evolve. We have presented a series of models, each building on what has been learned from previous versions. To some degree, this series represents a progression, an evolution toward better models. But it also represents a diversification, where a single model becomes a family of related models, with each individual model adapted to better handle a certain class of problems or applications. This process of model evolution and diversification is a response to the requirements of new and different applications for clients with particular needs and concerns. As in recursive validation, when validation results are used to improve the structure of a model, the validation becomes part of the process of model evolution.

The need to adapt a model to handle new problems or phenomena drives model evolution. In this respect, planning applications are particularly important because they pose a wide variety of problems, many of them "messy"—just the sort of problems a modeler would prefer to avoid. But these problems force us to build realism into the model. In this connection, Richard Hewett advocates participatory modeling involving the public (Hewett, 2014; Hewett and Escobar, 2011), and Daniel Sarewitz (2012, p. 149) observes that "scientists rightly extol the capacity of research to self-correct. But the lesson...is that this self-correction depends not just on competition between researchers, but also on the close ties between science and its application that allow society to push back against biased and useless results." Practical applications force a serious consideration of the complicated nature of reality, and complication is the neglected dimension of complexity theory. The result is ultimately a family of models with better performance, greater reliability, and a wider range of applicability. And the greater the number and variety of applications, the more effective is the evolutionary process that is improving and diversifying the models.

On the other hand, this evolutionary process only leads to more powerful and reliable models if the selection criteria are appropriate and if they are appropriately used. In reality, there are several criteria that can occasionally lead to *worse* models. The two most important of these are ease of use and conventional scientific respectability. Clients rightfully want a model that is easy to use because, for them, the model is simply a tool to help them solve a problem; their focus is necessarily on solving their problem, not on using the model. Of course, other things being equal, they would prefer a better model—one that is more powerful and reliable. But if the better model is difficult or time consuming to use, they may well choose an inferior model that is easier to use. For the selection process to operate in favor of more powerful models, those models must also be at least relatively easy to use. Nevertheless, even though the models described in this book have been designed as much as possible to be user friendly, inevitably, a complex integrated model will be more difficult to apply, and will require greater resources in terms of data and expert knowledge than a simple model requiring only limited, easily available data.

Scientific respectability, though important, can also hinder the evolution of better models. There are cases where a client has switched from a dynamic simulation model of land use change to a static statistical model because simulation did not seem scientifically respectable, even though the simulation model would clearly have been more appropriate. For the same reason, many other potential users never adopt a simulation model in the first place. In the eyes of many, simulation models seem to lack objectivity. Parameters cannot usually be fit using a standard statistical technique with known properties, and results cannot be validated with a conventional test of significance. In the absence of a widely accepted protocol for calibrating and validating simulation models, the objectivity that seems to be associated with statistical approaches appears as an important advantage. This is especially the case if use of the model must be justified to the public, to a third party—or in court. In discussing the legal issue, Marks (2007) points out that even when the European Competition Commission and the U.S. Federal Trade Commission have admitted evidence based on simulation models (in this case, market models) in regulatory hearings, they have done so only for models meeting strict criteria. Furthermore, their decisions are frequently challenged in court, where other, similarly strict criteria come into play. For example, in the United States, under the Daubert criteria, a simulation model must be predictive, all assumptions and simplifications must be clearly justified, and sensitivity analysis must show how the predictions depend on the assumptions. Furthermore, the models must adhere fully to the standards of the scientific method. These criteria sound reasonable, but they pose real problems for complex systems models. In view of the many doubts expressed in the modeling literature about the feasibility of validating land use models, the lack of a basis in probability theory, and the general methodological experimentation that characterizes urban and regional simulation modeling, it might be difficult to establish the admissibility of an urban simulation model in a legal case. The legal issue points again to the need for a formal methodological protocol for complex systems models in order to establish them in the eyes of the user community as fully "scientific," and hence safe to use.

It is unlikely that urban models will seek standing in a court case in the near future. But the possibility that they might brings into focus the need for explicit methodological standards. Urban modeling, especially land use modeling, is currently in a fluid, experimental stage, as shown by the wide variety of models that continue to be developed, and by the lack of attention to methodological issues related to modeling complex systems. There is much experimentation with cell size and shape, neighborhood definition, and especially calibration techniques. But almost no attention is paid to technical issues related to validation. For example, the Kappa statistic continues to be the only measure of correspondence between simulated and actual land use maps that is used in most studies, even though it is both inappropriate in principle and essentially uninterpretable in practice. In this context, it is essentially a number used to give the appearance of validation while hiding the fact that the issue is being avoided. The work aimed at providing appropriate methods being undertaken by Alex Hagen-Zanker, Xia Li, Daniel Brown, and a few others, as discussed in chapter 9, remains largely ignored by those engaged in modeling land use change. And yet this is the sort of work that will gradually resolve the issues around validation and lead to an appropriate methodology. The fact that at least some researchers are addressing these issues is a hopeful sign, however.

Of course, the issue of justifying a model is much broader than the problem of validation. Although validation is the ultimate test because it addresses the question of model performance, performance itself is generally assessed within the very limited context of a particular application. Cumulative validation through multiple applications broadens this context. But an integrated model such as the multiple activity variable grid CA discussed in chapter 8 is endowed with a much broader context, the context of the other models and empirical relationships that have been incorporated in it. These borrowed components together provide a degree of ready-made verification of the model because they have already been validated by both explicit tests and, in some cases, years of widespread, successful use. For example, the activity-based model defines the neighborhood effect on the basis of the principle of spatial interaction. When the model is calibrated, and the long tail of the neighborhood influence function is found to approximate an inverse power law, we are reassured because, in thousands of applications of spatial interaction models, interactions of a wide variety have been found to follow an inverse power relationship. Contrast this with the case of a simple CA-based land use model with a small neighborhood. Once calibrated, the model may perform well in a particular case, but the transition rule depends entirely on the data for that case, and we have no larger context providing additional information that would allow us to judge whether the model is inherently plausible. More generally, the broader context provided by the borrowed components of an integrated model adds greatly to the explanatory content of the model.

Paths to the Future

One of the most frequently encountered problems in a new model application is a lack of data, and this has tended to hinder the widespread use of the models we have been discussing. Fortunately, this problem is likely to fade as geocoded data proliferate, and so we might expect increased interest in the use of high resolution models. Paradoxically, however, the explosion in the quantity and use of geocoded data seems to be diverting attention from the future to the present. Indeed, the economics of the ecosystem of social media, geocoding, and app development works to focus attention on the immediate present, with interest shifting from models that show us possible futures and allow us to evaluate the likely consequences of present actions to apps that support current actions on the basis of current data. For example, websites that show current traffic conditions allow drivers who access them to alter their routes to avoid red zones of serious congestion. Both the data and the actions taken in response to the data are essentially in real time, and presumably the overall result is lower average trip times. But even simple future-oriented modeling could improve that result. If all of the cars on the road were Google cars, for example, it would be a simple matter to track not only their current position and speed, but also their planned route and destination—that is, their current plans for the near future. With this information, it would be possible to predict the traffic problems before they arose and determine changes to planned routes that would prevent the red zones from appearing in the first place.

Of course, this example describes a very straightforward modeling problem, one in which the consequences of current actions in terms of route changes could be predicted with a high degree of certainty. But, qualitatively, the Google cars model is essentially the same as an urban simulation model: both give us a view of the future as it depends on current conditions and our current actions, and both therefore give us some ability to shape that future. It is true that the futures shown to us by the urban model are hazier and less certain, with consequences that are less urgent in our lives, consequences that are years in the future and that may not happen anyway, whereas if we are caught in a traffic jam, we may miss our flight or be late for work. On the other hand, the issues that urban and regional models are designed to anticipate, though less urgent, are generally larger and more important—for example, given the likely future spatial structure of a city, will congestion be widespread and unavoidable, even with the best Google cars model?

If the future retains its interest, and urban and regional models become easier to use, more versatile, and more reliable, and if they earn a reputation for being scientifically legitimate, then we can expect that they will be more widely adopted. It is easy to imagine them becoming a sort of add-on to the GIS capabilities of planning departments, so that planners routinely run a model to check the possible consequences of proposed infrastructure projects, zoning changes, or private sector developments. Perhaps more important is the potential for the models to be used in participatory settings to facilitate agreement among stakeholders, as was illustrated in the case involving the location of areas to be designated for protection of biodiversity in Flanders. In fact, once a model is set up and calibrated, anyone can use it. It is, after all, a game, and anyone can play Urban Futures.

Ultimately, we do not know what the future holds for urban modeling. We are all of us living in a complex, self-organizing system, one with many possible futures. And as evolutionary epistemology has shown, we create the bifurcation tree of possible futures as we move through it, so the future is doubly open. The poet Antonio Machado realized this long ago:

Walking, you make a path.
And when you turn,
You look back at the path
You will never follow again.

References

ADSEI (Directorate-General Statistics and Economic Information). 2011. Pendelaars Verdienen Meer (Commuters Earn More). Press release, June 15, 2011.

Agostinho, J. 2007. The Use of a Cellular Automaton Land Use Model as a Tool for Urban Planning. Unpublished Master's thesis, Memorial University of Newfoundland.

Al-Ahmadi, K., L. See, and A. Heppenstall. 2013. Validating Spatial Patterns of Urban Growth from a Cellular Automata Model. In *Emerging Applications of Cellular Automata*, ed. A. Salcido, 23–52. Rijeka, Croatia: InTech.

Al-Ahmadi, K., L. See, A. Heppenstall, and J. Hogg. 2009. Calibration of a Fuzzy Cellular Automata Model of Urban Dynamics in Saudi Arabia. *Ecological Complexity* 6:80–101.

Alfasi, N., J. Almagor, and I. Benenson. 2012. The Actual Impact of Comprehensive Land-Use Plans: Insights from High Resolution Observations. *Land Use Policy* 29:862–877.

Allen, P. 1997. *Cities and Regions as Self-Organizing Systems: Models of Complexity*. Amsterdam: Gordon and Breach.

Allen, P., and M. Sanglier. 1979. A Dynamic Model of Growth in a Central Place System. *Geographical Analysis* 11:269–278.

Allen, P., and M. Sanglier. 1981. Urban Evolution, Self-Organization and Decision Making. *Environment & Planning A* 13:167–183.

Allen, P., M. Sanglier, G. Engelen, and F. Boon. 1984. Evolutionary Spatial Models of Urban and Regional Systems. *Sistemi Urbani* 1:3–36.

Alonso, W. 1964. *Location and Land Use: Toward a General Theory of Land Rent*. Cambridge, MA: Harvard University Press.

Anas, A., R. Arnott, and K. Small. 1998. Urban Spatial Structure. *Journal of Economic Literature* 36:1426–1464.

Andersson, C., K. Lindgren, S. Rasmussen, and R. White. 2002. Growth Simulation from "First Principles." *Physical Review E* 66. 0260204.

Andersson, C., S. Rasmussen, and R. White. 2002. Urban Settlement Transitions. *Environment & Planning B* 29:841–865.

Angel, S., and G. Hyman. 1976. *Urban Fields: A Geometry of Movement for Regional Science*. London: Pion Press.

Applebaum, W., and S. Kaylin. 1974. *Case Studies in Shopping Center Development and Operation*. New York: International Council of Shopping Centers.

Bak, P. 1994. Self-Organized Criticality: A Holistic View of Nature. In *Complexity: Metaphors, Models, and Reality*, ed. G. Cowan, D. Pines, and D. Meltzer, 447–496. Reading, MA: Addison-Wesley.

Bak, P. 1996. *How Nature Works: The Science of Self-Organized Criticality*. New York: Springer.

Bak, P., K. Chen, and K. Wisenfeld. 1988. Self-Organized Criticality. *Physical Review A*. 38:364–374.

Barredo, J., L. Demicheli, C. Lavalle, M. Kasanko, and N. McCormick. 2004. Modelling Future Urban Scenarios in Developing Countries: An Application Case Study in Lagos, Nigeria. *Environment & Planning B* 32:65–84.

Barredo, J., and M. Gómez Delgado. 2008. Towards a Set of IPCC SRES Urban Land Use Scenarios: Modelling Urban Land Use in the Madrid Region. In *Modelling Environmental Dynamics: Advances in Geomatic Solutions*, ed. M. Paegelow and M. Camado Olmedo, 363–386. Berlin: Springer.

Barredo, J., M. Kasanko, N. McCormick, and C. Lavalle. 2003. Modelling Dynamic Spatial Processes: Simulation of Urban Future Scenarios through Cellular Automata. *Landscape and Urban Planning* 64:145–160.

Barredo, J., C. Lavalle, V. Sagris, and G. Engelen. 2005. Representing Future Urban and Regional Scenarios for Flood Hazard Mitigation. In *Proceedings of the 45th Congress of the European Regional Science Association*. Amsterdam.

Bartley, W. 1987. Philosophy of Biology versus Philosophy of Physics. In *Evolutionary Epistemology, Rationality, and the Sociology of Knowledge*, ed. G. Radnitzky and W. Bartley, 7–46. La Salle, IL: Open Court.

Batty, M. 1976. *Urban Modelling: Algorithms, Calibrations, Predictions*. Cambridge: Cambridge University Press.

Batty, M. 2013. *The New Science of Cities*. Cambridge, MA: MIT Press.

Batty, M., and P. Longley. 1994. *Fractal Cities: A Geometry of Form and Function*. London: Academic Press.

Batty, M., and Y. Xie. 1994. From Cells to Cities. *Environment & Planning B* 21:S31–S48.

Beavon, K. 1977. *Central Place Theory: A Reinterpretation*. London: Longman.

Benenson, I. 2007. Warning! The Scale of Land-Use CA Is Changing! *Computers, Environment and Urban Systems* 31:107–113.

Benenson, I., and P. Torrens. 2004. *Geosimulation: Automata-Based Modeling of Urban Phenomena*. Chichester, UK: Wiley.

Benevolo, L. 1980. *The History of the City*. Trans. G. Culverwell. Cambridge, MA: MIT Press.

Berry, B. 1967. *Geography of Market Centers and Retail Distribution*. Englewood Cliffs, NJ: Prentice Hall.

Berry, B., and J. Parr. 1988. *Market Centers and Retail Location: Theory and Applications*. Englewood Cliffs, NJ: Prentice Hall.

Bettencourt, L., J. Lobo, D. Helbing, C. Kuhnert, and G. West. 2007. Growth, Innovation, Scaling, and the Pace of Life in Cities. *Proceedings of the National Academy of Sciences of the United States of America* 104:7301–7306.

Boots, B., ed. 2006. Special issue. *Journal of Geographical Systems* 8 (2).

Bretagnolle, A., Daudé, E. and Pumain, D. 2003. From Theory to Modelling: Urban Systems as Complex Systems. *Cybergeo: European Journal of Geography.* Dossiers, 335. http://cybergeo.revues.org/2420

Brimberg, J., P. Hansen, N. Mladenovic, and S. Salhi. 2008. A Survey of Solution Methods for the Continuous Location-Allocation Problem. *International Journal of Operations Research* 5:1–12.

Brockmann, D., L. Hufnagel, and T. Geisel. 2006. The Scaling Laws of Human Travel. *Nature* 439:462–465.

Broekx, S., De Nocker, L., Liekens, I., Poelmans, L., Staes, J., Van der Biest, et al. Raming van de Batengeleverd door het Vlaamse NATURA 2000-Netwerk. VITO-Rapport 2013/RMA/R/0087.

Brown, D., S. Page, R. Riolo, M. Zellner, and W. Rand. 2005. Path Dependence and the Validation of Agent-Based Spatial Models of Land Use. *International Journal of Geographical Information Science* 19:153–174.

Bunge, W. 1966. *Theoretical Geography*. 2nd ed. Lund: Gleerup.

Campbell, D. 1987. Evolutionary Epistemology. In *Evolutionary Epistemology, Rationality, and the Sociology of Knowledge*, ed. G. Radnitzky and W. Bartley. La Salle, IL: Open Court.

Carey, H. 1858. *Principles of Social Science*. Philadelphia: Lippincott.

Caruso, G., D. Peeters, J. Cavailhès, and M. Rounsevell. 2007. Spatial Configurations in a Periurban City: A Cellular Automata–Based Microeconomic Model. *Regional Science and Urban Economics* 37:542–567.

Caruso, G., M. Rounsevell, and G. Cojocaru. 2005. Exploring a Spatio-Dynamic Neighbourhood-Based Model of Residential Behaviour in the Brussels Periurban Area. *International Journal of Geographical Information Science* 19:103–123.

Chaudhuri, G., and K. Clarke. 2013. The SLEUTH Land Use Change Model: A Review. *International Journal of Environmental Resources Research* 1:89–104.

Christaller, W. 1966 [1933]. *Central Places in Southern Germany*. C. Baskin, trans. Englewood Cliffs, NJ: Prentice Hall.

Christaller, W. 1972. How I Discovered the Theory of Central Places: A Report about the Origin of Central Places. In *Man, Space and Environment*, ed. P. English and R. Mayfield, 601–610. New York: Oxford University Press.

Clarke, K., and L. Gaydos. 1998. Loose-Coupling a Cellular Automaton Model and GIS: Long-Term Urban Growth Prediction for San Francisco and Washington/Baltimore. *International Journal of Geographical Information Science* 12:699–714.

Clarke, K., N. Gazulis, C. Dietzel, and N. Goldstein. 2007. A Decade of SLEUTHing: Lessons Learned from Applications of a Cellular Automaton Land Use Change Model. In *Classics from IJGIS. Twenty Years of the International Journal of Geographical Information Systems and Science*, ed. P. Fisher, 413–425. Boca Raton, FL: Taylor and Francis.

Clarke, K., S. Hoppen, and L. Gaydos. 1997. A Self-Modifying Cellular Automaton Model of Historical Urbanization in the San Francisco Bay Area. *Environment & Planning B* 24:247–261.

Coelho, J., and A. Wilson. 1976. The Optimum Location and Size of Shopping Centres. *Regional Studies* 10:413–421.

Coffey, W. 1981. *Geography: Towards a General Spatial Systems Approach*. London: Methuen.

Crols, T., R. White, I. Uljee, G. Engelen, F. Canters, and L. Poelmans. 2015. A Travel-Time Based Variable Grid Approach for an Urban Cellular Automata Model. *International Journal of Geographical Information Science* 29: doi: 10.1080/13658816.2015.1047838.

De Decker, P. 2011. Understanding Housing Sprawl: The Case of Flanders, Belgium. *Environment & Planning A* 43 (7): 1634–1654.

De Keersmaecker, M.-L., P. Frankhauser, and I. Thomas. 2003. Using Fractal Dimensions for Characterizing Intra-Urban Diversity: The Example of Brussels. *Geographical Analysis* 35:310–328.

de Kok, J.-L., G. Engelen, R. White, and H. Wind. 2001. Modelling Land-Use Change in a Decision-Support System for Coastal-Zone Management. *Environmental Modeling and Assessment* 6:123–133.

de Nijs, T. 2009. *Modelling Land Use Change: Improving the Prediction of Future Land Use Patterns*. Netherlands Geographical Studies 386. Utrecht: Utrecht University; Royal Dutch Geographic Society.

Derex, M., M.-P. Beugin, B. Godelle, and M. Raymond. 2013. Experimental Evidence for the Influence of Group Size on Cultural Complexity. *Nature* 503:389–391.

Desmet, R., B. Hertveldt, I. Mayeres, P. Mistiaen, and S. Salimata. 2008. The PLANET Model: Methodological Report. PLANET 1.0. Working Paper 10–08. Brussels: Federaal Planbureau.

Dietzel, C., and K. Clarke. 2006. The Effect of Disaggregating Land Use Categories in Cellular Automata during Model Calibration and Forecasting. *Computers, Environment and Urban Systems* 30:78–101.

Domosh, M. 1990. Shaping the Commercial City: Retail Districts in Nineteenth-Century New York and Boston. *Annals of the Association of American Geographers* 80:268–284.

Dumortier, M., L. De Bruyn, M. Hens, J. Peymen, A. Schneiders, T. Van Daele, and W. Van Reeth, eds. 2009. *Natuurverkenning 2030: Natuurrapport Vlaanderen: NARA 2009*. INBO.M.2009.7. Brussels: Instituut voor Natuur- en Bosonderzoek (INBO). http://www.inbo.be/files/Bibliotheek/03/185803.pdf.

EEA (European Environment Agency). 2006. Urban Sprawl in Europe: The Ignored Challenge. EEA Technical Report 10/2006. Copenhagen.

EEA (European Environment Agency). 2007. Land-Use Scenarios for Europe: Qualitative and Quantitative Analysis on a European Scale. EEA Technical Report 9/2007. Copenhagen.

Engelen, G., H. Hagen-Zanker, A. de Nijs, A. Maas, J. van Loon, B. Straatman, et al. 2005. Formal Model Description. Bijlage [Appendix] B of *Kalibratie en Validatie van de LeefOmgevingsVerkenner*, 51–70. Bilthoven, Netherlands: Milieu- en Natuurplanbureau.

Engelen, G., C. Lavalle, J. Barredo, M. van der Meulen, and R. White. 2007. The MOLAND Modelling Framework for Urban and Regional Land use Dynamics. In *Modelling Land-Use Change: Progress and Applications*, ed. E. Koomen, J. Stillwell, A. Bakema, and H. J. Scholten, 297–320. Dordrecht: Springer.

Engelen, G., R. White, I. Uljee, M. van der Meulen, and B. Hahn. 2002. Sustainable Development of Islands: A Policy Support Framework for the Integrated Assessment of Socio-Economic and Environmental Development. In *Sustainable Development for Island Societies: Taiwan and the World*, ed. H.-H. Hsiao, C.-H. Liu, and H.-M. Tsai, 251–287. Taipei: Academia Sinica.

Engelen, G., R. White, and S. Wargnies. 1996. Numerical Modelling of Small Island Socio-Economics to Achieve Sustainable Development. In *Small Islands: Marine Science and Sustainable Development,* ed. G. Maul, 437–463. Coastal and Estuarine Studies series, vol. 51. Washington, D.C.: American Geophysical Union. http://onlinelibrary.wiley.com/doi/10.1002/9781118665237.fmatter/pdf

Filatova, T., D. Parker, and A. Van Der Veen. 2009. Agent-Based Urban Land Markets: Agents Pricing Behavior, Land Prices and Urban Land Use Change. *Journal of Artificial Societies and Social Simulation* 12 (7). http://jasss.soc.surrey.ac.uk/12/1/3.html

Forrester, J. 1969. *Urban Dynamics*. Cambridge, MA: MIT Press.

Fotheringham, S., and M. O'Kelly. 1989. *Spatial Interaction Models: Formulations and Applications*. Dordrecht: Kluwer Academic.

FPB/ADSEI (Federal Planning Bureau and Directorate-General Statistics and Information). 2008. Bevolkingsvooruitzichten 2007–2060 (Population projections 2007–2060), Planning Paper 105. Brussels. http://www.plan.be/press/communique-649-nl-bevolkingsvooruit zichten+2007+2060.

Frankhauser, P. 1988. Fractal Aspects of Urban Structures. In *Proceedings of the International Colloquium of the Sonderforschungsbereich 230: Naturlich Konstruktionen-Leichtbau in Architektur und Natur*. Stuttgart: University of Stuttgart.

Frankhauser, P. 1990. Aspects fractals des structures urbaines. *L'Espace géographique*(1): 45–69.

Frankhauser, P. 1994. *La fractilité des structures urbaines*. Paris: Anthropos.

Frankhauser, P. 2008. Fractal Geometry for Measuring and Modelling Urban Patterns. In *The Dynamics of Complex Urban Systems*, ed. S. Albeverio, D. Andrey, P. Giordano, and A. Vancheri, 213–243. Heidelberg: Physica.

Frankhauser, P., and R. Sadler. 1991. Fractal Analysis of Agglomerations. In *Natural Structures: Principles, Strategies, and Models in Architecture and Nature*, ed. M. Hilliges, 57–65. Stuttgart: University of Stuttgart.

Fujita, M. 1986. Urban Land Use Theory. In *Location Theory*, ed. J. Gabszewicz, J.-J. Thisse, M. Fujita, and U. Schweizer. Chur, Switzerland: Harwood Academic.

Fujita, M. 1989. *Urban Economic Theory: Land Use and City Size*. Cambridge: Cambridge University Press.

Gabaix, X., and Y. M. Ioannides. 2004. The Evolution of City Size Distributions. In *Handbook of Regional and Urban Economics*. 1st ed. Vol. 4, ed. J. Henderson and J. Thisse, 2341–2378 Amsterdam: Elsevier.

Gallego, J., and S. Peedell. 2001. Using CORINE Land Cover to Map Population Density. In *Towards Agri-Environmental Indicators: Integrating Statistical and Administrative Data with Land Cover Information,* 92–104. Topic Report 6/2001. Copenhagen: EEA.

Gavilan, J., S. Overloop, K. Carels, T. D'Heygere, K. Van Hoof, J. Helming, and D. Van Gijseghem. 2007. *Toekomstverkenning Landbouw en Milieu, het SELES-Model*. Brussels: Vlaamse MilieuMaatschappij en Departement Landbouw & Visserij Afdeling Monitoring en Studie.

Geldof, C., L. Goedertier, T. Lagast, I. Leenders, H. Leinfelder, G. Lievois, et al. 2013. Planning in Uitvoering: Strategische Projecten in het Vlaams Ruimtelijk Beleid. Brussels: Vlaamse Overheid, Departement Ruimte Vlaanderen. http://rsv.vlaanderen.be/Portals/121/documents/publicaties/RWO_strategische%20projecten.pdf.

Geurs, K. 2006. *Accessibility, Land Use and Transport: Accessibility Evaluation of Land-Use and Transport Developments and Policy Strategies*. Published Ph.D. thesis, Utrecht University. Delft: Uitgeverij Eburon.

Geurs, K., and B. van Wee. 2006. Ex post Evaluation of Thirty Years of Compact Urban Development in the Netherlands. *Urban Studies* (Edinburgh) 41:139–160.

Ghosh, A., and S. Craig. 1984. A Location Allocation Model for Facility Planning in a Competitive Environment. *Geographical Analysis* 16:39–51.

Gobin, A., I. Uljee, L. Van Esch, G. Engelen, J. de Kok, H. van der Kwast, et al. 2009. *Landgebruik in Vlaanderen*. Wetenschappelijk rapport, MIRA 2009 en NARA 2009, VMM, INBO. R.2009.20, www.milieurapport.be, www.nara.be.

Goodchild, M. 1984. ILACS: A Location Allocation Model for Retail Site Selection. *Journal of Retailing* 60:84–100.

Haedrich, R. 1985. Species Number-Area Relationship in the Deep Sea. *Marine Ecology Progress Series* 24:303–306.

Hagen, A. 2003. Fuzzy Set Approach to Assessing Similarity of Categorical Maps. *International Journal of Geographical Information Science* 17:235–249.

Hagen-Zanker, A. 2008. *Measuring the Performance of Geosimulation Models by Map Comparison*. Published Ph.D. thesis, University of Maastricht. Maastricht: Alex Hagen-Zanker.

Hagen-Zanker, A., and G. Lajoie. 2008. Neutral Models of Landscape Change as Benchmarks in the Assessment of Model Performance. *Landscape and Urban Planning* 86:284–296.

Hagen-Zanker, A., B. Straatman, and I. Uljee. 2005. Further Developments of a Fuzzy Set Map Comparison Approach. *International Journal of Geographical Information Science* 19:769–785.

Hägerstrand, T. 1952. *The Propagation of Innovation Waves. Lund Studies in Geography: Series B, Human Geography*. Lund: Royal University of Lund, Department of Geography.

Hägerstrand, T. 1967. The Computer and the Geographer. *Transactions of the Institute of British Geographers* 42:1–19.

Hägerstrand, T. 1970. What about People in Regional Science? *Papers of the Regional Science Association* 24 (1): 6–21.

Hägerstrand, T. 1975. Space, Time and Human Conditions. In *Dynamic Allocation of Urban Space*, ed. A. Karlqvist, L. Lundqvist, and F. Snickers, 3–14. Lexington, MA: Lexington Books.

Hahn, B., I. Uljee, M. Van der Meulen, and R. Vanhout. 2006. TiGS: Generic Program Interface and Spatio-Temporal Database. In *Time-GeographicalApproaches to Emergence and Sustainable Societies (TiGrESS): Final Report to the Commission of the EU*, ed. N. Winder. Newcastle upon Tyne: Newcastle University.

Haken, H. 1973. *Synergetics: Cooperative Phenomena in Multi-Component Systems.* Vieweg+Teubner Verlag.

Haken, H. 1983. *Advanced Synergetics.* Berlin: Springer.

Hanjoul, P., and D. Peeters. 1985. A Comparison of Two Dual-Based Procedures for Solving the *P*-Median Problem. *European Journal of Operational Research* 20:387–396.

Harvey, J. 2002. Estimating Census District Populations from Satellite Imagery: Some Approaches and Limitations. *International Journal of Remote Sensing* 23:2071–2095.

Helbing, D. 2001. Traffic and Related Self-Driven Many-Particle Systems. *Reviews of Modern Physics* 73:1067–1141.

Helbing, D., and B. Tilch. 1998. Generalized Force Model of Traffic Dynamics. *Physical Review E* 58:133–138.

Hewett, R. 2014. Integrating Stakeholder Knowledge in Cellular Automata Models of Land Use Change. Unpublished Ph.D. thesis, Universidad de Alcalá.

Hewett, R., and F. Escobar. 2011. The Territorial Dynamics of Fast-Growing Regions: Unsustainable Land Use Change and Future Policy Challenges in Madrid, Spain. *Applied Geography (Sevenoaks, England)* 31:650–657.

Hodgson, J. 1981. A Location-Allocation Model Maximizing Consumers' Welfare. *Regional Studies* 15:493–506.

Huang, J., and D. Turcotte. 1989. Fractal Mapping of Digitized Images: Application to the Topography of Arizona and Comparisons with Synthetic Images. *Journal of Geophysical Research* 94:7491–7495.

Huser, B., D. Rutledge, H. Van Delden, M. Wedderburn, M. Cameron, S. Elliott, et al. 2009. Creating Futures: Towards an Integrated Spatial Decision Support System for Local Government in New Zealand. In *Proceedings of the 18th World IMACS Congress and MODSIM09: International Congress on Modelling and Simulation*, ed. R. Anderssen, R. Braddock, and L. Newham, 2370–2376. Cairns, Australia: Modelling and Simulation Society of Australia and New Zealand and International Association for Mathematics and Computers in Simulation.

Isard, W. 1956. *Location and Space Economy: A General Theory Relating to Industrial Location, Market Areas, Land Use, Trade, and Urban Structure.* Cambridge, MA: MIT Press.

Isard, W., and T. E. Smith. 1969. *General Theory: Social, Political, Economic and Regional: With Particular Reference to Decision Making Analysis.* Cambridge, MA: MIT Press.

Jacobs, J. 1961. *The Death and Life of Great American Cities.* New York: Vintage Books.

Jantz, C., and S. Goetz. 2005. Analysis of Scale Dependencies in an Urban Land-Use-Change Model. *International Journal of Geographical Information Science* 19:217–241.

Jantz, C., S. Goetz, and M. Shelley. 2003. Using the SLEUTH Urban Growth Model to Simulate the Impacts of Future Policy Scenarios on Urban Land Use in the Baltimore-Washington Metropolitan Area. *Environment & Planning B* 30:251–271.

Jin, X., and R. White. 2012. An Agent-Based Model of the Influence of Neighbourhood Design on Daily Trip Patterns. *Computers, Environment and Urban Systems* 36:398–412.

Kauffman, S. 1989. Principles of Adaptation in Complex Systems. In *Lectures in the Science of Complexity*, ed. D. Stein, 619–712. Reading, MA: Addison-Wesley.

Kauffman, S. 1993. *The Origins of Order*. New York: Oxford University Press.

Kauffman, S. 1994. Whispers from Carnot: The Origins of Order and Principles of Adaptation in Complex Nonequilibrium Systems. In *Complexity: Metaphors, Models, and Reality*, ed. G. Cowan, D. Pines, and D. Meltzer, 83–160. Reading, MA: Addison-Wesley.

Kirchner, J., X. Feng, and C. Neal. 2000. Fractal Stream Chemistry and Its Implications for Contaminant Transport in Catchments. *Nature* 403:524–527.

Koh, N.-P. 1990. Modelling Retail System Dynamics: An Application to the System of Major Retail Centres in the St. John's Metropolitan Area 1960–1980. Unpublished Master's thesis, Memorial University of Newfoundland.

Kostof, S. 1991. *The City Shaped: Urban Patterns and Meanings Through History*. Boston: Bulfinch Press.

Kramer, A., R. Sabath, and R. Buchmeier. 2004. *Dollars and Cents of Shopping Centers: A Study of Receipts and Expenses in Shopping Center Operations*. Washington, DC: Urban Land Institute.

Krugman, P. 1998. What's New about the New Economic Geography? *Oxford Review of Economic Policy* 14:7–17.

Kuhn, H., and R. Kuenne. 1962. An Efficient Algorithm for the Numerical Solution of the Generalized Weber Problem in Spatial Economics. *Journal of Regional Science* 4:21–34.

Langton, C. 1992. Life at the Edge of Chaos. In *Artificial Life II*, ed. C. Langton, C. Taylor, D. Farmer, and S. Rasmussen, 41–91. Redwood City, CA: Addison-Wesley.

Lauwerier, H. 1991. *Fractals: Images of Chaos*. Princeton: Princeton University Press.

Levins, R. 1968. *Evolution in Changing Environments*. Princeton: Princeton University Press.

Li, X., C. Lao, X. Liu, and Y. Chen. 2011. Coupling Urban Cellular Automata with Ant Colony Optimization for Zoning Protected Natural Areas under a Changing Landscape. *International Journal of Geographical Information Science* 25:783–802.

Li, X., J. Lin, Y. Chen, X. Liu, and B. Ai. 2013. Calibrating Cellular Automata Based on Landscape Metrics by Using Genetic Algorithms. *International Journal of Geographical Information Science* 27:594–613.

Li, X., and X. Liu. 2006. An Extended Cellular Automaton Using Case-Based Reasoning for Simulating Urban Development in a Large Complex Region. *International Journal of Geographical Information Science* 20:1109–1136.

Li, X., Q. Yang, and X. Liu. 2008. Discovering and Evaluating Urban Signatures for Simulating Compact Development Using Cellular Automata. *Landscape and Urban Planning* 86:177–186.

Li, X., and A. Yeh. 2000. Modelling Sustainable Urban Development by the Integration of Constrained Cellular Automata and GIS. *International Journal of Geographical Information Science* 14:131–152.

Li, X., and A. Yeh. 2002. Neural Network–Based Cellular Automata for Simulating Multiple Land Use Changes Using GIS. *International Journal of Geographical Information Science* 16:323–343.

Liu, X., X. Li, X. Shi, S. Wu, and T. Liu. 2008. Simulating Complex Urban Development Using Kernel-Based Non-Linear Cellular Automata. *Ecological Modelling* 211:169–181.

Liu, X., X. Li, X. Shi, X. Zhang, and Y. Chen. 2010. Simulating Land-Use Dynamics under Planning Policies by Integrating Artificial Immune Systems with Cellular Automata. *International Journal of Geographical Information Science* 24:783–802.

Lorenz, E. 1963. Deterministic Nonperiodic Flow. *Journal of the Atmospheric Sciences* 20:130–141.

Lösch, A. 1954 [1940]. *The Economics of Location*. W. Woglom and W. Stolper, trans. New Haven: Yale University Press.

Lynch, K. 1960. *The Image of the City*. Cambridge, MA: MIT Press.

Machado, A. 1989. *Poesía y Prosa, Tomo II: Poesías Completas*. Edición Crítica de Oreste Macrí con la Coloboración de Gaetano Chiappini. Madrid : Espasa-Calpe and the Fundación Antonio Machado. Quoted poem first published in A. Machado, 1917, *Campos de Castilla*; excerpts translated by the author, R. White.

Maene, S. 2011. *Nieuwe Bevolkingsprojecties en Huishoudens Projecties 2009–2030: Een Vergelijking met Projecties Federaal Planbureau 2007–2060 Gebruikt in Milieuverkenning 2030*. Brussels: Studiedienst Vlaamse Regering.

Maes, F., S. Overloop, A. Gobin, J.-L. de Kok, G. Engelen, I. Uljee, et al. 2009.Land Use. In *Flanders Environment Report 2009: Environment Outlook 2030.*, ed. M. Van Steertegem, M. Bossuyt, J. Brouwers, C. De Geest, S. Maene, F. Maes, et al., 259–282. Erembodegem, Flanders: Flemish Environment Agency. http://www.milieurapport.be/Upload/main/MIRA_2009_english[1].pdf.

Makgill, R., and H. Rennie. 2012. A Model for Integrated Coastal Management Legislation: A Principled Analysis of New Zealand's Resource Management Act 1991. *International Journal of Marine and Coastal Law* 27:135–165.

Mandelbrot, B. 1975. *Les objets fractals: Forme, hazard, et dimension*. Paris: Flammarion.

Mandelbrot, B. 1982. *The Fractal Geometry of Nature*. San Francisco: W. H. Freeman.

Marceau, D., and I. Benenson, eds. 2011. *Advanced Geosimulation Models*. Sharjah, United Arab Emirates: Bentham Science. http://www.casa.ucl.ac.uk/Advanced%20 Geosimulation%20Models.pdf.

Maritan, A., F. Colaiori, A. Flammini, M. Cieplak, and J. Banavar. 1996. Universality Classes of Optimal Channel Networks. *Science* 272:984–986.

Marks, R. 2007. Validating Simulation Models: A General Framework and Four Applied Examples. *Computational Economics* 30:265–290.

Markus, M., and B. Hess. 1990. Isotropic Cellular Automaton for Modelling Excitable Media. *Nature* 347:56–58.

McGarigal, K., S. Cushman, M. Neel and R. Erne. 2002. FRAGSTATS: Spatial Pattern Analysis Program for Categorical Maps. http://www.umass.edu/landeco/research/fragstats/fragstats.html.

Mennis, J. 2003. Generating Surface Models of Population Using Dasymetric Mapping. *Professional Geographer* 55:31–42.

Minar, N., R. Burkhart, C. Langton, and M. Askenazi. 1996. The Swarm Simulation System: A Toolkit for Building Multi-Agent Simulations. Santa Fe Institute Working Paper 96-06-042.

Mitchell, M., J. P. Crutchfield, and P. Hraber. 1994. Dynamics, Computation, and the "Edge of Chaos": A Re-Examination. In *Complexity: Metaphors, Models, and Reality*, ed. G. Cowan, D. Pines, and D. Meltzer, 497–514. Reading, MA: Addison-Wesley.

Montgomery, D., T. Abbe, J. Buffington, P. Peterson, K. Schmidt, and J. Stock. 1996. Distribution of Bedrock and Alluvial Channels in Forested Mountain Drainage Basins. *Nature* 381:587–588.

Moreno, N., F. Wang, and D. Marceau. 2010. A Geographic Object–Based Approach in Cellular Automata Modelling. *Photogrammetric Engineering and Remote Sensing* 76:183–191.

Morris, A. 1972. *History of Urban Form*. London: Longmans.

Mumford, L. 1961. *The City in History: Its Origins, Its Transformations, and Its Prospects*. New York: Harcourt Jovanovich.

Muth, R. 1969. *Cities and Housing: The Spatial Pattern of Urban Residential Land Use*. Chicago: University of Chicago Press.

Nicolis, G., and I. Prigogine. 1989. *Exploring Complexity: An Introduction*. New York: W. H. Freeman.

Niedercorn, J., and B. Bechdoldt. 1969. An Economic Derivation of the "Gravity Law" of Spatial Interaction. *Journal of Regional Science* 9:273–281.

Nuzzo, R. 2014. Statistical Errors. *Nature* 506:150–152.

O'Sullivan, D. 2001. Graph-Cellular Automata: A Generalized Discrete Urban and Regional Model. *Environment & Planning B* 28:687–705.

Papageorgiou, Y. 1990. *The Isolated City State: An Economic Geography of Urban Spatial Structure*. London: Routledge.

Parker, D., T. Berger, and M. Manson. 2002. Agent-Based Models of Land-Use and Land-Cover Change. In *LUCC Report Series No. 6: Report and Review of an International Workshop October 4–7, 2001*. Berkeley: University of California.

Parker, D., and T. Filatova. 2008. A Conceptual Design for a Bilateral Agent-Based Land Market with Heterogeneous Economic Agents. *Computers, Environment and Urban Systems* 32:454–463.

Parker, D., S. Manson, M. Janssen, M. Hoffmann, and P. Deadman. 2003. Multi-Agent Systems for the Simulation of Land-Use and Land-Cover Change: A Review. *Annals of the Association of American Geographers* 93:314–337.

Passonneau, J., and R. Wurman. 1966. *Urban Atlas: 20 American Cities*. Cambridge, MA: MIT Press.

Peeters, D., J.-F. Thisse, and I. Thomas. 1998. Transportation Networks and the Location of Human Activities. *Geographical Analysis* 30:355–371.

Pelfrene, E. 2005. *Ontgroening en Vergrijzing in Vlaanderen, 1990–2050 (Growing Up and Aging in Flanders, 1990–2050): Verkenningen op Basis van de*

NIS-Bevolkingsvooruitzichten, Stativaria 36. Brussels: Administratie Planning en Statistiek, Ministerie van de Vlaamse Gemeenschap.

Pérez, L., S. Dragićević, and R. White. 2013. Model Testing and Assessment: Perspectives from a Swarm Intelligence, Agent-Based Model of Forest Insect Infestations. *Computers, Environment and Urban Systems* 39:121–135.

Petrov, L., C. Lavalle, and M. Kasanko. 2009. Urban Land Use Scenarios for a Tourist Region in Europe: Applying the MOLAND Model to Algarve, Portugal. *Landscape and Urban Planning* 92:10–23.

Petrov, L., H. Shahumyan, B. Williams, and S. Convery. 2013. Applying Spatial Indicators to Support a Sustainable Urban Future. *Environmental Practice* 15:19–32.

Peymen, J., M. Hens, A. Gobin, I. Uljee, L. Van Esch, G. Engelen, et al. 2009. Landgebruik. In *Natuurverkenning 2030. Natuurrapport Vlaanderen, NARA 2009*, ed. M. Dumortier, L. De Bruyn, M. Hens, J. Peymen, A. Schneiders, T. Van Daele, and W. Van Reeth, 69–101. INBO.M.2009.7. Brussels: Instituut voor Natuur- en Bosoderzoek (INBO).

Pinto, N., and A. Antunes. 2010. A Cellular Automata Model Based on Irregular Cells: Application to Small Urban Areas. *Environment & Planning B* 37:1095–1114.

Pirenne, H. 1937. *Economic and Social History of Medieval Europe*. New York: Harcourt, Brace & World.

Pontius, R. G. 2000. Quantification Error versus Location Error in Comparison of Categorical Maps. *Photogrammetric Engineering and Remote Sensing* 66:1011–1016.

Pontius, R. G. 2002. Statistical Methods to Partition Effects of Quantity and Location during Comparison of Categorical Maps at Multiple Resolutions. *Photogrammetric Engineering and Remote Sensing* 68:1041–1049.

Popper, K. 1959 [1934]. *The Logic of Scientific Discovery*. London: Hutchinson.

Popper, K. 1963. *Conjectures and Refutations*. London: Routledge and Kegan Paul.

Popper, K. 1982. *The Open Universe*. Totowa, NJ: Rowman and Littlefield.

Portugali, J. 2000. *Self-Organization and the City*. Berlin: Springer.

Portugali, J., and I. Benenson. 1994. Competing Order Parameters in a Self-Organizing City. In *Managing and Marketing of Urban Development and Urban Life*, ed. G. Braun, 669–681. Berlin: Dietrich Reimer.

Portugali, J., and I. Benenson. 1995. Artificial Planning Experience by Means of a Heuristic Cell-Space Model: Simulating International Migration in the Urban Process. *Environment & Planning A* 27:1647–1665.

Portugali, J., and I. Benenson. 1997. Human Agents between Local and Global Forces in a Self-Organizing City. In *Self-Organization of Complex Structures: From Individual to Collective Dynamics*, ed. F. Schweitzer, 537–546. Boca Raton, FL: CRC Press.

Portugali, J., I. Benenson, and I. Omer. 1994. Socio-Spatial Residential Dynamics: Stability and Instability within a Self-Organizing City. *Geographical Analysis* 26:321–340.

Portugali, J., I. Benenson, and I. Omer. 1997. Spatial Cognitive Dissonance and Sociospatial Emergence in a Self-Organizing City. *Environment & Planning B* 24:263–285.

Poston, T., and A. Wilson. 1977. Facility versus Distance Travelled: Urban Services and the Fold Catastrophe. *Environment & Planning A* 9:681–686.

Poundstone, W. 1985. *The Recursive Universe: Cosmic Complexity and the Limits of Scientific Knowledge*. Oxford: Oxford University Press.

Power, C. 2009. A Spatial Agent-Based Model of N-Person Prisoner's Dilemma Cooperation in a Socio-Geographic Community. *Journal of Artificial Societies and Social Simulation* 12 (1). http://jasss.soc.surrey.ac.uk/12/1/8.html.

Power, C. 2014. A Spatial Agent-Based Model of Social Relationality: Emergent Cooperation and Leadership in Community Development. Unpublished Ph.D. thesis, Memorial University of Newfoundland.

Power, C., A. Simms, and R. White. 2001. Hierarchical Fuzzy Pattern Matching for the Regional Comparison of Land Use Maps. *International Journal of Geographical Information Science* 15:77–100.

Price, R. 2007. Cellular Automata Land Use Change Model. White paper. Hamilton, New Zealand: Landcare Research.

Prigogine, I. 1980. *From Being to Becoming*. San Francisco: W. H. Freeman.

Prigogine, I. 1997. *The End of Certainty: Time, Chaos, and the New Laws of Nature*. New York: Free Press.

Prigogine, I., and I. Stengers. 1979. *La Nouvelle Alliance*. Paris: Éditions Gallimard.

Prigogine, I., and I. Stengers. 1984. *Order out of Chaos: Man's New Dialogue with Nature*. New York: Bantam Books.

Prokop G., H. Jobstmann, and A. Schönbauer. 2011. Report on Best Practices for Limiting Soil Sealing and Mitigating Its Effects. Technical Report 2011-050. Brussels: European Commission, DG Environment.

Pumain, D. 1997. Pour une théorie évolutive des villes. *L'Espace géographique* 26:119–134.

Pumain, D. 2006. An Alternative Explanation of Hierarchical Differentiation in Urban Systems. In *Hierarchy in Natural and Social Sciences*, ed. D. Pumain, 169–222. Dordrecht: Springer Netherlands.

Pumain, D., T. Saint-Julien, and L. Sanders. 1986. Applications of a Dynamic Urban Model. *Geographical Analysis* 19:152–166.

Refsgaard, J., and H. Henriksen. 2004. Modelling Guidelines: Terminology and Guiding Principles. *Advances in Water Resources* 27:71–82.

Ren, J., and R. White. 1995. The Simulation of Urban System Dynamics in Atlantic Canada, 1951–1991. *Canadian Geographer* 39:252–262.

Rennie, H. 2011. Effects-Based Planning and Property Rights: Reflections on New Zealand's Resource Management Act. Paper 735 in *Track 15 (Planning Law, Administration & Property Rights)*, World Planning Schools Congress 2011. Perth: University of Western Australia.

Richardson, F. 1926. Atmospheric Diffusion Shown on a Distance-Neighbour Graph. *Proceedings of the Royal Society of London. Series A* 110:709–737.

Richardson, F. 1961. The Problem of Contiguity: An Appendix of Statistics of Deadly Quarrels. *General Systems Yearbook* 6:139–187.

RIKS (Research Institute for Knowledge Systems). 2007. *MOLAND Transport Model*. Maastricht.

Rosen, R. 1991. *Life Itself: A Comprehensive Inquiry into the Nature, Origin, and Fabrication of Life*. New York: Columbia University Press.

Rossi, A. 1982. *The Architecture of the City*. Cambridge, MA: MIT Press.

Rouleau, B. 1967. *Le Tracé des Rues de Paris: Formation, Typologie, Fonctions*. Paris: Éditions du CNRS.

Rutledge, D., M. Cameron, S. Elliott, T. Fenton, B. Huser, G. McBride, et al. 2008. Choosing Regional Futures: Challenges and Choices in Building Integrated Models to Support Long-Term Regional Planning in New Zealand. *Regional Science Policy & Practice* 1:85–108.

Rutledge, D., G. McDonald, M. Cameron, G. McBride, J. Poot, F. Scrimgeour, et al. 2007. Development of Spatial Decision Support Systems to Support Long-Term, Integrated Planning. In *Proceedings of MODSIM 2007: International Congress on Modelling and Simulation*, ed. L. Oxley and D. Kulasiri, 308–314. Christchurch, New Zealand: Modelling and Simulation Society of Australia and New Zealand.

RWO (Department for Spatial Planning, Housing Policy, and Built Heritage). 2011. *Ruimtelijk Structuurplan Vlaanderen*. Brussels. http://rsv.vlaanderen.be/Portals/121/documents/publicaties/RSV2011.pdf.

RWO (Department for Spatial Planning, Housing Policy, and Built Heritage). 2012. *Green Paper Spatial Policy Plan: Flanders in 2050: Human Scale in a Metropolis? Spatial Policy Plan*. Brussels. http://www2.vlaanderen.be/ruimtelijk/docs/groenboek%20ruimtelijke%20ordening%20EN%20DEF.pdf.

Rykiel, E. 1996. Testing Ecological Models: The Meaning of Validation. *Ecological Modelling* 90:229–244.

Sarewitz, D. 2012. Beware the Creeping Cracks of Bias. *Nature* 485:149.

Schroeder, M. 1991. *Fractals, Chaos, Power Laws: Minutes from an Infinite Paradise*. New York: W. H. Freeman.

Shahumyan, H., S. Convery, and E. Casey. 2010. Exploring Land Use–Transport Interactions in the Greater Dublin Region Using the Moland Model. In *Proceedings of ITRN 2010*. Dublin: University College Dublin.

Shahumyan, H., R. White, L. Petrov, B. Williams, S. Convery, and M. Brennan. 2011. *Urban Development Scenarios and Probability Mapping for the Greater Dublin Region: The MOLAND Model Applications*. Lecture Notes in Computer Science, vol. 6782, Part 1, 119–134. New York: Springer.

Shahumyan, H., R. White, B. Twumasi, S. Convery, B. Williams, M. Critchley, et al. 2009. The MOLAND Model Calibration and Validation for the Greater Dublin Region. Urban Institute Ireland Working Paper Series. Dublin: University College Dublin.

Silva, E. 2004. The DNA of Our Regions: Artificial Intelligence in Regional Planning. *Futures* 36:1077–1094.

Silva, E., and K. Clarke. 2002. Calibration of the SLEUTH urban growth model for Lisbon and Porto, Portugal. *Computers, Environment and Urban Systems* 26:525–552.

Sims, D., E. Southall, N. Humphries, G. Hays, C. Bradshaw, J. Pitchford, et al. 2008. Scaling Laws of Marine Predator Search Behaviour. *Nature* 451:1098–1102.

Smith, T. R. 1977. Continuous and Discontinuous Response to Smoothly Decreasing Effective Distance: An Analysis with Special Reference to "Overbanking" in the 1920s. *Environment & Planning A* 9:461–475.

Smolin, L. 2013. *Time Reborn: From the Crisis in Physics to the Future of the Universe.* New York: Houghton Mifflin Harcourt.

Solé, R., S. Manrubia, M. Benton, and P. Bak. 1997. Self-Similarity of Extinction Statistics in the Fossil Record. *Nature* 388:764–767.

Stanilov, K., and M. Batty. 2011. Exploring the Historical Determinants of Urban Growth Patterns through Cellular Automata. *Transactions in GIS* 15:253–271.

Stanley, M., L. Amaral, S. Buldyrev, S. Havlin, H. Leschhorn, P. Maass, et al. 1996. Scaling Behaviour in the Growth of Companies. *Nature* 379:804–806.

Straatman, B., R. White, and W. Banzhaf. 2008. An Artificial Chemistry-Based Model of Economies. In *Artificial Life XI: Proceedings of the Eleventh International Conference on the Simulation and Synthesis of Living Systems*, ed. S. Bullock, J. Noble, R. Watson, and M. Bedau, 592–599. Cambridge, MA: MIT Press.

Straatman, B., R. White, and G. Engelen. 2004. Toward an Automatic Calibration Procedure for Constrained Cellular Automata. *Computers, Environment and Urban Systems* 28:149–170.

Tellier, L.-N. 1992. From the Weber Problem to a "Topodynamic" Approach to Locational Systems. *Environment & Planning A* 24:793–806.

Tellier, L.-N. 1993. *Économie spatiale: Rationalité économique de l'espace habité*. Quebec: Gilles Morin.

Thomas, I., P. Frankhauser, and C. Biernacki. 2008. The Morphology of Built-Up Landscapes in Wallonia (Belgium): A Classification Using Fractal Indices. *Landscape and Urban Planning* 84:99–115.

Thomas, I., P. Frankhauser, B. Frenay, and M. Verleysen. 2010. Clustering Patterns of Urban Built-Up Areas with Curves of Fractal Scaling Behaviour. *Environment and Planning. B, Planning & Design* 37:942–954.

Thomas, I., C. Tannier, and P. Frankhauser. 2008. Is There a Link between Fractal Dimension and Residential Environment at a Regional Level. *Cybergeo: European Journal of Geography*. Dossiers, 413. http://cybergeo.revues.org/16283

Thornes, J. 1990. Big Rills Have Little Rills.... *Nature* 345:764–765.

Timmermans, H. 1984. Decompositional Multi-Attribute Preference Models in Spatial Choice Analysis: A Review of Some Recent Developments. *Progress in Human Geography* 8:189–221.

Torrens, P. 2012. Moving Agent Pedestrians through Space and Time. *Annals of the Association of American Geographers* 102:35–66.

Uljee, I., G. Engelen, and R. White. 1996. RamCo Demo Guide: Version 1.10. Work Document CZM-C 96.08. Hague: National Institute for Coastal and Marine Management.

U.S. Census Bureau. 1958, 1963, 1967, 1972, 1977. *Census of Retail Trade: Major Retail Centers in Standard Metropolitan Statistical Areas*. Washington, DC: GPO.

Urban Land Institute. 1969. *The Dollars and Cents of Shopping Centers: A Study of Receipts and Expenses*. Washington, DC: Urban Land Institute.

Uyttenhove, P. 1989. Architectuur, Stedenbouw en Planologie Tijdens de Duitse Bezetting: De Moderne Beweging en het Comissariaat-Generaal voor's Lands Wederopbouw (1940–1944). *BTNG-RBHC* 20:465–510.

Van Claude, M. 2009. Economisch Belang van de Belgische Havens: Vlaamse zeehavens, Luiks havencomplex en haven van Brussel, Verslag 2007, Working Paper Document Nr 172, Juli 2009, Nationale Bank van België.

Van de Voorde, T., J. van der Kwast, I. Uljee, G. Engelen, and F. Canters. 2010. Improving the Calibration of the MOLAND Urban Growth Model with Land-Use Information Derived from a Time-Series of Medium Resolution Remote Sensing Data. In *Computational Science and Its Applications: Proceedings of the ICCSA 2010 International Conference*, ed. D. Taniar, O. Gervasi, B. Mugante, E. Pardede, and B. O. Apduhan. Fukuoka, Japan. Berlin: Springer.

van Delden, H., I. Uljee, and A. Dominguez. 2006. Herramientas y Modelos de Simulación para Apoyar la Toma de Decisiones sobre Desarrollo Sostenible: Un Modelo Dinámico de Planificación Espacial Aplicado a Vitoria-Gasteiz. *IV Encuentro Iberoamericano de Desarrollo Sostenible*. CONANA 8, Cumbre de Desarrollo Sotenible, Madrid.

van Delden, H., J. van Vliet, D. Rutledge, and M. Kirkby. 2011. Comparison of Scale and Scaling Issues in Integrated Land-Use Models for Policy Support. *Agriculture, Ecosystems & Environment* 142:18–28 vvan.

Vandermeer, J., I. Perfecto, and S. Philpott. 2008. Clusters of Ant Colonies and Robust Criticality in a Tropical Agroecosystem. *Nature* 451:457–459.

Van Esch, L., G. Engelen, A. Gobin, and I. Uljee. 2010. *Landgebruikskaart Vlaanderen en Brussel: Intern rapport 2010/RMA/R/158*. Mol, Belgium: Vlaamse Instelling voor Technologisch Onderzoek.

van Loon, J. 2004. Towards Model-Specific Automated Calibration Procedures for the LeefOmgevingsVerkenner Model. Unpublished Master's thesis, University of Maastricht.

Van Steertegem, M., M. Bossuyt, J. Brouwers, C. De Geest, S. Maene, F. Maes, et al., eds. 2009. *Flanders Environment Report 2009: Environment Outlook 2030*. Erembodegem, Flanders: Flemish Environment Agency. http://www.milieurapport.be/Upload/main/MIRA_2009_english[1].pdf.

van Vliet, J., R. White, and S. Dragićević. 2009. Modeling Urban Growth Using a Variable Grid Cellular Automaton. *Computers, Environment and Urban Systems* 33:35–43.

Voets, J., B. De Peuter, B. Vandekerckhove, D. Broeckaert, M. Leroy, P. Maes, et al. 2010. *Evaluererend Onderzoek naar de Effectiviteit van de Uitvoering van het Ruimtelijk Beleid in Vlaanderen: Voorbereidend Onderzoek voor het Beleidsplan, Instituut voor de Overheid*. K. U. Leuven, Sum Research; Departement Architectuur, Sint-Lucas Hogeschool W&K; Nijmegen School of Management, Radboud Universiteit Nijmegen. Brussels: Ministerie Vlaamse Gemeerschlap.

von Thünen, J. 1966 [1826]. *Von Thünen's "Isolated State."* C. Wartenberg, trans. Oxford: Pergamon.

Warntz, W. 1965. *Macrogeography and Income Fronts*. Philadelphia: Regional Science Research Institute.

Warntz, W. 1967. Global Science and the Tyranny of Space. *Papers / Regional Science Association. Regional Science Association. Meeting* 19:7–19.

Warntz, W. 1973–1974. Pressure Surfaces, Critical Elements and Network Representations for Description, Analysis and Prediction of Structures and Flows. *Atmosphere* (Toronto) 12:44–45.

Weber, A. 1957 [1909]. *Alfred Weber's "Theory of the Location of Industries."* C. Friedrich, trans. Chicago: University of Chicago Press.

White, R. 1974. Sketches of a Dynamic Central Place Theory. *Economic Geography* 50:219–227.

White, R. 1975. Simulating the Dynamics of Central Place Systems. *Proceedings of the Association of American Geographers* 7:279–282.

White, R. 1976. A Generalization of the Utility Theory Approach to the Problem of Spatial Interaction. *Geographical Analysis* 8:39–46.

White, R. 1977. Dynamic Central Place Theory: Results of a Simulation Approach. *Geographical Analysis* 9:226–243.

White, R. 1978. The Simulation of Central Place Dynamics: Two Sector Systems and the Rank-Size Distribution. *Geographical Analysis* 10:201–208.

White, R. 1983. Chaotic Behaviour and the Self-Organization of the Urban Retail System. Brussels Working Papers on Spatial Analysis, Series A: Human Systems, no. 3. *Brussels: Service de Chimie Physique II, Université Libre de Bruxelles.*

White, R. 1989. The Artificial Intelligence of Urban Dynamics: Neural Network Modeling of Urban Structure. *Papers/Regional Science Association. Regional Science Association. Meeting* 67:43–53.

White, R. 2005. Modelling Multi-Scale Processes in a Cellular Automata Framework. In *Complex Artificial Environments*, ed. J. Portugali, 165–178. Berlin:Springer.

White, R. 2006. Pattern Based Map Comparisons. *Journal of Geographical Systems* 8:145–164.

White, R., and G. Engelen. 1993. Cellular Automata and Fractal Urban Form: A Cellular Modelling Approach to the Evolution of Urban Land Use Patterns. *Environment & Planning A* 25:1175–1199.

White, R., and G. Engelen. 1997. Cellular Automata as the Basis of Integrated Dynamic Regional Modelling. *Environment & Planning B* 24:235–246.

White, R., and G. Engelen. 2000. High-Resolution Integrated Modelling of the Spatial Dynamics of urban and Regional Systems. *Computers, Environment and Urban Systems* 24:383–400.

White, R., G. Engelen, and I. Uljee. 1997. The Use of Constrained Cellular Automata for High-Resolution Modelling of Urban Land-Use Dynamics. *Environment and Planning. B, Planning & Design* 24:323–343.

White, R., G. Engelen, and I. Uljee. 2000. Modelling Land Use Change with Linked Cellular Automata and Socio-Economic Models: A Tool for Exploring the Impact of Climate Change on the Island of St. Lucia. In *Spatial Information for Land Use Management*, ed. M. Hill and R. Aspinall, 189–204. Amsterdam: Gordon and Breach.

White, R., G. Engelen, I. Uljee, C. Lavalle, and D. Ehrlich. 2000. Developing an Urban Land Use Simulator for European Cities. In *Proceedings of the 5th EC GIS Workshop: GIS of*

Tomorrow, ed. K. Fullerton, 179–190. Brussels: European Commission Joint Research Centre.

White, R., H. Shahumyan, and I. Uljee. 2011. Activity Based Variable Grid Cellular Automata for Urban and Regional Modelling. In *Advanced Geosimulation Models*, ed. D. Marceau and I. Benenson, 14–29. Sharjah, United Arab Emirates: Bentham Science. http://www.casa.ucl.ac.uk/Advanced%20Geosimulation%20Models.pdf.

White, R., G. Straatman, and G. Engelen. 2004. Planning Visualization and Assessment: A Cellular Automata Based Integrated Spatial Decision Support System. In *Spatially Integrated Social Science*, ed. M. Goodchild and D. Janelle, 420–442. Oxford: Oxford University Press.

White, R., I. Uljee, and G. Engelen. 2012. Integrated Modelling of Population, Employment, and Land Use Change with a Multiple Activity Based Variable Grid Cellular Automaton. *International Journal of GIS* 26:1251–1280.

Williams, B., H. Shahumyan, I. Boyle, S. Convery, and R. White. 2012. Utilizing an Urban-Regional Model (MOLAND) for Testing the Planning and Provision of Wastewater Treatment Capacity in the Dublin Region 2006–2026. *Planning Practice and Research* 27:227–248.

Williams, R. 1973. *The Country and the City*. London: Chatto & Windus.

Wilson, A. 1970. *Entropy in Urban and Regional Modelling*. London: Pion.

Wilson, A. 1976. Toward Models of the Evolution and Genesis of Urban Structure. Working paper no. 166. Leeds: School of Geography, University of Leeds.

Wilson, A. 1977. Spatial Interaction and Settlement Structure: Toward an Explicit Central Place Theory Working Paper 200. School of Geography, University of Leeds.

Wolfram, S. 2002. *A New Kind of Science*. Champaign, IL: Wolfram Media.

Wouters, K. 2013. In de ban van het lint. Lintbebouwing in Vlaanderen. EindverhandelingVerkeerskunde 3HSV. Diepenbeek: Universiteit Hasselt. www.tmleuven.be/thesisprijs/laureates/2013WoutersKim_thesis.pdf.

Wu, C., and A. Murray. 2007. Population Estimation Using Landsat Enhanced Thematic Mapper Imagery. *Geographical Analysis* 39:26–43.

Yasenovskiy, V., and J. Hodgson. 2007. Hierarchical Location-Allocation with Spatial Choice Interaction Modeling. *Annals of the Association of American Geographers* 97:496–511.

Yeh, A., and M. Chow. 1996. An Integrated GIS and Location-Allocation Approach to Public Facilities Planning: An Example of Open Space Planning. *Computers, Environment and Urban Systems* 20:339–350.

Yeh, A., and X. Li. 2006. Errors and Uncertainties in Urban Cellular Automata. *Computers, Environment and Urban Systems* 30:10–28.

Zipf, G. 1949. *Human Behavior and the Principle of Least Effort: An Introduction to Human Ecology*. Cambridge, MA: Addison-Wesley.

Index

Accessibility, 56, 107, 109, 113, 121, 123, 139, 145, 146, 148, 150, 151, 155, 158, 161, 176, 181, 184, 185, 186, 192, 195, 207, 219, 239, 243, 262, 263, 264, 282, 284, 285
 calculations, 105, 151–153
 parameters, 106, 151, 284
Activity-based approach, 176, 193, 194, 202, 204, 208, 211, 212, 223, 224, 225, 301
Agency for Forest and Nature (ANB), 291, 292
Agent-based approach, 33, 43, 58, 60, 215, 230, 231, 242, 243
Agents, 13, 32, 33, 34, 39, 58, 60, 77, 112, 139, 219, 230, 231, 241, 242, 243, 244, 246, 248
Agentschap Ondernemen, 263
Agglomeration, diseconomies and economies of, 45, 48, 49, 67, 68, 72, 75, 77, 80, 180, 185–188, 193, 194, 224, 225, 226, 237–239, 310. *See also* Diseconomies exclusion band
Agglomerations (urban), 186, 266, 269, 276, 280
Agostinho, Joaquim, 222
Agriculture, 8, 9, 65, 82, 131, 132, 133, 135, 211, 220, 251, 253, 254, 255, 257, 258, 259, 261, 277, 290, 291
Algorithms, 1, 2, 15, 16, 21, 22, 26, 30, 36, 39, 50–52, 59, 81, 93, 138, 190, 228, 248, 260, 283, 287, 289, 291
Alleles, 27, 28
Allen, Peter, 57–58, 66, 132, 135

Allocation module, 142, 147, 148, 282–284, 286, 287
Allées, 5
Alonso, William, 14, 32, 48, 56, 114, 213, 235, 240
Alonso-Muth model, 32, 38, 53, 114, 240, 248
Âme de la cité, 13, 14
Andersson, Claes, 176
Angel, S., 14, 48
Artificial neural network (ANN). *See* Neural network
Animations, 116, 193
Antwerp (Belgium), 192, 201, 209, 210, 266, 269, 272, 277, 278, 280
Area-radius relationship, 91, 92, 97, 118, 120, 240. *See also* Fractal dimension, radial dimension
Atlanta (Georgia), 62, 94, 99
Attractivity, 56, 124, 143, 145–147, 153, 161. *See also* Potential
Attractors, 16, 17, 27, 32
Auckland (New Zealand), 173
Australia, 92

Babylov model, 171
Bak, Per, 29, 98, 241
Banzhaf, Wolfgang, 81, 231
Baroque urban patterns, 5, 6, 7
Batty, Michael, 22, 55, 59, 88, 94, 143, 245
Beavon, Keith, 45, 77, 78
Beijing (China), 92
Beleidsplan Ruimte Vlaanderen (BRV), 253, 257

Belfast (Northern Ireland), 153
Belgium, 99, 153, 192, 201, 204, 207, 208, 211, 241, 242, 251, 254, 255, 258–260, 263, 266. *See also* Flanders; Wallonia
Belinstown (Ireland), 163
Belousov-Zhabotinsky reaction, 3
Benenson, Izhak, 33, 40, 60, 82, 243, 246, 295
Berlin, 92, 93, 240
Berry, Brian, 51, 52, 73, 74
Bid rent curves, 114
Bifractal, 91, 93, 94, 237, 240, 248
Bifurcation, 16, 18, 19, 21, 29, 31, 33, 36, 37, 41, 51, 70, 72, 73, 81–85, 113, 115, 127, 166, 214–216, 231, 233, 236–238, 248, 249, 252, 297, 299, 303
Big box store, 80, 143
Biodiversity, 172, 173, 251, 290–292, 303
Biological Valuation Map (BWK), 263
Bohr, Neils, 213
Boolean networks, 22, 27, 28, 29, 31, 32, 33, 241
Boston (Massachusetts), 92
Brasilia (Brazil), 5
Brown, Daniel, 37, 39, 215, 301
Brownian motion, 17, 242
Brussels (Belgium), 15, 90, 207–209, 241, 255, 258, 259, 265–267, 269–271, 278, 280, 281, 312
Brussels-Antwerp corridor, 192, 201, 209, 269, 277
Brussels school, 22, 57
Built-up area, 87, 89, 90, 94, 158, 273

Calibration, 28, 33, 37–39, 52, 58, 62, 87, 90, 91, 113, 118, 121, 122, 124, 127, 128, 135, 138, 144, 145, 154, 156, 158, 160, 161, 163, 169, 180, 182, 184, 192, 193, 201, 202, 204, 207, 212, 228, 231, 233, 243, 244, 257, 258, 260, 262, 297, 298, 300, 301. *See also* Overcalibration; Validation; Verification
 procedures, 54, 55, 59, 96, 102, 212–216, 218–227, 229, 230, 236, 240–242, 245, 261, 263, 264, 300, 301
Camera obscura, 5, 6
Canoe metaphor, 17–21, 216

Canterbury (New Zealand), 77
Cardiff (Wales), 88
Cellular automata (CA). *See also* Game of life
 activity based, 63, 175–177, 179, 180, 186, 192, 202, 204, 211, 212, 237, 238
 classical, 22, 23 26, 29, 32, 33, 116
 definition, 23, 34, 35
 Flanders application, 251, 258, 262–264, 283, 292, 295, 297
 land use, 32–34, 37, 40, 41, 54, 58–61, 85, 103–105, 110, 113, 114, 122, 129, 130, 135, 137–139, 141–143, 145, 148, 151, 153, 154, 157, 161, 168, 169, 171, 184, 202, 213, 229, 235, 243, 248, 251
Cell. *See also* Activity potential; Transition potential
 demands, 124, 134, 138, 143, 148–150, 179, 187
 neighborhood, 23, 27, 34, 35, 59, 61, 109, 110, 124, 139, 141, 175, 177, 182, 184, 189, 190, 243
 space, 23, 26, 34, 61, 65, 67, 105, 106, 108, 110, 117, 118, 139, 175, 177, 228, 238, 239, 301
 space, inhomogeneous, 23, 34, 61, 75, 76, 105, 295
 state, 2, 25, 27, 28, 43, 55, 65, 93, 181, 183, 185, 187, 189, 191, 193, 195, 197, 199, 201, 203, 205, 207, 209, 219, 220, 222, 228, 230, 236, 239, 240, 242, 244, 246, 301
 state transitions, 35, 61, 104, 177
Center of gravity. *See* Gravity equation
Central business district (CBD), 71, 72
Central Statistical Office of Ireland (CSO), 156, 157
Centroid, 144, 262
Chaotic dynamics, 16, 17, 26–28, 32, 33, 87, 230, 298
Chicago (Illinois), 4
China, 7, 59, 62
Christaller, Walter, 43, 44, 45, 46, 47, 48, 51, 56, 65, 66, 77
Cincinnati (Ohio) 94, 99, 100, 121
Clarke, Keith, 60, 62, 295
Class IV behavior, 26, 29

Clustering-dispersal bifurcation, 72, 75, 77, 78, 85, 214, 237, 238, 244, 248
Cluster size–frequency relationship, 87, 91, 96, 98–102, 112, 115, 118, 120, 121, 124, 127, 169, 198, 200, 204, 207, 222, 225, 227, 237, 240–242, 248, 264
Cluster size indicator, 265, 269–272, 277, 278, 289
Coevolution and coadaptation, 28, 29
Compatibility factors, 179, 180, 198
Complex systems, 1–4, 10, 11, 13–15, 20, 22, 25, 27–31, 33, 35–39, 41, 42, 54, 55, 65, 80, 81, 83, 85–87, 98, 103, 121, 129, 141, 166, 213, 214, 218, 228–231, 233–237, 246, 249, 295–301, 303
Complexity, 10, 11, 13, 14, 23, 29, 36–38, 54, 55, 82, 87, 103, 236, 241, 249, 292, 297, 299
Complicated reality, 11, 19, 20, 33, 66, 228, 230, 299
CORINE, 122
Correlation dimension. *See under* Fractal dimension
Côte d'Azur, 153
Coupled models, 28, 230, 282, 295
Critical values, 26–29, 32, 84, 98, 185, 241, 242
Crutchfield, James, 17, 26

Dasymetric mapping, 182, 207, 279
Daubert criteria, 300
De Lijn, 262
Demographic models, 2, 4, 8, 57, 113, 129, 130, 131, 134–136, 141, 143, 144, 153, 156, 173, 228, 295
De Nijs, Ton, 152, 168, 217, 220
De Taeye law, 254
Diffusion-limited aggregation (DLA), 30, 61, 88
Diffusive growth, 61, 62
Digital elevation model (DEM), 108, 109, 114
Dijkstra algorithm, 190
Dilation dimension. *See under* Fractal dimension
Dimension. *See* Fractal dimension
Disamenity, 124, 151
Diseconomies of scale and agglomeration. *See* Agglomeration, diseconomies and economies of; Externalities
Diseconomies exclusion band, 185, 194
Dispersal. *See* Clustering-dispersal bifurcation
Distance
  cell (Euclidian), 109, 118, 124, 176, 177, 180, 182–184, 189, 203, 209, 307
  interregional, 144, 145, 163, 175, 262
  network, 188–191, 194–197, 201, 203, 204, 209, 210, 305, 307
  zero, 110, 111 (*see also* Inertia factor)
Distance-decay, 73, 77, 81–86, 106, 144–146, 151, 152, 182, 184, 188, 195, 219, 237, 243, 248, 285
Dublin (Ireland), 76, 77, 154
  activity based application, 177, 180, 188, 192–194, 196–206, 223, 224, 226
  fractal structure, 92–97, 99–101, 240
  Murbandy model application, 106–108, 115, 117, 122, 123, 125–128, 137
  Moland model applications, 144, 151, 153, 155–161, 163, 165, 166, 229, 235, 244, 245
Dublin Regional Authority (DRA), 163

Economic activity and sectors, 1–3, 8, 9, 20, 46, 57, 58, 67, 103, 129, 131, 137, 138, 144, 148–156, 169, 179, 180, 182, 193, 207, 228, 252, 256, 258, 259–263, 266, 297, 302
Economic models, 9, 80, 81, 85, 113, 129, 130, 132, 133–136, 138, 139, 141, 143, 145, 153, 168, 173, 175, 208, 211, 228
Economics (discipline, theory), 4, 10, 14, 21, 44–46, 48, 52, 53, 65, 66, 232, 237, 238, 248, 295
Economies of scale and agglomeration. *See* Agglomeration, diseconomies and economies of; Externalities
Emergence, 1, 3, 4, 13, 15, 22, 23, 28, 29, 33, 45, 53, 70, 118, 124, 127, 242, 244, 246, 296
Energy barrier, 216

Engelen, Guy, 57, 59, 118, 121, 130, 139, 141, 143, 144, 153, 171, 177, 194, 208, 220
Enterprise Flanders. *See* Agentschap Ondernemen
Environment explorer (LeefOmgevingsVerkenner, LOV), 154, 168, 171, 218
Epistemology, 35, 39, 42, 228, 232–234, 296, 303
Error propagation, 59, 129
Errors
 in activity data, 156, 158, 180
 in land use maps, 93, 169
 in simulation predictions, 159, 160, 169, 181, 195, 197, 198, 202–206, 218, 220, 221, 223, 224, 226, 261, 309, 310
Essen (Germany), 92
European Union (EU), 157, 207, 255, 261, 262, 275, 290, 291
Exclusion band. *See* Diseconomies exclusion band

Falsification, 38, 39
Far-from-equilibrium, 3, 4, 15, 20–22, 29, 33, 82, 87, 236
Fitness landscape, 27, 28, 31, 233, 284
Flanders (Belgium), 99, 153, 154, 189, 191, 204, 206, 208, 211, 229, 241, 242, 251–268, 270–282, 284, 290–292, 303, 312
Flanders Spatial Policy Plan. *See* Beleidsplan Ruimte Vlaanderen
Flemish Diamond, 269, 272, 273, 277
Flemish Ecological Network (VEN), 263
Flemish Environment Agency (VMM), 258, 292
Flemish Institute for Nature and Forest Research (INBO), 261, 291
Forestalling, 72, 76, 77, 80
Fotheringham, Stewart, 53, 55
Fractal dimension, 101, 103, 117
 cluster size–frequency dimension (*see* Cluster size–frequency relationship)
 correlation dimension, 89–91, 93, 99, 228
 dilation dimension, 90
 grid dimension (*see* Correlation dimension)
 radial dimension, 87, 89–96, 98, 99, 103, 118, 222, 227, 237, 240

Fractals, 17, 26, 29–32, 38, 39, 88, 95, 98, 118, 228

Game of Life, 22, 23, 24, 25, 26
Genk (Belgium), 269, 285
Germany, 44, 45, 48, 50
Ghent (Belgium), 209, 266, 280
GIS (Geographic Information System), 34, 54, 59, 217, 258, 263, 284, 302
Glider, 24, 25
Gobin, 253, 261, 263
Goodchild, Michael, 51, 52
Gravity equation, 50, 56, 62, 68, 70, 176, 237, 238, 243
Graphical user interface (GUI), 130, 132
Greater Dublin Region (GDR). *See* Dublin
Guangzhou (China), 59

Hagen-Zanker, Alex, 38, 221, 222, 227, 301
Hägerstrand, Torsten, 53, 54
Haken, Hermann, 15, 236, 246
Halting theorem, 22, 29
Hamilton (New Zealand), 171
Hasselt (Belgium), 266, 277, 280
Herentals (Belgium), 269
High-n. *See* Low-order goods
High-order goods, 45, 46, 60, 70, 71–73, 75–77, 79, 80, 83, 84, 238
Hinterland, 65, 144
Houston (Texas), 62, 94, 99, 100, 120

Île de France, 6
Implementation of models, 9, 40, 58, 122, 168, 208, 221
Implementation of plans, 41, 154, 173, 216, 252, 254–257, 263, 264, 290–292
Individual-based model, 33–34, 43, 54, 58, 80, 82, 86, 116, 246, 248
Inertia factor, 110, 114, 127, 147, 180, 182, 187, 218, 263. *See also* Distance, zero
Influence function, 110, 111, 118, 124, 125, 138, 146, 148, 183, 193, 194, 217–220, 237–239, 243–246, 248, 263, 264, 283, 287, 301. *See also* Weights in influence functions
Inner zone, 92, 93, 94, 95, 96, 97, 120, 127, 240, 243

Innovation, 29, 57, 58, 79, 80, 85
Input-output, 9, 131, 132, 133, 134, 135, 139
Institute for Nature and Forest Research (INBO). *See* Flemish Institute for Nature and Forest Research
Integrated modeling, 2, 4, 8, 9, 11, 40, 60, 63, 65, 129, 130, 141, 144, 145, 152, 153, 154, 161, 163, 168, 171, 173, 178, 211, 212, 219, 222, 230, 246, 248, 251, 253, 255, 293, 295–297, 300, 301
Interaction
 among land uses, 110, 118, 142, 173, 176, 177, 182, 184, 242
 spatial, 4, 52, 53, 55–58, 63, 65–68, 70, 79, 81–83, 139, 141, 142–143, 175–177, 182, 219, 237, 242, 248, 260, 262, 297, 301 (*See also* Gravity equation)
Intersectoral flows matrix 133, 134
Interventions, 40, 116, 121, 214, 249
Ireland, 154, 156, 157, 198
Isard, Walter, 53
Italy, 13, 123, 245

Jacobs, Jane, 13, 14

Kappa, fuzzy, 221, 222
Kappa statistic, 37, 39, 128, 129, 221, 222, 227, 301
Kauffman, Stuart, 22, 27, 28, 29, 31, 32, 33, 233, 241
Kink (in area-radius relationship), 91, 92, 118, 240, 243
Koh, Ngiap-Puoy, 66, 69, 75
Kuenne, Robert, 50, 52
Kuhn, Harold, 50, 52

Lagos (Nigeria), 123, 244, 245
Land take–neutral scenario (LTN) 275, 276, 277, 278, 279, 280, 281
Land use–transportation interaction models (LUTI), 40, 41, 262
Langton, Christopher, 22, 26, 27, 28, 29, 33
LeefOmgevingsVerkenner (LOV). *See* Environment explorer
Le Nôtre, André, 5
Leuven (Belgium), 266, 269, 280

Levins, Richard, 235, 236, 248, 249
Liege (Belgium), 201
Limits-to-growth, 55
Liu, Xiaoping, 59, 60
Location-allocation, 51, 52
London (England), 40, 76, 77, 92, 245, 246, 247, 311
Longley, Paul, 88, 94
Los Alamos National Laboratory, 15, 22
Lösch, August
LOV. *See* Environment explorer
Low-n. *See* High order goods
Low-order goods, 45, 72, 73, 75, 79, 80

Maastricht (Netherlands), 100, 102
Machado, Antonio, 11, 303
Macro-scale model, 130, 131, 132, 135, 138, 139, 141, 143, 147
Macro-scale structures, 3, 17, 33
Madrid (Spain), 123
Major retail center (MRC), 71, 72, 75–78, 80, 81
Makassar (Indonesia), 139
Mall, shopping, 79, 80, 81, 85, 94, 143
Mandelbrot, Benoit, 29, 30, 88
Manhattan (New York City), 76
Map Comparison Kit (MCK), 222
Marceau, Danielle, 33, 59
Marketing principle, 47, 53, 68
Mechelen (Belgium), 266, 269, 272, 280
Melbourne (Australia), 92
Memorial University of Newfoundland, 50
Methodology, 11, 14, 39, 217, 228, 229, 231, 232, 234, 289, 292, 297, 298, 301
Mexico, 15, 92
Migration, 57, 131, 134–136, 138, 143, 147, 248, 252, 259
Milan (Italy), 95
Milwaukee (Wisconsin), 94, 99, 100
Mitchell, Melanie, 17, 26
MOLAND model, 153, 154, 156, 161, 163, 168, 171, 173, 175, 177, 184, 194, 201–204, 211, 212, 218, 219, 225, 243, 248
Monte Carlo mode, 116, 166
Montreal (Canada), 76, 77
Moore neighborhood, 23, 177

Moscow (Russia), 92
MRC. *See* Major retail center
Multiactivity, 176
Multiagent model, 58
Multicriterion approach, 62, 216, 222, 225, 298
Multiobjective approach, 216, 225
Murbandy project, 121, 122, 124, 139, 154, 156, 193
Muth, Richard, 32, 48, 114, 240

NACE classification system, 157, 158, 263
Natura 2000, 263, 282, 284, 286, 290, 292, 293
Nature Outlook 2030 NARA-S-2009, 253, 258, 261
Neerpelt (Belgium), 269
Neighborhood effect, 110, 111, 113, 115, 118, 124, 142, 143, 145, 146, 148, 150, 176, 177, 185, 186, 188, 191, 192, 211, 218, 237–239, 243, 248, 301
Neoclassical theory, 14, 38, 48
Neopositivist approach, 6
Netherlands, 40, 100, 101, 102, 145, 153, 154, 168, 169, 170, 171, 172, 218, 229, 254
Neural Network, 22, 32, 33, 43, 59, 297
New York (city), 14, 66, 76, 77
New Zealand, 77, 153, 154, 171, 257
Niedercorn, John, 52, 53, 81
Nigeria, 123

Omer, Itzhak, 60, 82, 243
Optimization, 7, 28, 35, 37, 39, 43, 51, 59, 60, 212, 220, 223–225, 235, 256, 281–283, 286, 287, 290–292, 309
OptimizationTool, 282, 283, 287, 290–292
Ostend (Belgium), 280
Outer zone, 91–97, 118, 120, 127, 243
Overcalibration, 60, 91, 102, 127, 204, 215–217, 225, 229, 230, 235, 298

Papageorgiou, Yorgos, 14, 48, 56
Pareto optimality, 287–289
Paris (France), 4, 5, 6, 7, 58, 79, 92
Parr, John, 52, 73
Passonneau, Joseph, 81, 94, 99, 100, 121
Peeters, Dominique, 51, 52

Penn-Jersey model, 40
Philadelphia (Pennsylvania), 40
Phoenix (Arizona), 198
Picturescape, 88
Pittsburgh (Pennsylvania), 92
Planners, 3, 8, 14, 39–41, 59, 88, 204, 211, 214, 228, 249, 252, 253, 257, 289, 290, 293, 295, 296, 302
Planning interventions, 40, 116, 121, 214, 249
Pontius, Gil, 221, 227
Popper, Karl, 38, 39, 219, 225, 232, 233, 295
Pordenone (Italy), 244, 245
Portugal, 123
Portugali, Juval, 60, 82, 243, 246, 295
Potential, 56, 143, 146, 189
  activity potential, 16, 18, 20, 146, 150, 180–182, 184–188, 193–195, 198, 201, 225, 226, 239, 305, 310
  potential energy, 16, 18, 20
  transition potential, 104, 109, 111, 113–116, 118, 124, 125, 175–177, 186, 187, 194, 220, 238, 283 (*See also* Transition rules)
Power, Conrad 33, 222, 227
Power centers, 80
Power law, 28, 29, 56, 81, 89, 240, 241, 301
Predator-prey model, 173
Predictability, 17–20, 33, 35, 36, 38, 41, 51, 212, 214–217, 225, 229, 231, 236, 249, 296–298. *See also* Quasi-predictability
Prigogine, Ilya, 3, 4, 15, 17, 20, 57, 83, 85, 232, 236, 242
Productivity, 44, 135, 138, 179, 211
Puerto Rico, 142, 153, 154, 229
Pumain, Denise, 58
P-values, 223

Quasi-predictability, 296–298
Quasi-principle, 29

Radial dimension. *See under* Fractal dimension
Radial symmetry, 5, 51, 248
Random Boolean networks. *See* Boolean networks

Random perturbation. *See* Stochastic perturbation
Rank-size distribution, 73–76, 81, 99, 264
Rayon de segregation, 91
Regionalized model, 130, 138, 142, 143
Registered agricultural land, 261, 262, 266. *See also* Unregistered agricultural land
Remote sensing data, 8, 54, 58, 59, 93, 122, 217, 227, 297
Rent, 48, 77, 90, 114
Repulsion effect, 105, 110, 113, 118, 124, 220, 286
Resonance, stochastic. *See* Stochastic resonance
Retail centers, 63, 65–67, 69–73, 75–81, 85
Ribbon development, 99, 204, 206, 242, 254
Ricardian rent theory, 48
Richardson, Fry, 30, 88
Riskiness, Popperian, 219, 225, 229, 295
RIVM (National Institute for Health and Environment, the Netherlands), 168, 169, 170
Road gravity. *See* Gravity equation
Roeselare (Belgium), 269
Rossi, Aldo, 5, 13
RUBELIM application, 282, 290
RuimteModel, 154, 251, 253, 257–264, 273, 276, 281–283, 285, 287, 289, 290, 292, 293

Saint Lucia, 130, 131, 133, 137, 141
Sandpile model, 98, 241
Sanglier, Michelle, 57, 66
Santa Fe Institute, 15, 22, 27
Scale free, 30, 90, 130, 161
Scaling. *See* Scale free
Sealed surface, 138, 211
Seattle (Washington), 62, 81, 216
Secondary activity, 179–182, 187, 188, 193, 198, 211
Self-distance, 144
Self-organization, 1–4, 7, 10, 11, 13–17, 20–23, 26, 29–31, 33, 35–38, 39, 41, 42, 52–54, 56, 57, 60, 65, 79, 83, 85, 87, 88, 91, 98, 101, 124, 127, 166, 186, 214, 218, 228, 229, 231, 234, 236, 240, 246, 248, 249, 264, 296–298, 303

Senegal, 58
Sensitivity analysis, 50, 70, 75, 76, 184, 300
Shahumyan, Harutyun, 144, 163, 164, 177
Shannon entropy, 26
Shopping goods. *See* High-order goods
Silva, Elisabete, 60, 62
Simms, Alvin, 222, 227
SLEUTH model, 60–62
Snohomish county (Washington), 77
Solvay Institute, 15
Spain, 123, 251
Spokane (Washington) 77
Sprawl, urban, 6, 62, 135, 154, 207, 208, 253, 254, 273, 276–278
Stanilov, Kiril, 245, 247, 311
Stationarity, 216, 225, 231, 236, 240, 241
Stengers, Isabelle, 15, 17, 232, 242
Stochastic perturbation, 112–118, 127, 139, 166, 181, 186, 195, 220, 235, 242
Stochastic resonance, 14, 113, 115, 116, 127
Straatman, Bas, 81, 171, 220, 221, 231
Stuttgart (Germany), 15, 92, 246
Suburbanization, 254, 255, 266, 272, 273, 276, 278
Suitability, 105, 106, 109, 110, 113, 114, 116–118, 121, 123, 137–139, 143, 145, 146, 148, 150, 155, 157, 158, 161, 166, 176, 179, 181, 186, 219, 239, 261–264, 282, 284, 285
Sulawesi (Indonesia), 139
Supercell, 176, 177, 178, 182, 184, 189, 190, 191
Swarm intelligence, 33
Synergetics, 15, 246

Tannier, Cécile, 90, 228
Tel Aviv (Israel), 40, 82, 246
Tellier, Luc-Normand, 50, 52
Template, neighborhood, 109, 177, 178, 184
Testability, 17, 37, 48, 214
Theory, 1–4, 6, 10, 11, 13–15, 17, 19, 21–23, 27, 29, 31, 33, 35–39, 41, 43–46, 48, 49, 51, 52–55, 65, 70, 75, 76, 81, 82, 85, 86, 221, 225, 228, 229, 231, 233, 235–237, 239, 241, 243–249, 295, 297, 299, 300

Thermodynamics, 15–18, 20, 82, 83, 85, 232, 236
Thomas, Isabelle, 52, 90, 228
Threshold size, 44, 45, 69, 83, 287
Tongeren (Belgium), 280, 287, 288, 289
Torrens, Paul, 53, 60
Transients, 26, 29
Transit, 13, 28, 76, 154, 163
Transition potential. *See* Potentials, transition
Transition rules, 22, 23, 26, 32, 34, 35, 54, 59, 61, 113, 114, 187, 242, 248, 297, 301. *See also* Potentials, transition
Turing machine, 23, 26
Turnhout (Belgium), 266

Ucello, Paolo, 5
Ulam, Stanislaw, 22, 23
Uljee, Inge, 59, 121, 123, 130, 139, 141, 177, 194, 208, 221
Universality, 63, 219, 244–246, 249, 298
Université Libre de Bruxelles, 15
University of Puerto Rico, 142
University of Stuttgart, 246
Unpredictability, 20, 249
Unregistered agricultural land, 261, 262, 267, 312
Urban centered regions, 144, 145, 168, 169
Urban Environment Project (UEP), 154–156, 158, 163, 193, 194, 201, 202, 204, 218, 219
Urbanization, 61–63, 76, 91, 93, 94, 96, 118, 127, 161, 207, 240, 252, 256, 265, 266, 268, 269, 272, 273, 276, 277, 280, 290, 297
Urban sprawl. *See* Sprawl, urban
Utility theory, 14, 53, 81

Validation, 11, 31, 33, 46, 87, 90, 91, 121, 122, 127, 129, 154, 156, 158, 169, 184, 192, 201, 212–215, 217, 219, 220–223, 225, 227–229, 246, 264, 295–301

Varignon frame, 48, 50, 52
VEN. *See* Flemish Ecological Network
Verification, 31, 35, 39, 212, 213, 224, 246, 298, 301
Vitoria-Gasteiz (Spain), 123
Von Thünen, Johann, 44, 48, 56

Waikato (New Zealand), 154, 171
Wallonia (Belgium), 90, 207, 208, 255, 259
Waregem (Belgium), 269
Warntz, William, 55, 143, 230
Wastewater application, 154, 163, 165, 166, 204
Wavelet analysis, 38, 222
Weber model, 48–52, 56
Weights in influence functions, 110, 111, 118, 124, 125, 151, 152, 182–185, 188, 189, 192, 194, 219, 221, 238, 239, 243, 245, 263. *See also* Influence function
Wellington (New Zealand), 173
White, Roger, 32, 33, 53, 59, 66, 71, 73–75, 81, 117, 121, 130, 139, 141, 171, 176, 177, 194, 198, 208, 220, 222, 227, 231, 298
Wicklow County (Ireland), 117, 123, 159–161, 167, 198, 203
Williams, Brendan, 163, 165, 166, 167
Wilson, Alan, 52, 53, 66, 81
WISE model, 154, 171, 173
Wolfram, Stephen, 52, 53, 66, 81
Wurman, Richard, 81, 94, 99, 100, 121

Xplorah model, 142, 154

Yeh, Anthony, 52, 59

Zipf, George, 264, 265
Zipf law, 265
Zoning, 60, 106, 108, 113, 114, 116–118, 121, 123, 139, 145, 155, 157, 158, 171, 176, 181, 186, 198, 239, 261, 263, 264, 284, 285, 303